Guidelines
For Oncology
Nursing Practice

Oncology Nursing Society

Guidelines For Oncology Nursing Practice

Second Edition

Edited by

Joan C. McNally, RN, MSN, OCN
Michigan Cancer Foundation
Detroit, Michigan

Eileen T. Somerville, RN, MS
University of Arkansas
Medical Science Campus
Little Rock, Arkansas

Christine Miaskowski, RN, PhD, OCN
Department of Physiological Nursing
School of Nursing
University of California, San Francisco
San Francisco, California

Marcia Rostad, RN, MS, NS, OCN
University Medical Center
Tucson, Arizona

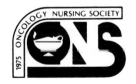

W. B. SAUNDERS COMPANY
Harcourt Brace Jovanovich, Inc.
Philadelphia London Toronto Montreal Sydney Tokyo

W. B. SAUNDERS COMPANY
Harcourt Brace Jovanovich, Inc.

The Curtis Center
Independence Square West
Philadelphia, PA 19106

Library of Congress Cataloging-in-Publication Data

Guideline for oncology nursing practice / editors, Joan C.
  McNally . . . [et al.]. — 2nd ed.
    p.   cm.
    "The revised ANA/ONS Standards of Oncology Nursing
Practice have been integrated into this edition"—Pref.
    Includes bibliographical references and index.
    ISBN 0-7216-3419-2
    1. Cancer—Nursing.   2. Cancer—Nursing—
Standards.   I. McNally, Joan C.   II. American Nurses'
Association. Standards of oncology nursing practice.
[DNLM: 1. Neoplasms—nursing.   2. Nursing
Process.   3. Outcome and Process Assessment (Health
Care)—methods.   4. Patient Care]
RC266.A64   1991
610.73'698—dc20
DNLM/DLC   90-9189

Editor: Thomas Eoyang

Production Manager: Frank Polizzano

Manuscript Editor: Elisa Costanza Affanato

Indexer: Dennis Dolan

GUIDELINES FOR ONCOLOGY NURSING PRACTICE   ISBN   0-7216-3419-2

Contributors

E. JOYCE ALEXANDER, RN, MSN, OCN

Emory University Hospital
Atlanta, Georgia

Injury, Potential for, Related to Thrombocytopenia

CAROL PAPPAS APPEL, RN, MSN, OCN

Harper Hospital
Detroit, Michigan

*Nutrition, Alteration in: More Than Body
Requirements Related to Disease Process and
Treatment*

PAT ASCHEMAN, RN, OCN

Johnson County Radiation Therapy
Overland Park, Kansas

*Nutrition, Alteration in: Less Than Body
Requirements Related to Dysphagia*

LAURA M. BENSON, RN, BSN, OCN

The Jack D. Weiler Hospital of the Albert Einstein
College of Medicine
Bronx, New York

*Ineffective Airway Clearance; Alteration in
Breathing Patterns: Diversional Methods*

MARY ANNE BORD, RN, MA, MN, OCN

Mercy Hospital and Medical Center
San Diego, California

Alteration in Comfort: Pruritus

ANNE CALAFATO, RN, OCN

Monmouth Hematology-Oncology Associates
Long Branch, New Jersey

*Body Fluid Composition, Alteration in:
Hypercalcemia*

MARGARET M. CAWLEY, RN, MS, OCN

Booth Memorial Medical Center
Flushing, New York

*Alteration in Cardiac Output, Decreased: Related to
Superior Vena Cava Syndrome*

BERNADINE CIMPRICH, PhD, RN, CS

University of Wisconsin-Madison
Madison, Wisconsin

*Knowledge Deficit Related to Prevention and Early
Detection of Lung Cancer*

JANE C. CLARK, MN, RN, OCN, CGNP

Emory University Hospital
Atlanta, Georgia

*Mucous Membrane Integrity, Impairment of,
Related to Vaginal Changes*

CATHERINE M. COLEMAN, RN

Long Beach Memorial Breast Center
Long Beach, California

*Knowledge Deficit Related to Prevention and Early
Detection of Breast Cancer*

**PATRICIA MANDA COLLINS, RN, MSN,
OCN**

South Miami Hospital
Miami, Florida

*Mobility, Impaired Physical, Related to
Amputation*

REBECCA CRANE, RN, MN

Harbor-UCLA Medical Center
Torrance, California

*Knowledge Deficit Related to Prevention and Early
Detection of Breast Cancer*

Contributors

KATHLEEN CUSHMAN, RN, MSN

University of Virginia Health Sciences Center
Charlottesville, Virginia

Knowledge Deficit Related to Prevention and Early Detection of Bladder Cancer

RUTH BOPE DANGEL, RN, MN, OCN

Formerly of Riverside Methodist Hospitals
Columbus, Ohio

Injury, Potential for, Related to Disseminated Intravascular Coagulopathy (DIC)

DEBRYNDA BREWER DAVEY, EdD, RN

Delta State University School of Nursing
Cleveland, Mississippi

Self-Care Deficit, Related to Disease Process and Treatment

BEVERLY VINCENT DAVIS, RN, MSN, OCN

University of Washington Medical Center
Seattle, Washington

Injury, Potential for, Related to Graft Versus Host Disease (GVHD)

JOANNE DOUBLSKY, RN, MSN

St. Francis Medical Center
Trenton, New Jersey

Ineffective Individual Coping

SR. KARIN DUFAULT, SP, PhD, RN

St. Elizabeth Medical Center
Yakima, Washington

Ineffective Family Coping; Mobility, Impaired Physical, Related to Disease Process and Treatment

JAN M. ELLERHORST-RYAN, RN, MSN, CS

Bethesda Oak Hospital
Cincinnati, Ohio

Ineffective Breathing Pattern

JULIA FANSLOW, EdD, RN, OCN, ONS

St. Joseph Hospital Cancer Center
Tacoma, Washington

Knowledge Deficit Related to Prevention and Early Detection of Cervical and Uterine (Endometrial) Cancer

JUANITA FARNEN, RN, BSN, MA, OCN

Trinity Lutheran Hospital
Kansas City, Missouri

Nutrition Alteration in: Less Than Body Requirements Related to Dysphagia

SHARON CANNELL FIRSICH, RN, MS, OCNS

Providence Medical Center
Portland, Oregon

Ineffective Family Coping; Mobility, Impaired Physical, Related to Disease Process and Treatment

BARBARA FLYNN, RN, BSN

Northwestern Memorial Hospital
Chicago, Illinois

Knowledge Deficit Related to Unproven Methods of Cancer Treatment

MARY C. FRASER, RN, MA

Cancer Nursing Service
Clinical Center and Family Studies
National Cancer Institute
National Institutes of Health
Bethesda, Maryland

Knowledge Deficit Related to Prevention and Early Detection of Skin Cancer

MARIANNE FRENCH, RN, CANP, OCN

University of Southern California
Los Angeles, California

Bowel Elimination, Alteration in: Constipation

ANNE GARDNER, RN, BSN, OCN

St. Vincent Hospital and Medical Center
Portland, Oregon

Ineffective Family Coping; Mobility, Impaired Physical, Related to Disease Process and Treatment

SUSAN GELBARD, RN, MSN

Miami, Florida

Knowledge Deficit Related to Contraception

PAMELA GENTZSCH, RN, MN, OCN

St. Jude Medical Center
Fullerton, California

Mobility, Impaired Physical, Related to Spinal Cord Compression

MICHELLE GOODMAN, RN, MS

Rush-Presbyterian-St. Luke's Medical Center
Chicago, Illinois

Mucous Membrane Integrity, Impairment of, Related to Stomatitis

ROSEMARY GRADY, RN, BSN, OCN, MA

Kansas University Medical Center
Kansas City, Kansas

Nutrition, Alteration in: Less Than Body Requirements Related to Dysphagia

SUSAN JANE HAGAN, ARNP, MS

James A. Haley V.A.M.C.
Tampa, Florida

Elimination, Alteration in: Enterocutaneous Fistula Formation; Elimination, Alteration in: Nonenterocutaneous Fistula Formation

BARBARA HALL, MSN, RN, OCN

University Hospitals-Cleveland
Cleveland, Ohio

Nutrition, Alteration in: Less Than Body Requirements Related to Nausea and Vomiting

JAMES P. HALLORAN, JR., MSN, RN, OCN

Park Plaza Hospital
Houston, Texas

Knowledge Deficit Related to Prevention and Early Detection of HIV Disease

INA J. HARDESTY, RN, MA, OCN

Cleveland Clinic Foundation
Cleveland, Ohio

Nutrition, Alteration in: Less Than Body Requirements Related to Nausea and Vomiting

CATHERINE D. HARVEY, RN, MSN

Oncology Services
Grossmont Hospital
La Mesa, California

Grieving

SUE P. HEINEY, MN, RN, CS

Center for Cancer and Blood Disorders
Children's Hospital at Richland Memorial
Columbia, South Carolina

Grieving

CATHERINE M. HOGAN, MN, RN, OCN

New England Deaconess Hospital and
Dana Farber Cancer Institute
Boston, Massachusetts

Sexual Dysfunction Related to Disease Process and Treatment

ROSEMARIE HOGAN, MSN, RN

Frances Payne Bolton School of Nursing
Case Western Reserve University
Cleveland, Ohio

Nutrition, Alteration in: Less Than Body Requirements Related to Nausea and Vomiting

ANNE M. HUGHES, MN, RN, C

San Francisco General Hospital
San Francisco, California

Knowledge Deficit Related to Prevention and Early Detection of HIV Disease

CATHERINE A. HYDZIK, RN, MS, OCN

Jack D. Weiler Hospital of the Albert Einstein
College of Medicine
Bronx, New York

Alteration in Cardiac Output, Decreased: Related to Cardiac Tamponade

Contributors

PATRICIA F. JASSAK, MS, RN, CS

Foster G. McGaw Hospital
Loyola University Medical Center
Maywood, Illinois

Knowledge Deficit Related to Biotherapy

ANN L. JESSUP, BSN, MPA, OCN

Riverview Medical Center Hospice/Oncology
Support
Red Bank, New Jersey

*Body Fluid Composition, Alteration in:
Hypercalcemia*

MARGARET B. JONES, RN, BS

St. Vincent Hospital and Medical Center
Portland, Oregon

*Ineffective Family Coping; Mobility, Impaired
Physical, Related to Disease Process and Treatment*

**CATHERINE M. KELLEY, RN, MSN,
OCN**

Northwestern Memorial Hospital
Chicago, Illinois

*Knowledge Deficit Related to Unproven Methods of
Cancer Treatment*

LINDA FAUTH KENNELLY, RN, MA

Division of Nursing, New York University
New York, New York

*Altered Tissue Perfusion, Peripheral, Related to
Lymphedema*

MAUREEN LARKIN, RN, MA, OCN

Jack D. Weiler Hospital of the Albert Einstein
College of Medicine
Bronx, New York

*Ineffective Airway Clearance; Alteration in
Breathing Patterns: Diversional Methods*

JUNE P. MARTIN, RN, MSN, CS

North Carolina Baptist Hospital
Winston-Salem, North Carolina

*Knowledge Deficit Related to Prevention and Early
Detection of Prostate Cancer; Knowledge Deficit
Related to Prevention and Early Detection of
Testicular Cancer*

**NOELLA DEVOLDER McCRAY, RN, MN,
OCN**

Kansas City Clinical Oncology Program
Kansas City, Missouri

Alteration in Comfort: Pruritus

PATRICIA McFARLAND, RN, CETN

J.A. Haley VA Hospital
Tampa, Florida

*Elimination, Alteration in: Enterocutaneous Fistula
Formation; Elimination, Alteration in:
Nonenterocutaneous Fistula Formation*

JOAN C. McNALLY, RN, MSN, OCN

Michigan Cancer Foundation
Detroit, Michigan

*Potential for Infection; Skin Integrity, Impairment
of, Related to Radiation Therapy*

**CHRISTINE MIASKOWSKI, RN, PhD,
OCN**

Department of Physiological Nursing
School of Nursing
University of California, San Francisco
San Francisco, California

*Knowledge Deficit Related to Surgery; Body Fluid
Composition, Alteration in: Tumor Lysis Syndrome*

JEAN R. MOSELEY, RN, MN, OCN

Portland, Oregon

*Ineffective Family Coping; Mobility, Impaired
Physical, Related to Disease Process and Treatment*

MARY OGRINC, MS, MBA, RN

Cleveland Clinic Foundation
Cleveland, Ohio

*Sensory/Perceptual Alterations Related to
Peripheral Neuropathy*

PATTI OWEN, RN, MN, OCN

Northside Hospital
Atlanta, Georgia

*Skin Integrity, Impairment of, Related to
Malignant Skin Lesions*

MICHAELYN A. PAGE, MS, RN, OCN

University of Michigan Medical Center
Ann Arbor, Michigan

Alteration in Comfort: Sleep Pattern Disturbance

JUDITH PAICE, RN, MS

Rush-Presbyterian-St. Luke's Medical Center
Chicago, Illinois

Alteration in Comfort: Acute Pain

CATHERINE PANOURYAS, RN, MS

New York Hospital/Cornell Medical Center
New York, New York

*Alteration in Breathing Patterns: Mechanical
Ventilation*

MARY JO PEARL, RN, BSN, OCN

St. Vincent Hospital and Medical Center
Portland, Oregon

*Mobility, Impaired Physical, Related to Disease
Process and Treatment*

BARBARA F. PIPER, RN, MS

University of California, San Francisco
Mt. Zion Hospital Medical Center
San Francisco, California

Alteration in Comfort: Fatigue

MARY BETH RILEY, RN, MSN, OCN

Arkansas Cancer Research Center
Little Rock, Arkansas

*Knowledge Deficit Related to Unproven Methods of
Cancer Treatment*

MARCIA ROSTAD, RN, MS, NS, OCN

University Medical Center
Tucson, Arizona

*Injury, Potential for, Related to Anemia; Bowel
Elimination, Alteration in: Constipation; Bowel
Elimination, Alteration in: Bowel Obstruction*

ELLEN L. ROTH, RN, MSN

Northwestern University/Northwestern Memorial
Hospital
Chicago, Illinois

*Knowledge Deficit Related to Unproven Methods of
Cancer Treatment*

CAROL SANDOR, MSN, RN, OCN

Audie L. Murphy Memorial Veterans Hospital
San Antonio, Texas

*Nutrition, Alteration in: Less Than Body
Requirements Related to Disease Process and
Treatment*

GAIL EGAN SANSIVERO, RN, MS, OCN

Albany Medical Center
Albany, New York

*Knowledge Deficit Related to Prevention and Early
Detection of Colorectal Cancer*

JOAN R. SCHLEPER, RN, OCN

Formerly of M.D. Anderson Cancer Center
Houston, Texas

*Knowledge Deficit Related to Prevention and Early
Detection of Head and Neck Cancer*

JUDITH A. SCHREIBER, MSN, RN

Harper Hospital
Detroit, Michigan

Impaired Gas Exchange

SUZANNE SHAFFER, RN, MN, OCN

Department of Nursing Services
University of Kansas Medical Center
Kansas City, Kansas

Alteration in Comfort: Pruritus

JUDITH A. SHELL, RN, MS, OCN

Butterworth Hospital
Grand Rapids, Michigan

Knowledge Deficit Related to Radiation Therapy

Contributors

EILEEN T. SOMERVILLE, RN, MS

University of Arkansas Medical Science Campus
Little Rock, Arkansas

*Knowledge Deficit Related to Chemotherapy;
Knowledge Deficit Related to Bone Marrow
Transplant*

**MARY McCARTY SPENCER, RN, MSN,
CETN**

Carrollton, Texas

*Urinary Elimination, Alteration in: Diversional
Methods*

JOY STAIR, RN, MS

Catherine McAuley Health System
Ann Arbor, Michigan

*Potential for Infection; Sexual Dysfunction:
Infertility*

SANDRA STONE, RN, MS

Oregon State Hospital
Salem, Oregon

*Ineffective Family Coping; Mobility, Impaired
Physical, Related to Disease Process and Treatment*

CAROL STONER, MS, RN

Valparaiso, Indiana

*Mucous Membrane Integrity, Impairment of,
Related to Stomatitis*

ROBERTA A. STROHL, RN, MN

Department of Radiation Oncology
University of Maryland at Baltimore
Baltimore, Maryland

*Knowledge Deficit Related to Brachytherapy
(Implants); Skin Integrity, Impairment of, Related
to Radiation Therapy*

PATRICIA A. STUCKEY, MSN, RN, OCN

Medical College of Virginia
Virginia Commonwealth University School of
    Nursing
Richmond, Virginia

*Urinary Elimination, Alteration in: Bladder
Irritation*

**LINDA KRATCHA SVENINGSON, RN,
MS, OCN**

Roger Maris Cancer Center
Fargo, North Dakota

*Body Fluid Composition, Alteration in: Syndrome
of Inappropriate Antidiuretic Hormone (SIADH)*

INGA TOKAR, BSN, RN

Cancer Nursing Service/Dermatology Clinic
National Cancer Institute
National Institutes of Health
Bethesda, Maryland

*Knowledge Deficit Related to Prevention and Early
Detection of Skin Cancer*

HAIDEE F. WATERS, DNSc, RN

Medical College of Virginia
Virginia Commonwealth University School of
    Nursing
Richmond, Virginia

*Urinary Elimination, Alteration in: Bladder
Irritation*

JENNIFER S. WEBSTER, MN, RN, OCN

Emory University Hospital
Atlanta, Georgia

Bowel Elimination, Alteration in: Diarrhea

**SAUNDRA J. WILLOUGHBY, RN, BSN,
OCN**

Amicare Home Health Care, Inc.
Subsidiary of Sisters of Mercy Health Corporation
Farmington Hills, Michigan

Alteration in Comfort: Chronic Pain

**KAREN WOJTALEWICZ-FRIEDBERG,
MS, RN**

Bloomingdale, Illinois

*Knowledge Deficit Related to Unproven Methods of
Cancer Treatment*

HILARY ANN WOOD

Franklin Square Hospital Center
Baltimore, Maryland

Ineffective Breathing Pattern

SHEILA K. WROBLEWSKI, RN, BSN, MN

Half Moon Bay, California

Bowel Elimination, Alteration in: Constipation

CAROL A. YURKOVIC, RN, BSN

Livingston, New Jersey

Altered Tissue Perfusion, Peripheral, Related to Lymphedema

CAROL A. ZABINSKI, MSN, RN, CS, OCN

Providence Hospital
Southfield, Michigan

Fluid Volume Deficit Related to Disease Process and Treatment; Alteration in Cardiac Output, Decreased: Related to Third Space Syndrome

Preface

This revised edition represents the substantial changes that have occurred in oncology nursing practice during the past 5 years. The original framework for the Guidelines for Cancer Nursing Practice has been modified to reflect changes in the levels of care and revisions made in the ONS/ANA Outcome Standards for Cancer Nursing Practice and the Nursing Diagnosis Taxonomy.

Many of the original guidelines in the previous edition have been consolidated and all have been substantially revised to reflect current clinical practice. New guidelines have been added, including Knowledge Deficit Related to Prevention and Early Detection of Bladder Cancer, Prostate Cancer, and HIV; Knowledge Deficit Related to Biotherapy and Bone Marrow Transplant; Alteration in Comfort: Fatigue; Potential for Injury: Graft Versus Host Disease (GVHD); and Alteration in Breathing Patterns: Mechanical Ventilation. A new section on Decreased Cardiac Output, including Superior Vena Cava Syndrome, Cardiac Tamponade, and Third Space Syndrome has been added. The 67 topics covered emphasize the more common clinical and psychological problems experienced by cancer patients and their families. In addition, the guidelines emphasize the concepts of adaptation and promotion of self-care and rehabilitation of the patient and family.

The editors wish to point out that the revised ANA/ONS Standards of Oncology Nursing Practice have been integrated into this edition. The guidelines were revised in collaboration with the Clinical Practice Committee of the Oncology Nursing Society.

In each of the guidelines, in Levels 1 and 2 the term patient includes patient, family, and significant other. However, in the guidelines relating to Knowledge Deficit in Level 1A, the term client has been substituted to reflect the individual's state of wellness. The term patient/caregiver is used in Level 3 because the patient usually requires assistance with nursing during this phase of illness.

Readers are encouraged to use this manual to develop standards of patient care, to formulate educational programs, to develop criteria for quality assurance programs, and to stimulate researchable questions in cancer nursing practice.

1. ANA/ONS Division on Medical Surgical Nursing Practice: Outcome Standards for Cancer Nursing Practice. Kansas City, MO, American Nurses' Association, 1979.
2. North American Nursing Diagnosis Association Taxonomy I with Complete Diagnosis. St. Louis, North American Nursing Diagnosis Association, 1987.
3. ANA and ONS Standards of Oncology Nursing Practice. Kansas City, MO, American Nurses' Association, 1987.

Acknowledgments

This manual represents the contributions of many dedicated Oncology Nursing Society members. The editors would like to recognize the following individuals:

- The core members of the Clinical Practice Committee involved in the content review and facilitation of the review process:
  - Kathryn Caudell, RN, MN, OCN
    Thousand Oaks, CA
  - Kimberly Rumsey, RN, MSN, OCN
    Spring, TX
  - Nancy Hayes, RN, MS, OCN
    Tampa, FL
  - Marie Whedon, RN, MSN, OCN
    West Lebanon, NH
  - Jill Fiscus, RN, MSN, OCN
    Milwaukee, WI
- The corresponding members of the Clinical Practice Committee participating in the content review:
  - Kathryn Conrad, RN, MSN, OCN
    Monroeville, PA
  - Amy Antle, RN, BSN, MPH, OCN
    Albuquerque, NM
  - Sheila Wroblewski, RN, MN, OCN
    Irvine, CA
  - Lynne Brophy, RN, BSN
    Chapel Hill, NC
  - Kathleen Keane, RN, MS
    Boston, MA
  - Dawn Camp-Sorrell, RN, MSN, OCN
    Hermitage, TN
  - Regina Schmitt, RN, MS, OCN
    Englewood, CO
  - Mary Gullatte, RN, MN
    Marietta, GA

Acknowledgments

- Marcia Caruso-Bergman, RN, BA, MSN, OCN
  Kensington, CT
- Victoria Hargrave-Koertge, RN, BSN, OCN
  Cincinnati, OH
- Janis M. Petree, RN, BS, BSN, PHN, OCN
  Mountain View, CA
- Ann Dose, RN, BSN, OCN
  Lake City, MN
- June Eilers, RN, MN, OCN
  Overland Park, KS
- Thomas J. Szopa, RN, MS, CETN, OCN, New Boston, NH, who practices in surgical oncology and volunteered to review guidelines in this area.
- Bridget Culhane, RN, MN, OCN, Director of Education, and Becky Nelson, Education Secretary, for their support and coordination of our efforts in the ONS office.

The editors wish to acknowledge the original authors of the following guidelines:

- Phyllis Heft: Knowledge Deficit Related to Prevention and Early Detection of Cervical and Uterine (Endometrial) Cancer.
- Linda Delaney: Knowledge Deficit Related to Prevention and Early Detection of Lung Cancer.
- Janis Faehnrich: Knowledge Deficit Related to Prevention and Early Detection of Head and Neck Cancer.
- David Buchanan: Knowledge Deficit Related to Early Detection of Testicular Cancer.
- Joy Stair: Knowledge Deficit Related to Prevention and Early Detection of Malignant Melanoma; Knowledge Deficit Related to Prevention and Early Detection of Nonmelanoma Skin Cancers; Skin Integrity, Impairment of: Related to Malignant Skin Lesions.
- Barbara Nettles: Grieving.
- Josie Howard-Rubin: Nutrition, Alteration in: Less Than Body Requirements Related to Disease Process and Treatment; Sexual Dysfunction Related to Disease Process and Treatment.
- Priscilla Houck, Karen Taylor, and Maureen Gallagher: Fluid Volume Deficit Related to Disease Process and Treatment.
- Anna Curry Sanford: Injury, Potential for, Related to Thrombocytopenia.
- Jean Andejeski: Injury, Potential for, Related to Anemia.
- Arlene Fleck: Mobility, Impaired Physical, Related to Disease Process and Treatment.
- Kathy Jacobs: Self-Care Deficit, Related to Disease Process and Treatment.
- Mary Davis: Bowel Elimination, Alteration in: Diarrhea.
- Juanita Swihart: Bowel Elimination, Alteration in: Bowel Obstruction.
- Linda H. Johnston and Joy Stair: Sexual Dysfunction: Infertility.

- Martha Bangs: Ineffective Airway Clearance.
- Andrea Krzysko, Sally Erdel, Mary Greiner, and Anita Lawrance: Impaired Gas Exchange.
- Terese Cagney Burch: Altered Breathing Patterns: Diversional Methods.
- Linda Dolan, Theresa Beck, and Susan Quinn: Body Fluid Composition, Alteration in: Hypercalcemia.

Contents

Contents

Contents

Contents

Contents

Introduction

THEORETICAL FRAMEWORK

The theoretical framework for the guidelines utilizes a concept of levels of care, a nursing diagnosis taxonomy, the application of the nursing process, and the standards of oncology nursing practice.

The Stair and McNally Levels of Care framework depicted in Table 1 has been adapted from Leavell and Clark's Levels of Prevention and describes the levels of care required by the oncology patient. Level 1 includes potential health problems or problems that can be prevented through nursing education; Level 2 addresses nursing management of patients having a mild to moderate degree of illness; and Level 3 focuses on nursing management and rehabilitation of severe or chronic conditions. Each level within the guideline includes nursing assessment parameters, patient expected outcomes, and nursing interventions or patient teaching strategies.

The first edition of the guidelines was structured using the 1979 Outcome Standards of Cancer Nursing Practice. This second edition has been modified to reflect the revised ANA/ONS Standards of Oncology Nursing Practice and includes the additional high incidence problem areas. The critical indicators and outcome of criteria listed for each high incidence problem area are taken from the ANA/ONS Standards for Oncology Nursing Practice.

SCOPE OF ONCOLOGY NURSING PRACTICE

The recognition of cancer as a major health problem has led to the development of oncology nursing as a specialty. The practice of oncology nursing encompasses the roles of direct caregiver, educator, administrator, and researcher; it extends to all care settings in which individuals with an actual or potential diagnosis of cancer receive health care, screening, and/or preventive education. The promotion of cancer prevention and early detection practices and the facilitation of optimal individual and family functioning throughout the disease process are primary goals of oncology nursing practice.

The oncology nurse achieves these primary goals by diagnosing and treating human responses exhibited by individuals and families actually experiencing or at risk of developing cancer. Human responses can include physical symptoms, functional limitations, psychosocial disruptions, and knowledge deficits associated with

TABLE 1. LEVELS OF CARE: GUIDELINES FOR CANCER PRACTICE

Characteristics of Altered Health Status	Expected Outcome Focus	Nursing Management
Level 1—Potential, Prevention		
• "At risk" populations • Minor signs/ symptoms of altered health status • Minor interruptions in life activities • Able to continue normal activities with minimal effort/ assistance	• Prevent/correct altered health status • Prevent complications/ sequelae of altered health status • Prevent/minimize disability • Achieve/maintain normal functioning	• Monitoring/assessment • Teaching • Emotional support • Coordination of services • Referral • Assistance in home adaptation • Evaluation
Level 2—Mild to Moderate		
• Progressive signs/ symptoms of altered health status • Presence of minor complications/ sequelae of altered health status • Unable to carry on normal activity • Requires varying amounts of assistance	• Correct/control/ improve altered health status • Prevent further complications/sequelae • Prevent/minimize prolonged disability • Achieve normal/ improved functioning	• As in Level 1 • Direct physical care
Level 3—Severe/Chronic		
• Advanced signs/ symptoms of altered health status • Presence of complications/ sequelae of altered health status • Unable to care for self • Without strong caregiver support, consider institutionalization	• Control/improve/ manage altered health status • Control complications/ sequelae of altered health status • Restoration of the individual to optimal level of functioning within constraints of disability	• As in Levels 1 and 2 • Rehabilitative strategies

the diagnosis of cancer and/or life style patterns known to increase cancer risk. Treatment of these responses involves the delivery of physical care to manage the disease and treatment-related symptomatology; psychosocial support to build or sustain coping capacity; and education to encourage active participation in decision-making and self-care.

General Oncology Nursing Practice

In addition to basic preparation as a registered professional nurse, oncology nursing practice at the generalist level requires a cancer-specific knowledge base and demonstrated clinical expertise in cancer care beyond that acquired in a basic nursing program. Oncology nurses base their practice on philosophic tenets that recognize:

1. the uniqueness of individuals and their responses to cancer and its treatment;
2. the relationship between physiologic and psychosocial life processes relative to the dynamic nature of the cancer experience and its impact on the individual and family network;
3. the individual's desire for autonomy and the right to self-determination in decision-making relative to health and illness;
4. the existence of complementary health care goals in which nursing is primarily responsible for effecting the care goals but participatory for achieving the cure goals.

The oncology nurse acts as a coordinator of care, collaborating with other health team members to implement required care and to mobilize appropriate family and community resources. The oncology nurse is an advocate for the patient, securing information, obtaining sufficient answers to questions, and helping the patient to maintain a maximal level of independence. The oncology nursing role as advocate extends to supporting the patient's informed decisions regarding care and treatment.

The oncology nurse is accountable for delivering care within the framework of the nursing process. In keeping with the ONS Standards for Oncology Nursing Practice, the oncology nurse gathers data in 11 high-incidence problem areas and uses those assessment findings to formulate relevant nursing diagnoses and to prioritize the identified problems according to need acuity. Collaborating with both client and family members, the oncology nurse engages in mutual goal setting, develops and implements a plan of care designed to achieve the identified goals, and evaluates the effectiveness of the plan by examining client and family outcomes.

The oncology nurse actively participates in professional role development activities, including continuing education, quality assurance, ethical decision-making, and review and clinical application of research findings.

Advanced Oncology Nursing Practice

Advanced oncology nursing practice requires substantial theoretical knowledge in oncology nursing and proficient use of this knowledge in providing expert care to individuals diagnosed with cancer and their families, as well as the at-risk community-at-large. This advanced practice may include the roles of direct caregiver, coordinator, consultant, educator, researcher, and administrator. Consistent with the American Nurses' Association Social Policy Statement and the Position on Advanced Clinical Nursing Practice issued by the National Council of State Boards of Nursing, the basis for advanced nursing practice in oncology requires a minimum of a master's degree.

Oncology nurses practicing at the advanced level must be able to assess, conceptualize, diagnose, and analyze complex clinical and nonclinical problems related to an actual or potential diagnosis of cancer. In addition, advanced practice implies the ability to consider a wide range of theory and research relevant to understanding cancer-related problems and the ability to select and justify the application of the most meaningful theory or research to assist in problem-solving.

Advanced nursing practice in oncology is actualized through a variety of roles. The role of direct caregiver implies mastery of the nursing process and the ability to provide, guide, and evaluate nursing practice delivered to individuals diagnosed with cancer, their families, and the community. The coordinator role involves the expert use of the change process with the multidisciplinary oncology team to determine and achieve realistic health care goals for a particular individual or for an entire community.

The consultant role in advanced oncology nursing practice involves providing expertise about oncology to colleagues, allied health personnel, and all health care consumers. The educator role is exemplified by the expert design, implementation, and evaluation of educational activities after the learning needs of the client or the community have been assessed. The role of the researcher at the advanced level implies at least beginning skills in the use of the process that includes the ability to identify current researchable problems in cancer nursing, collaborate in research, and evaluate and implement research findings that have an impact on cancer care or cancer nursing. The administrative role involves use of the managerial process to create an environment that is conducive to the good health of the public and to professional nursing practice.

Advanced oncology nursing practice is best defined as expert competency and leadership in the provision of care to individuals with an actual or potential diagnosis of cancer.

IMPLEMENTATION OF GUIDELINES

Nursing Practice

The guidelines in this manual are intended to provide direction for the nurse in individualizing the care of the cancer patient and family. They are not intended to be used as standardized nursing care plans.

First, the nurse must choose the level of care required by the patient. It is important to read the definition/description of the level, as some levels have, of necessity, been approached differently. For example, the Guidelines for Prevention and Early Detection and Knowledge Deficit address Level 1 only, and nursing management is written as a comprehensive patient teaching plan.

Expected outcomes for the guidelines have been written for each level and address several distinct areas: patient knowledge/learning, patient skills/resources necessary to adapt to or correct/manage the problem, and patient physiologic status related to the problem. These outcomes correspond with specific nursing management strategies. For example, if nursing care is directed at patient teaching, the outcome is written to measure the patient's learning. When the nursing management addresses assessment, monitoring, or intervention, the patient outcome describes the physiologic status to be achieved.

Nursing management is comprehensive, and all interventions may not be relevant for all patients. It is the responsibility of the nurse to select the appropriate nursing interventions for individual patients and families. Nursing care is identified in three major areas: assessment, direct care/supervision, and patient education.

Staff Development

It is envisioned that this manual will be utilized in staff development activities. It may be incorporated as core content in orientation programs for oncology nurses, and specific content may be used in staff education programs. This book may serve as a resource in preparation for the ONS certification examination.

Patient Education

The Patient Teaching sections and the Patient Education Materials and Community Resources sections should be used to design patient education programs and resource references. They can be adapted for use in all settings.

Quality Assurance

Nursing process and patient outcomes are incorporated into these guidelines. Thus, content may be used as a framework for quality assurance monitoring tools or incorporated into existing monitoring tools. It is also envisioned that the nurse will utilize the expected outcomes in the evaluation of patient and family care.

Research

It is expected that use of these guidelines will encourage research to validate nursing practice and stimulate questions for nursing research.

REFERENCES

ANA-ONS Division on Medical-Surgical Nursing Practice. Outcome Standards for Cancer Nursing Practice. Kansas City, MO, American Nurses' Association, 1979.

ANA-ONS Standards of Oncology Nursing Practice. Kansas City, MO, American Nurses' Association, 1987.

Leavell, H., and Clark, E.G.: Preventive Medicine for the Doctor in His Community. New York, McGraw-Hill, 1965.

North American Nursing Diagnosis Association Taxonomy I with Complete Diagnosis. St. Louis, North American Nursing Diagnosis Association, June, 1987.

PREVENTION AND EARLY DETECTION

The nurse assesses the patient's personal risk factors and early detection practices to formulate actual or potential nursing diagnoses.

Appropriate patient outcomes to consider in planning nursing interventions will specify the patient's ability to:

1. recognize factors that place an individual at risk and may lead to cancer, such as the use of tobacco, improper nutrition, treatment with immunosuppressive agents, aging, and exposure to carcinogens.
2. describe high-risk behaviors, health-promoting activities (such as smoking cessation), and early detection techniques (such as breast self-examination, self-oral examination, and self-guaiac testing).
3. describe cancer warning signals.
4. identify a plan for seeking health care assistance whenever any alteration in health status occurs.
5. describe applicable cancer self-detection measures.

Evaluation of the patient's responses to nursing care is based on whether the patient possesses adequate information about cancer prevention and detection.

Excerpted from the ANA/ONS Standards of Oncology Nursing Practice.

Knowledge Deficit Related to Prevention and Early Detection of Bladder Cancer

Kathleen Cushman

Population at Risk

- Tobacco smokers
- In industrialized nations: workers in the dye, rubber, leather, paint, and organic chemical industries, especially prior to 1970. Janitors and cleaners, mechanics, truck drivers, mining machine operators, printing machine operators. Others with a history of occupational exposure to benzidine, 2-naphthylamine (chemical intermediates of aniline dye), or 4-aminobiphenyl
- In developing nations: people infected with *Schistosoma haematobium,* a parasitic organism endemic in African and Mediterranean countries causing urinary tract infections, particularly among males in agricultural occupations

LEVEL 1A: Prevention

EXPECTED OUTCOME

1. Patient demonstrates knowledge related to prevention of bladder cancer:
   - identifies personal risk factors for bladder cancer.
   - identifies smoking cessation as a means to prevent bladder cancer.
   - participates in a program for smoking cessation if applicable.
   - takes appropriate precautions to prevent exposure to carcinogens in the work place.
   - identifies methods to limit exposure to industrial carcinogens if in a high-risk occupation.
   - identifies hygienic measures to prevent schistosomiasis if at risk for exposure.
   - complies with prescribed therapy for schistosomiasis if applicable.

NURSING MANAGEMENT

Assessment

1. Evaluate knowledge level related to risk factors.
2. Obtain smoking and occupational histories.

3. For patients at risk for schistosomiasis, assess personal hygiene and environmental sanitation.

3

Knowledge Deficit Related to Prevention and Early Detection of Bladder Cancer

Patient Teaching

1. Define and describe the bladder cancer disease process, giving rationale for prevention and early detection measures.
2. Encourage smoking cessation as a measure to reduce risk for many illnesses, including bladder cancer. Provide referrals to smoking cessation programs.
3. Emphasize the importance of compliance with measures deemed appropriate by industry and government standards to protect against exposure to industrial carcinogens.
4. For patients at risk for schistosomiasis, health education should be presented related to hygiene and sanitation to reduce the risk of infection and increase participation in programs to treat infection and eradicate the water snails that transmit the organism.

LEVEL 1B: Early Detection

EXPECTED OUTCOME

1. Patient demonstrates knowledge related to early detection of bladder cancer:
   - lists signs and symptoms that should be brought to the attention of a health care professional.
   - identifies bladder cancer screening programs available.
2. Patient applies knowledge of prevention and early detection methods for bladder cancer to self-care:
   - initiates discussion of personal risk factors with primary health care provider.
   - participates in bladder cancer screening programs as available.

NURSING MANAGEMENT

Assessment

1. Evaluate level of motivation to participate in prevention and screening programs.
2. Access urinary habits and check urine for presence of blood.

Patient Teaching

1. List risk factors for bladder cancer, stressing that the disease has a long latency period. Emphasize that potential for developing bladder cancer may persist for twenty years or more after exposure to identified risk factors, and that observation for early signs and symptoms and participation in screening programs should continue.
2. Identify hematuria, with or without dysuria and urinary frequency, as the most common early sign of bladder cancer may be microscopic.
3. Discuss the benefits of participating in a bladder cancer screening program if available through work place.

4. Discuss measures used to detect early bladder cancer:
    - cytology (total voided urine specimen obtained in late morning and sent immediately to laboratory).
    - flow cytometry (examines DNA content of urine cells).
    - excretory urogram (intravenous pyelogram) evaluates upper tracts of ureters as well as bladder.
    - cystoscopy (visualizes bladder, opportunity to biopsy and bimanual examination).
    - carcinoembryonic antigen (CEA) serum level.
    - computed tomography, ultrasound, magnetic resonance imaging.

SUGGESTED READINGS

Brownson, R.C., Chang, J.C., and Davis, J.R.: Occupation, smoking, and alcohol in the epidemiology of bladder cancer. American Journal of Public Health 77(10):1298–1300, 1987.

Carpenter, A.A.: Clinical experience with transitional cell carcinoma of the bladder with special reference to smoking. Journal of Urology 141 (3):527–528, 1989.

Koroltchouk, V., Stanley, K., Stjernsward, J., and Mott, K.: Bladder cancer: Approaches to prevention and control. Bulletin of the World Health Organization 65(4):513–520, 1987.

Morrison, A.S., Buring, J.E., Verhoek, W.G., et al.: An international study of smoking and bladder cancer. Journal of Urology 131(2):650–654, 1984.

Rubin, P. (Ed.): Urologic and Male Genital Cancers in Clinical Oncology: A Multidisciplinary Approach. New York, American Cancer Society, 1983.

Wallace, D.M.A.: Occupational urothelial cancer. British Journal of Urology 61(3):175–182, 1988.

PATIENT EDUCATION MATERIALS AND COMMUNITY RESOURCES

Lewis, A.: Research Report: Cancer of the Bladder. National Cancer Institute, 1987.

What You Need to Know About Cancer of the Bladder. National Cancer Institute, 1981.

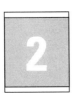

Knowledge Deficit Related to Prevention and Early Detection of Breast Cancer

Catherine M. Coleman and Rebecca Crane

Population at Risk

- All women, especially those over 40 (including pregnant and lactating women)
- Women with personal history of noninvasive or invasive breast carcinoma
- Women with biopsy-proven benign breast disease with hyperplasia or atypia
- Women with maternal or paternal family history of breast cancer
- Women who had early menses (before age 12), late menopause (after age 50), late first pregnancy (after age 30), or who have never had children

EXPECTED OUTCOME

1. Patient discusses individual thoughts and fears related to breasts and breast cancer:
   - verbalizes personal feelings about body image and breasts.
   - identifies personal, cultural, religious, or other factors that may influence self-care regarding prevention and early detection of breast disease.
   - expresses questions, fears, and concerns related to perceived risk of developing breast cancer.
2. Patient demonstrates understanding of general concepts related to breast health, and general facts related to breast disease in the United States:
   - verbalizes knowledge of breasts as site of normal physiologic changes throughout the life cycle.
   - identifies major anatomic structures of the breast.
   - identifies breast as most common site of cancer incidence in American women.
   - identifies definitions for the terms benign, malignant, in situ, invasive.
   - states that most breast abnormalities are benign.
   - acknowledges that most women discover their own breast changes.
   - verbalizes how to access major national and community resources related to breast health and breast cancer.
   - states that prognosis for breast cancer is most favorable when the tumor size is one-third of an inch (1 cm) or smaller.
   - describes options for treatment of early breast cancer.

"Women with no risk factors may develop breast cancer and women with many risk factors may not" (American Cancer Society, 1988c)

3. Patient states personal risk for developing breast cancer:
   - defines personal meaning of risk.
   - describes necessity of discerning facts from conflicting information on risk factors.
   - identifies significant risk factors in relation to self.
4. Patient defines three effective methods of early detection appropriate to age and personal history:
   - states the three most effective methods of early detection of breast cancer (mammography, clinical breast examination, and breast self-examination [BSE]).
   - defines the rationale for use of the three methods concurrently.
   - acknowledges lack of proven preventive methods.
   - identifies the ACS screening guidelines for breast cancer.
5. Patient describes usefulness of mammography as one method of early detection of breast cancer:
   - states that mammography is the most reliable method of finding breast cancer before it can be palpated.
   - defines the rationale for regular mammography.
   - differentiates between a screening and diagnostic mammogram.
   - states four components of quality assurance relative to mammography.
   - describes guidelines for frequency of mammography relative to age and risk status.
6. Patient describes importance of clinical breast examination as one method of early detection of breast cancer:
   - defines the rationale for regular clinical breast examination.
   - identifies both visual inspection and thorough palpation as major components of a regular clinical breast examination.
   - describes guidelines for frequency of clinical breast examinations relative to age and risk status.
   - schedules appointment for clinical breast examination through primary health care provider.
7. Patient demonstrates ability to perform a thorough breast self-examination:
   - defines the rationale for monthly BSE.
   - expresses understanding of normal visual and physical characteristics of own breasts.
   - defines abnormal breast changes that should be reported.
   - states appropriate time of month for BSE relative to current menstrual status.
   - redemonstrates to nurse a proficient BSE.
8. Patient applies knowledge about methods of early detection to self-care, appropriate to age and personal history:
   - initiates referral and schedules appointment for clinical breast examination, mammography, and BSE instruction through appropriate health care provider.
   - discusses personal concerns and needs related to risk factors, further individualized instruction in BSE, frequency and proficiency of clinical examinations, and quality mammography.
   - defines and adheres to self-care schedule of mammography, BSE, and clinical breast examination.

- verbalizes willingness to seek prompt attention from a health professional if a change occurs.

NURSING MANAGEMENT

Assessment

1. Establish level of knowledge related to breast health and breast cancer detection:
   - determine knowledge of common facts related to breast health and disease.
   - assess knowledge relative to prevention and early detection methods (dietary risk reduction, mammography, clinical breast examination, and breast self-examination (BSE)).
   - ascertain frequency and proficiency of BSE practice, preferably with direct observation of BSE technique (visual inspection and palpation).
   - ask if and when patient has had prior mammography; discuss patient perception of examination.
   - ask if and when patient has had prior clinical breast examination; discuss patient perception of examination.
   - obtain nursing history relative to cosmetic or therapeutic breast surgery.
2. Identify readiness to learn:
   - assess educational level, preferred learning methods, and barriers to learning (anxiety level, medical history of breast problems or breast cancer, level of comfort, excessive fatigue, expressions of denial).
   - observe verbal and nonverbal behavior.
   - assess level of interest for learning both information and skills related to frequency and proficiency of BSE.
   - determine willingness to schedule 15–30 minutes for breast health instruction.
3. Evaluate level of motivation or anxiety.
4. Identify other factors that may influence instruction or compliance (e.g., physical limitations, financial constraints, cultural taboos, religious beliefs, personal beliefs, feelings).

Patient Teaching

1. Provide comfortable, quiet, and private environment for teaching and learning.
2. Utilize a variety of audiovisual aids to assist in instruction:
   - videotapes.
   - slide and tape programs.
   - breast palpation models.
   - pamphlets in English or other languages are useful tools (see Teaching Aids).
3. Encourage patient to express fears and feelings related to breasts and breast cancer.
4. Explore common misconceptions and associations surrounding the words "cancer" and "breast" in our society.
5. Provide information that defines the terms: tumor, benign, malignant, cancer, biopsy.
6. Define concept of "risk"
   - one in ten women will develop breast cancer in their lifetime. Nine in ten will not.
7. Discuss nutritional factors that may contribute to development of breast cancer:
   - high-fat diet.
   - low-fiber diet.
   - diet low in vitamins A and C.
8. Encourage patient to develop and maintain good nutrition and health habits (e.g., regular exercise; low-fat, high-fiber diet rich in vitamins A and C; limited intake of caffeine; stress reduction).
9. Give rationale for early detection: increased cure rate if in situ or noninvasive

stage 0 or stage I cancer is detected; more breast-saving treatment options.

10. Share information regarding the most accepted and effective methods of early detection for breast cancer: mammography, BSE, and physical examination by a health professional.
    - mammography performed for appropriate age groups is single most accurate test available to find preclinical cancer.
    - rationale for combined methods to maximize detection of interval cancers between mammogram.

11. Discuss ACS screening guidelines for breast cancer:
    - monthly breast self-examination for all women over 20.
    - breast physical examination every 3 years for women ages 20 to 40.
    - breast physical examination every year for women over age 40.
    - one baseline mammogram for women 35 to 40 years of age.
    - a mammogram every 1 to 2 years for women aged 40 to 49.
    - annual mammography for women over age 50.
    - frequent exams and earlier mammogram for women with personal or family histories of breast cancer or who are at higher than average risk.

12. Describe for patient the components of quality assurance in mammography (e.g., low dose equipment, skilled radiologic technologist, expert physician interpretation, meticulous attention to x-ray film processing).

13. Instruct in normal anatomy and normal physiologic changes with age, menstrual cycle, pregnancy, and lactation.

14. Inform patient that BSE should be done monthly, one week after onset of menses for premenopausal women.

15. Demonstrate BSE including inspection and palpation using appropriate audiovisual-tactile teaching aids:
    - correct position for visual inspection.

- correct position for palpation to maximize exposure of upper outer quadrant where 50 per cent of all breast cancers develop.
- perimeter of breast tissue to be included in BSE.
- finger pads for palpation, and movement in dime-sized circles.
- three levels of pressure (light, medium, deep) during each palpation to maximize detection of superficial and deep lesions.
- systematic pattern for palpation of entire breast.

16. Encourage patient to disrobe from waist up to promote personalized instruction in visual inspection and palpation techniques of BSE.

17. Demonstrate to patient how to differentiate her own breast tissue and nodularity.

18. Observe patient's return demonstration and provide corrective feedback of BSE technique.

19. Instruct women with a history of silicone implants, radiation therapy to the breast, or prior cosmetic or therapeutic breast surgery to perform the same BSE technique to monitor normal areas for visual and palpable changes.

20. Discuss possible site of chest wall, lymph node, or incisional recurrence for women with a history of breast cancer.

21. Plan additional BSE training or instruction if needed or desired.

22. Encourage patient to initiate request for mammography and BSE instruction as appropriate at the time of clinical breast examination to promote correlation of normal anatomy and physiology, menstrual, or other changes.

23. Provide patient with written instructions for ongoing breast health care to include mammography and date of follow-up, BSE and time of month, and clinical breast examination with date of follow-up.

24. Assist patient to formulate and discuss questions and concerns with primary

Knowledge Deficit Related to Prevention and Early Detection of Breast Cancer

health care provider to reinforce personal plan of breast health care.

25. Refer patient or family to appropriate local, regional, or national resources for additional information (e.g., American Cancer Society, American College of Radiology, and National Cancer Institute).

SUGGESTED READINGS

American Cancer Society: Breast self-examination: A new approach. (Publication No. 6438.39). Oakland, CA, California Division, American Cancer Society, 1988a.

American Cancer Society: Breast self-examination: Proficiency criteria and guidelines. Oakland, CA, California Division, American Cancer Society, 1988b.

American Cancer Society: Cancer Facts & Figures—1990 (Publication 90-450m-No. 5008-LE). Atlanta, 1990.

American Cancer Society: Clinical breast examination: Proficiency criteria and guidelines. (Publication No. 6438.42). Oakland, CA, California Division, American Cancer Society, 1988c.

American Cancer Society: Special Touch Facilitator's Guide. (Publication 87-25M-No. 2415-LE). Atlanta, 1987.

American Cancer Society: Staging for breast carcinoma. (Publication No. 89-25M-No. 3485.05) Atlanta GA, American Cancer Society, 1989.

Assaf, A.R., Cummings, K.M., Graham, S., et al.: Comparison of three methods of teaching women how to perform breast self-examination. Health Education Quarterly 12:259–272, 1985.

Clarke, D.E., and Sandler, L.S.: Factors involved in nurses' teaching breast self-examination. Cancer Nursing 12(1):41–46, 1989.

Dorsay, R.H., Cuneo, W.D., Somkin, C.P., and Tekawa, I.S.: Breast self-examination: Improving competence and frequency in a classroom setting. American Journal of Public Health 78:520–522, 1988.

Dupont, W.D., and Page, D.L.: Risk factors for breast cancer in women with proliferative breast disease. New England Journal of Medicine 312:146–151, 1985.

Feig, S.A.: Decreased breast cancer mortality through mammographic screening: Results of clinical trials. Radiology 167:659–665, 1988.

Fletcher, S.W.E., O'Malley, M.S., and Bunce, L.A.: Physicians' abilities to detect lumps in silicone breast models. Journal of the American Medical Association 253:2224–2228, 1985.

Foster, R.S., and Costanza, M.C.: Breast self-examination practices and breast cancer survival. Cancer 53:999–1005, 1984.

Haughery, B.P., Marshall, J.R., Mettlin, C., et al.: Nurses' ability to detect nodules in silicone breast models. Oncology Nursing Forum 11:37–42, 1984.

Huguley, C.M., Brown, R.L., Greenberg, R.S., and Clark, W.S.: Breast self-examination and survival from breast cancer. Cancer 62:1389–1396, 1988.

Kegeles, S.S.: Education for breast self-examination: Why, who, what, and how. Preventive Medicine 14:702–720, 1985.

McGinn, K.: Keeping Abreast. Palo Alto, CA, Bull Publishing, 1987.

O'Malley, M.S., and Fletcher, S.W.: US Preventive Services Task Force. Screening for breast cancer with breast self-examination: A critical review. Journal of the American Medical Association 257:2196–2203, 1987.

Pennypacker, H.S., Criswell, E.L., Neelakantan, P., et al.: Toward an effective technology of instruction in breast self-examination. International Journal of Mental Health 11: 98–116, 1982.

Pennypacker, H.S., Goldstein, M.K., and Stein, G.H.: A precise method of manual breast self-examination. In Mettlin, C., and Murphy, G. (Eds.): Progress in Cancer Control. IV: Research in the Cancer Center. New York: Alan R. Liss, 1983, pp 305–311.

Sachs, B.C.: Breasts: Sex symbols and releasers. Breast—Diseases of the Breast 4(4):26–30, 1987.

Saunders, K.J., Pilgram, C.A., and Pennypacker, H.S.: Increased proficiency of search in breast self-examination. Cancer 58:2531–2537, 1986.

Wertheimer, M.D., Costanza, M.C., Dodson, T.F., et al.: Increasing the effort toward breast cancer detection. Journal of the American Medical Association 255:1311–1315, 1986.

PATIENT EDUCATION MATERIALS AND COMMUNITY RESOURCES

American Cancer Society
California Division
1710 Webster Street
P.O. Box 2061
Oakland, CA 94612
415-893-7900
1. BSE Skills Checklist
2. Breast Health materials in non-English languages.

Krames Communications
312 90th Street
Daly City, CA 94015–1898
800-223-5299
Breast series—print brochures

Lange Productions
7661 Curson Terrace
Hollywood, CA 90046
213-874-4730

Videotapes:
1. Breast Facts: The Basics (1989)
2. BSE: A New Approach (1988)
3. Imaging the Augmented Breast (1988)
4. Mammography: An Image for Life (1988)
5. Radiation Therapy: An Option for Early Breast Cancer (1989)

Mammatech Corporation
900 NW 8th Avenue
Gainesville, FL 32601
800-626-2273
1. Mammacare Learning System—interactive videotape of BSE with life-like breast model and lump simulations
2. Lump-Chart—3 Dimensional. Chart illustrates 3 mm to 5 cm lump sizes.
3. Simulated models with life-like breast nodularity and five lumps under 1 cm with different locations and textures illustrating normal, benign, and malignant characteristics.

National Telephone Information Service

American Cancer Society, Atlanta, GA. 800-227-2345

American College of Radiology, Mammography Accreditation Program, Reston, VA, 800-227-5463

National Alliance of Breast Cancer Organizations, New York, NY, 212-719-0154

National Cancer Institute, Bethesda, MD, 800-4-CANCER

National Coalition for Cancer Survivorship, 505-764-9956

Y-ME, Breast Cancer Support Program, Homewood, IL, 800-221-2141

Knowledge Deficit Related to Prevention and Early Detection of Cervical and Uterine (Endometrial) Cancer

Julia Fanslow

Population at Risk

- Females ages 18–70
- Cervical cancer; multiple sex partners; first intercourse at an early age; poor personal hygiene; history of viral infections, such as herpes II and papilloma; low socioeconomic strata
- Uterine (endometrial) cancer; obesity; nulliparity; irregular menses; diabetes mellitus; history of infertility or failure to ovulate; prolonged estrogen therapy

LEVEL 1A: Prevention of Cervical Cancer

EXPECTED OUTCOME

1. Patient states that a knowledge deficit exists.
2. Patient demonstrates knowledge related to prevention of cervical cancer:
   - identifies personal risk factors.
   - identifies measures to minimize risk factors.
   - identifies measures to prevent cervical cancer.

NURSING MANAGEMENT

Assessment

1. Obtain history of risk factors.
2. Assess gynecologic status:
   - menstrual history: date of menarche, regularity, any dysfunction.
   - pregnancies, miscarriages, abortions.
   - date of menopause.
3. Obtain most recent pelvic exam and Pap testing results.
4. Obtain relevant sexual history.
5. Assess beliefs and values that may affect compliance with recommended practices.
6. Assess hygiene practices, particularly related to genitourinary (GU) system. Include type of contraceptive used (barrier vs. nonbarrier).
7. Assess knowledge of prevention of cervical cancer.

Patient Teaching

1. Encourage active patient participation in goal setting, decision-making, and problem-solving.
2. Provide information on risk factors of cervical cancer and how to minimize them.
3. Assist the patient/family in assuming responsibility for maximizing physical and mental health potential.
4. Provide information about the disease of cervical cancer and appropriate preventative measures.
5. Explain importance of a complete gynecologic examination that includes pelvic examination and Pap test in preventing cervical cancer.
6. Discuss schedule of gynecologic check-ups; ACS Guidelines recommended:
   - having complete pelvic examination and Pap test at onset of sexual activity or by age 20.
   - pelvic examination and Pap test should be done annually until two consecutive normal exams and then at least every 3 years.
   - ACOG recommends annual pelvic examination and Pap test.
   - continue pelvic examination and Pap test after menopause.

LEVEL 1B: Early Detection of Cervical Cancer

EXPECTED OUTCOME

1. Patient states that a knowledge deficit exists.
2. Patient demonstrates knowledge related to early detection of cervical cancer.
   - states signs and symptoms of disease process, including those to be reported to health care professionals.
   - states individual risk factors.
   - demonstrates self-direction and self-management by carrying out appropriate health care follow-up related to gynecologic examination and Pap testing.
3. Patient preserves child-bearing ability and sexual function:
   - implements learned prevention and detection interventions.
   - verbalizes signs and symptoms of gynecologic dysfunction.
   - follows up appropriately on gynecologic dysfunction.

NURSING MANAGEMENT

Assessment

1. Assess gynecologic status:
   - menstrual history: date of menarche, regularity, dysfunction.
2. Obtain most recent results of pelvic examination, Pap test.
3. Obtain relevant sexual history.
4. Obtain history of signs and symptoms of cervical cancer:
   - early detection:
     - slight watery, purulent, or mucoid discharge.
     - slight bleeding after intercourse, exertion, travel, or douching.
   - late detection:
     - yellow vaginal discharge, frequently foul smelling.
     - peri-irritation, vulvitis.
     - pelvic pain.

5. Assess hygiene practices, particularly related to the GU system. Include type of contraceptive used (barrier and nonbarrier types).
6. Assess knowledge related to early detection of cervical cancer.

Patient Teaching

1. Implement Patient Teaching Level 1A.
2. Inform patient of direct relationship between cure and early detection (preinvasive disease is 100 per cent curative).
3. Define medical terms used in classification of Pap test:
   - Class I: smear is normal, no abnormal cells.
   - Class II: atypical cells are present below the level of cervical neoplasia.

- Class III: smear contains abnormal cells consistent with dysplasia.
- Class IV: smear contains abnormal cells consistent with carcinoma in situ.
- Class V: smear contains abnormal cells consistent with invasive carcinoma of squamous cell origin.

5. Discuss follow-up for Pap test:
   - Class I: after two consecutive (annual) negative tests, obtain Pap test every 3 years.
   - Class II–III: in consultation with physician may repeat Pap test in 3 to 6 months.
   - Class IV: in consultation with physician, may do colposcopy, biopsy, cryotherapy, carbon dioxide laser treatment, hysterectomy.
   - Class V: treatment is initiated and will depend on stage of disease, may include surgery, radiation, and chemotherapy.

LEVEL 1A: *Prevention of Uterine (Endometrial) Cancer*

EXPECTED OUTCOME

1. Patient states that a knowledge deficit exists.
2. Patient demonstrates knowledge related to prevention of uterine cancer:
   - identifies personal risk factors.
   - identifies measures to minimize risk factors.
   - identifies measures to prevent uterine cancer such as regular Pap testing, endometrial biopsy, pelvic examination.

NURSING MANAGEMENT

Assessment

1. Obtain history of risk factors.
2. Obtain most recent results of pelvic examination, Pap test, and endometrial biopsy at menopause.
3. Assess gynecologic status:

- menstrual history: date of menarche, regularity or dysfunction.
- history of pregnancy: miscarriages, abortions.
- date of menopause.
4. Assess knowledge related to prevention of uterine cancer.

Patient Teaching

1. Implement Patient Teaching Level 1A.
2. Discuss importance and components of regular health care check-ups.
3. Discuss role of diet and weight control in cancer prevention.
4. Emphasize importance of screening, especially for high-risk patients.

5. Discuss signs and symptoms of dysfunctional vaginal bleeding to be reported to health care providers:
   - changes in patterns of bleeding.
   - "breakthrough" bleeding.
   - irregular menses.
   - postmenopausal bleeding occurring 6 months or more after cessation of menses.

LEVEL 1B: Early Detection of Uterine (Endometrial) Cancer

EXPECTED OUTCOME

1. Patient states that a knowledge deficit exists.
2. Patient demonstrates awareness of knowledge needs:
   - verbalizes need for behavior changes to reestablish or maintain optimum health.
   - verbalizes need for self-management of health promotion and maintenance.
3. Patient demonstrates knowledge related to early detection of uterine cancer:
   - states signs and symptoms of disease process including those to be reported to health professionals.
   - gives verbal feedback of knowledge gained through teaching.
   - demonstrates self-direction and self-management by carrying out appropriate health care follow-up.
4. Patient preserves child-bearing ability and sexual function:
   - implements learned prevention and detection interventions.
   - verbalizes signs and symptoms of gynecologic dysfunction.
   - does follow-up on gynecologic dysfunction appropriately.

NURSING MANAGEMENT

Assessment

1. Obtain history of signs and symptoms of vaginal bleeding:
   - postmenopausal.
   - irregular menses.
   - irregular flow of menses.
   - unusual spotting.
   - changes in normal pattern of bleeding.
2. Obtain most recent results of pelvic examination, Pap test, endometrial biopsy, fractional curettage.
3. Note history of risk factors.
4. Assess gynecologic status:
   - menstrual history, date of menarche, regularity, dysfunction.
   - presence of endometrial hyperplasia.
5. Assess knowledge of early detection of uterine cancer.

Knowledge Deficit Related to Prevention and Early Detection of Cervical and Uterine (Endometrial) Cancer

Patient Teaching

1. Implement Patient Teaching in Level 1A.
2. Explain need for regular gynecologic checkups, especially for high-risk patients.
3. Discuss ACS Guidelines for uterine (endometrial) cancer:
   - pelvic examination every 3 years for women from 20 to 40 years of age and annually for women age 40 and older.
   - endometrial tissue sample at menopause if at higher risk.
4. Educate about usefulness of Pap test and endometrial biopsy:
   - Pap test is only 50 per cent effective in detecting uterine cancer.
   - endometrial biopsy is test of choice.
   - importance of continued screening after menopause.
5. Emphasize need for follow-up for abnormal symptoms if not resolved.
6. Teach classifications of uterine cancer when appropriate.
7. Discuss treatment options for uterine cancer when appropriate.

SUGGESTED READINGS

American Cancer Society: Cancer Facts and Figures, 1990. Atlanta, 1990.

Groenwald, S.: Cancer Nursing Principles and Practice. Boston, Jones & Bartlett, 1987.

Holleb, A.L. (Ed.): Early gynecologic cancers. CA: A Cancer Journal for Clinicians 39(3):133–192, 1989.

Holleb, A. (Ed.): Cancer statistics. CA: A Cancer Journal for Clinicians 39(1): 1–64, 1989.

Nelson, J., Averette, H., and Richart, R.: Cervical intra-epithelial neoplasia (dysplasia and carcinoma in situ) and early invasive cervical carcinoma. CA: A Cancer Journal for Clinicians 39(3):157–178, 1989.

PATIENT EDUCATION MATERIALS AND COMMUNITY RESOURCES

American Cancer Society Public Education materials related to prevention and early detection of cervical and uterine cancer. For example:
Cancer Facts for Women
Facts on Uterine Cancer
Cancer Facts and Figures 1990 (updated annually).

National Cancer Institute Public Education materials related to prevention and early detection of cervical and uterine cancer. For example:
Cancer of the Uterus
Cancer of the Cervix

Public Education materials related to prevention and early detection of cervical and uterine cancer available from major cancer centers. For example:
Pap Smear: Early Detection for Cervical Cancer (available from Fred Hutchison Cancer Center, Seattle, WA)

Knowledge Deficit Related to Prevention and Early Detection of Colorectal Cancer

Gail Egan Sansivero

Population at Risk

- Individuals over 40 years of age
- Individuals with high-fat or low-fiber dietary patterns
- Individuals with a personal or family history of adenomatous colonic polyps, familial adenomatous polyposis syndrome (Gardner's syndrome), hereditary nonpolyposis colorectal cancer syndrome (Messner, 1986; Winawer, 1987)
- Individuals with chronic ulcerative colitis (particularly if of 10 years' duration or longer), Crohn's disease, or Peutz-Jeghers syndrome, chronic granulomatous colitis (Messner, 1986)
- Individuals with a family history of colorectal cancer or sporadic colorectal adenomas
- Individuals with a history of colorectal cancer, breast, or endometrial cancer (Winawer, 1987)

LEVEL 1A: Prevention

EXPECTED OUTCOME

1. Patient states that a knowledge deficit exists.
2. Patient demonstrates knowledge of risk factors for colorectal cancer:
   - identifies diseases associated with colorectal cancer.
   - identifies types of diets associated with colorectal cancer.
   - identifies age of 40 years or more as risk factor.
   - identifies personal risk factors.
3. Patient identifies health and personal habits that promote bowel health:
   - inspects stools regularly.
   - restricts fat content in diet.
   - uses natural laxatives when needed.
   - includes fresh fruits and vegetables in diet regularly.
   - exercises regularly.
   - maintains adequate hydration status.

NURSING MANAGEMENT

Assessment

1. Evaluate readiness to learn (including motivating factors, impeding factors, attention span, and stress level).
2. Assess for presence and effect of any impediments to learning (illiteracy, sensory impairments, etc.).
3. Obtain history of colorectal cancer and polypotic disease. Diseases associated with in-

creased risk of colorectal cancer include adenomatous polyps, Crohn's disease, Peutz-Jeghers syndrome, villous adenomas, familial polyposis (Gardner's syndrome), and ulcerative colitis for 10 years or longer.

4. Assess risk factors: age over 40 years (highest risk is for those over 60 years), high-fat diet, low-fiber diet, previous history of cancer.

5. Assess personal habits affecting bowel health:
   - pattern of elimination: frequency, character of stool (color, texture, presence of excessive mucus or fat, presence of blood).
   - use of laxatives (types, frequency, response).
   - dietary pattern (amount and type of fat and fiber/bulk in daily foods); excessive use of butter, oil, animal fats, dairy products; limited use of whole grains, fresh fruits, vegetables.
   - assess fluid intake for adequacy.
   - assess activity level (quantity and frequency of exercise).

Patient Teaching

1. Help patient identify personal risk factors through education about:
   - bowel diseases associated with an increased risk of colorectal cancer.
   - age groups at high risk.
   - dietary habits that contribute to increased risk.

2. Ask patient to inspect stools on regular basis for abnormal color (red, tarry), blood, change in shape of stools such as pencil-shaped stools, or excessive mucus or fat, and to report any abnormalities to health care team.

3. Describe normal bowel pattern (for most individuals this is one to two stools every 1–2 days). See Patient Education and Resources List.

4. Identify and use available educational materials to teach signs and symptoms of colorectal cancer.

5. Explain dietary interventions to promote bowel health:
   - use bulk or fiber in daily diet as natural laxative to promote bowel health. Foods high in fiber include whole grains and fresh fruits and vegetables.
   - use all food groups to balance nutrition.
   - use natural laxatives (prune juice, senna, bran flakes/foods) if needed.
   - maintain adequate fat intake: about 25 per cent of total calories (average American consumes 40 per cent fat).
   - eat high-fiber diet. Diets lower in fiber lead to low-bulk stools and slow transmission of dietary components through the gut. This may permit longer time for formation of carcinogens in gut and longer contact time.
   - drink adequate fluid: about 2–3 L per day.
   - maintain adequate exercise level to promote bowel motility.

LEVEL 1B: Early Detection

EXPECTED OUTCOME

1. Patient recognizes symptoms that require health care evaluation:
   - identifies changes in bowel habits, abdominal pain with bloating, bloody stools, and black, tarry stools as symptoms to report to the health care team.

2. Patient seeks health care for symptoms of colorectal cancer:
   • participates in screening programs for colorectal cancer.
   • identifies an available physician or primary health care provider.
3. Patient describes detection measures to determine the presence of colorectal cancer, including:
   • Hemoccult testing.
   • inspection of stools.
   • rectal examination.
   • double-contrast barium enema.
   • sigmoidoscopy.
   • colonoscopy.
   • carcinoembryonic antigen (CEA).
4. Patient identifies appropriate community and personal resources that provide information and support.

NURSING MANAGEMENT

Assessment

1. Evaluate recent health history, paying particular attention to weight changes, appetite, energy, and activity level.
2. Assess personal and family risk factors.
3. Determine ability and willingness to participate in self-detection (e.g., guaiac stool testing, observation of stools).
4. Evaluate local resources for health care in the community. Assess resources for payment for health care. Determine options for choice of health care and of health care provider (i.e., clinic, private physician, etc.).
5. Identify resources for transportation to health care provider.
6. Evaluate previous patterns of patient/family behavior related to health maintenance.
7. Assess patient/family ability to make informed decision to seek treatment or not.

Patient Teaching

1. Establish relationship with high-risk patient/family.
2. Discuss need for high-risk patient/family to comply with screening, at early age (e.g., 40 years) when possible, without becoming "cancer phobic."
3. Indicate importance of early detection and immediate action in relation to disease course and outcome.
4. Explain symptoms to report to health care team:
   • changes in bowel habits (constipation, diarrhea).
   • weight loss.
   • abdominal pain (usually vague and crampy), indigestion, bloating.
   • fatigue, weakness.
   • anorexia.
   • sense of incomplete evacuation after bowel movement.
   • decrease in caliber of stool.
   • passage of blood or mucus in stool.
   • tenesmus (painful straining to produce stool).
   • black, tarry stools.
   • increased use of laxatives.
5. Offer instruction for recording signs and symptoms and bowel pattern (including frequency).
6. Explain ACS screening guidelines:
   • annual digital rectal examination after age 40 (75 per cent of rectal tumors are within reach of the examining finger).
   • guaiac stool testing annually after age 50; after age 40 if in high-risk group.
   • sigmoidoscopy every 3 to 5 years beginning at age 50 (ACS, 1989).

7. Provide written information on collection method for stool specimen to be brought to health care provider:
   - dietary restrictions 48 hours before and during testing: Avoid: red or rare meat, turnips, broccoli, cauliflower, cantaloupe, aspirin, tonics, nonsteroidal anti-inflammatory agents, ascorbic acid (vitamin C) (Messner, 1986).
   - two separate specimens for 3 consecutive days.
   - specimens should be returned to health care provider upon completion of sampling.
   - specimens should be stored no longer than 14 days before testing.
8. Explain that colonoscopy should be done when any of the tests in #6 are positive.
9. Explain purpose and procedure of all detection methods including barium enema and CEA levels.
10. Indicate that benign polyps may be removed during detection procedures to reduce incidence of cancer.
11. Offer instruction on available community health care resources (see Patient Education and Resources List).

tion and education. Oncology Nursing Forum 16(1):87–94, 1989.

Glasel, M.: Cancer prevention: Myths and realities. Cancer Nursing 10(Suppl 1):91–94, 1987.

Gralick, R., Macrae, F.A., and Fleisher, M.: How to perform the fecal occult blood test. CA: A Cancer Journal for Clinicians 34(3):134–145, 1984.

Messner, R.L., Gardner, S.S., and Webb, D.D.: Early detection—The priority in colorectal cancer. Cancer Nursing 9(1):8–14, 1986.

Mitchell-Beren, M.E., Beren, M.E., Dodds, M.E., et al.: A colorectal cancer prevention, screening, and evaluation program in community black churches. CA: A Cancer Journal for Clinicians 39(2):115–118, 1989.

Rose, M.A.: Health promotion and risk prevention: Applications for cancer survivors. Oncology Nursing Forum 16(3):335–340, 1989.

Stroenlein, J.R., Gaulston, K., and Hunt, R.H.: Diagnostic approach to evaluating the cause of a positive fecal occult blood test. CA: A Cancer Journal for Clinicians 34(3):148–157, 1984.

Wanebo, H.J., Fang, W.L., Mills, A.S., et al.: Colorectal cancer—A blueprint for disease control through screening by primary core physicians. Archives of Surgery 121(11):1347–1352, 1986.

White, L.N., and Taylor, D.: Prevention/detection: The nurse's role. Cancer Nursing 10(Suppl 1):72–78, 1987.

Winawer, S.J.: Screening for colorectal cancer. In DeVita, V.T., Hellman, S., and Rosenberg, S.A. (Eds.): Cancer: Principles and Practice of Oncology. Philadelphia, J.B. Lippincott, 1987.

Winchester, D.P., Sylvester, J., and Maher, M.L.: Risks and benefits of mass screening for colorectal neoplasia with the stool guaiac test. CA: A Cancer Journal for Clinicians, 33(6):333–334, 1983.

SUGGESTED READINGS

American Cancer Society: The health professional and cancer prevention and detection. No 3372-PE. Atlanta, American Cancer Society, 1989.

American Nurses' Association and Oncology Nursing Society. Standards of oncology nursing practice. Kansas City, MO, American Nurses Association, 1987.

Campbell, H.S.: Risk factors for cancer. Cancer Nursing 10(Suppl 1):79–87, 1987.

Crespi, M.D., Weissman, G.S., Gilbertson, V.A., et al.: The role of proctosigmoidoscopy in screening for colorectal neoplasia. CA: A Cancer Journal for Clinicians 34 (3):158–166, 1984.

Faulkenberry, J.E.: Cancer prevention and detection: Colorectal cancer. Cancer Nursing 7(5):415–423, 1984.

Fenoglio-Preiser, C.M., and Hutter, R.V.P.: Colorectal polyps: Pathologic diagnosis and clinical significance. CA: A Cancer Journal for Clinicians 35(6):322–344, 1985.

Fitzsimmons, M.L., Conway, T.A., Madsen, N., et al.: Hereditary cancer syndromes: Nursing's role in identifica-

PATIENT EDUCATION MATERIALS AND COMMUNITY RESOURCES

American Cancer Society Public Education Materials

#2051—English	Go For Early Detection (brochure)	
#2673—Spanish		
#2137	Go For the Best Protection (poster)	
#2666	Don't Miss Out on Your Sunset Years (brochure) (for Black Population)	
#2670	Ask Your Physician (pocket-size cards)	

#2675.02	You Can Protect Yourself Against Colorectal Cancer, 1988 (brochure) (English and Spanish)
#2004	Facts on Colorectal Cancer, 1988
#2729	Check Yourself, 1988

National Cancer Institute Public Education Materials

Good News, Better News, Best News . . . Cancer Prevention. 84-2671, 1984.

What You Need to Know About Colorectal Cancer. 88-1552, 1988.

Diet, Nutrition and Cancer Prevention: A Guide for Food Choices. 87-2878, 1987.

Cancer Facts for People Over 50. 84-456, 1984.

Everything Doesn't Cause Cancer. 85-2059, 1985.

Good News for Blacks About Cancer. 87-2956, 1987.

Facts on Cancer Sites (Spanish): Colon y Del Recto. 1988.

Cancer of Colon and Rectum: Research Report. 88-95, 1988.

Knowledge Deficit Related to Prevention and Early Detection of Head and Neck Cancer

Joan R. Schleper

Population at Risk

- Individuals, particularly white males, over age 60
- Individuals with a history of any form of tobacco use
- Individuals with a history of excessive ethanol alcohol consumption
- Individuals with poor oral and dental hygiene
- Individuals with occupational exposure to asbestos, coke, arsenic, nickel, chromium, cutting oils (used by machinists), mustard gas, and exposure to wood, textile, or leather dusts
- Individuals who have been overexposed to ultraviolet radiation
- Individuals who have received previous ionizing radiation for the treatment of benign conditions
- Individuals with a positive personal or family history of head and neck cancer
- Individuals who have been exposed to specific viruses: Epstein-Barr, human papilloma, or herpes simplex
- Immunosuppressed individuals

LEVEL 1A: *Prevention*

EXPECTED OUTCOME

1. Patient demonstrates knowledge of prevention of head and neck cancer:
   - identifies risk factors that cannot be altered: age, gender, race, past, personal and family history.
   - identifies risk factors that can be modified or reduced: those related to life style and personal habits, and environment and occupation.
2. Patient identifies and demonstrates measures to prevent or reduce the occurrence of head and neck cancer.

(The contents of this chapter in no way are meant to represent the views of the Department of Veterans Affairs.)

NURSING MANAGEMENT

Assessment

1. Assess patient/caregiver knowledge level and willingness to learn.
2. Assess the patient's risk factor profile for head and neck cancer as listed above in Population at Risk.
3. Assess life style and personal habits:
   - tobacco use: types used (combustible and smokeless forms), daily amount consumed, number of years used.
   - alcohol consumption: amount per day, number of years used.
   - frequency of dental visits, including those of patients who are edentulous.
   - dietary intake, particularly foods containing vitamins A, B, and C, and protein.

Patient Teaching

1. Teach that head and neck cancers (oral cavity, pharynx, and larynx) occur in white males over the age of 40 (peak incidence 60 to 70 years) who use tobacco and/or alcohol. An increase in incidence is also occurring in females and blacks with the same personal habits.
2. State that 90 per cent of head and neck cancers are related specifically to tobacco use. The tobacco risk is dose-dependent or proportional to:
   - amount of tobacco used daily.
   - types of tobacco used: cigarettes, cigars, pipes, snuff, chewing tobacco.
   - number of years used.
   - amount of tar in cigarettes.
3. Explain that excessive alcohol intake is defined as a quantity of six or more of any ethanol alcohol consumed daily (6 oz hard liquor, six 12 oz beers, six 5 oz glasses of wine). Alcohol use alone accounts for only 4 per cent of all cancer risks, but when used in combination with tobacco, there appears to be a compound irritating effect on the mucous membranes of the mouth and throat.
4. Discuss daily dietary intake. Diet should include foods from the four basic food groups, especially foods containing vitamins A, B, and C, and proteins. Dietary deficiencies are common in those who abuse alcohol.
5. Discuss the importance of annual dental visits if teeth are present, and visits every three years if patient is edentulous. The majority of head and neck cancer patients have poor oral and dental hygiene. Therefore, there may be a possible association between chronic irritation from jagged sharp teeth or ill-fitting dentures or partials, and the development of an oral cancer.
6. Discuss the importance of compliance with safety measures if exposure to carcinogenic agents occurs in the work place.
7. Inform patient of implications of a family history of cancer, specifically head and neck cancer. The risk may be increased somewhat, therefore factors within the patient's control such as tobacco and alcohol use should be avoided.
8. Discuss primary measures to reduce risks for head and neck cancer:
   - Optimally, avoid or stop tobacco use; minimally, reduce daily intake.
   - If patient does not abuse alcohol, limit daily alcohol intake to two drinks or less.
   - Identify local resources and various programs to help the patient/family eliminate tobacco and/or alcohol use.
   - Provide outlets to assist patient in coping with anxieties (e.g., support groups, counseling).
   - Perform daily oral hygiene, brushing and flossing (if teeth are present).
   - See a dentist annually or every three years if edentulous.
   - Eat a well-balanced diet.
   - Use protective measures in the work place.

- Limit sun exposure from 10 AM to 2 PM, cover skin, and use sunscreens daily with SPF of 15, particularly if fair-skinned.

LEVEL 1B: *Early Detection*

EXPECTED OUTCOME

1. Patient demonstrates knowledge of early detection modalities:
   - describes proper monthly self-inspection and palpation techniques of the skin, oral cavity, and cervical lymphatics.
   - identifies signs and symptoms to report to health care team.
   - describes importance of annual dental and physician visits, particularly to the otolaryngologist, or head and neck surgeon.

NURSING MANAGEMENT

Assessment

1. Inspect face and neck for asymmetry, masses, jugular distention, pain, numbness, or tingling.
2. Palpate bony surface above and below the eye, maxilla, and zygoma noting tenderness, asymmetry, or bone deformity.
3. Inspect and palpate the skin surfaces of the scalp, neck, and face. Observe any pigmented lesions for changes in:
   - color—various shades.
   - size—greater than 6 mm.
   - shape.
   - sudden increase in elevation.
   - maculopapular appearance; scaly, rough, or ulcerated surface.
   - firm consistency.
   - itching, burning, tingling, or bleeding.
   - persistent (longer than 3 weeks) ulcerations particularly with associated color changes.
4. Assess eyes for:
   - diplopia.
   - exophthalmos (may be due to tumor in the maxillary/ethmoid sinuses).
   - motor functions of CN III, IV, VI.
5. Assess the external auditory canal and, if able, tympanic membrane for:
   - color changes.
   - sores and lesions.
   - retraction.
   - bulging.
   - fluid.
   - intactness.
   - obstruction.
   - history of changes in hearing, ear pain, complaints of a "stopped up" ear, or dizziness and tinnitus.
6. Direct inspection with a light source of the nose and nasal cavity for the following:
   - marked asymmetry.
   - color changes.
   - persistent sores and lumps.
   - unilateral nasal obstruction, bleeding, discharge, odor.
   - loss of smell—deficit of CN I (cranial nerve I).
7. With a light source and gloves, inspect and palpate structures in the oral cavity and oropharynx: lips, buccal and labial gingivae, mucosa, hard and soft palate, all surfaces of tongue, floor of mouth, tonsillar pillars and regions, oropharyngeal wall. Observe oral cavity for:
   - leukoplakia—a persistent painless white patch that cannot be rubbed off.

- erythroplasia (erythroplakia), a painless, velvety, beefy red patch that cannot be rubbed off.
- speckled red and white color changes.
- pigment changes other than normal melanosis (pigment noted around gums and buccal mucosa in dark-skinned individuals).
- persistent ulceration or bleeding.
- asymmetry/masses.
- areas of abnormal thickening or induration.
- an unexplained loosened upper molar, usually a symptom of maxillary sinus cancer.
- sharp, jagged teeth or ill-fitting dentures or partials.
- motor deficits of cranial nerves V, (trismus), IX and X (asymmetry of the soft palate, tonsillar pillars), and XII (limited or inability to move tongue).

8. Inspect and palpate the cervical lymph nodes for:
   - enlargement > 1 cm.
   - firm to hard consistency.
   - fixed or limited mobility.
   - spheric, matted, or ill-defined shape.
   - nontenderness.

9. Inspect and palpate thyroid gland for:
   - asymmetry/enlargement.
   - nodules.
   - firmness or induration.
   - history of hoarseness.

10. Review symptomatology for indirect assessment of base of tongue, larynx, hypopharynx:
   - persistent hoarseness/voice change.
   - dysphagia (pain, difficulty swallowing).
   - persistent or specific sore throat.
   - referred ear pain.
   - stridor/dyspnea.
   - mass in neck.

Patient Teaching

1. Instruct patient to perform monthly examinations of the skin, mouth, and neck.

Particular attention should be directed to the high-risk sites in the mouth: lips, buccal mucosa (inside the cheek wall), gums, sides and underside of tongue, soft palate (nonbony part of the roof of the mouth and tonsil regions).

2. Inform the patient to look and feel for:
   - painless red or white color changes.
   - sores and ulcers that do not heal.
   - lumps or thickenings that do not go away within three weeks.
   - pigmented lesions that change in color, size, shape, surface, or elevation.

3. Other symptoms to teach the patient to observe for include:
   - hoarseness/voice change.
   - difficulty swallowing.
   - persistent sore throat.
   - ear pain.

4. Stress the importance of the patient seeing a dentist or ear, nose, and throat physician if a change is detected or if a symptom persists to ensure early detection and prompt treatment.

5. Inform the patient that self-examination practices promote patient responsibility that increases the control that he or she maintains over health.

6. Convey the importance of monthly self-examination practices particularly to those who refuse to avoid or cannot avoid the use of tobacco and alcohol. About 40 per cent of those individuals who continue to smoke will develop a second primary.

7. State the importance of annual professional examinations with the dentist and the ear, nose, and throat-head and neck physician.

8. Inform the patient of head and neck cancer prevention and early detection information available through Cancer Information Service, the National Cancer Institute, and the American Cancer Society.

SUGGESTED READINGS

Baker, K.H., and Feldman, J.E.: Cancers of the head and neck. Cancer Nursing 10:293–299, 1987.

Batsakis, G.: Tumors of the Head and Neck. Baltimore, Williams & Wilkins, 1979.

Decker, J., and Goldstein, J.C.: Current concepts in otolaryngology: Risk factors in head and neck cancer. New England Journal of Medicine 306:1151–1155, 1982.

Decoufle, P.: Occupation. In Schottenfeld, D., and Fraumeni, J.F. (Eds.): Cancer Epidemiology and Prevention. Philadelphia, J.B. Lippincott, 1982, pp. 318–335.

Gluckman, J.L., and Crissman, J.D.: Survival rates in 548 patients with multiple neoplasms of the upper aerodigestive tract. Laryngoscope 93:71–74, 1983.

Graham, S., Dayal, H., Rohrer, T., et al.: Dentition, diet, tobacco, and alcohol in the epidemiology of oral cancer. Journal of the National Cancer Institute 59:1611–1615, 1977.

Henningfield, J.E.: Side effects of nicotine dependence. New Jersey Medicine 85:108–112, 1988.

Mashberg, A., Garfinkel, L., and Harris, S.: Alcohol as a primary risk in oral squamous cell carcinomas. CA: A Cancer Journal for Clinicians 31:146–155, 1981.

Mashberg, A., and Meyers, H.: Anatomic site and size of 22 early asymptomatic oral squamous cell carcinomas. Cancer 37:2149–2157, 1976.

Rothman, K.J., Cann, C.I., Flanders, D., et al.: Epidemiology of laryngeal cancer. Epidemiology Review 2:195–209, 1980.

Schleper, J.R.: Prevention, detection, and diagnosis of head and neck cancers. Seminars in Oncology 5:1–11, 1989.

Schottenfeld, D.: Alcohol as a co-factor in etiology of cancer. Cancer 43:1962–1966, 1979.

Shillitoe, E.J.: Viruses in the etiology of head and neck cancer. Cancer Bulletin 39:82–85, 1987.

Spitz, M.R., and Newell, G.R.: Descriptive epidemiology of squamous cell carcinoma of the upper aerodigestive tract. Cancer Bulletin 39:79–81, 1987.

Southwick, H.: Head and neck cancer: Early detection. Cancer 47:1188–1192, 1981.

Suen, J., and Myers, E.: Cancer of the head and neck. New York, Churchill Livingstone, 1981.

Willett, W.C., and MacMahon, B.: Diet and cancer. New England Journal of Medicine 310:633–638, 1984.

PATIENT EDUCATION MATERIALS AND COMMUNITY RESOURCES

Cancer Information Service: 1-800-4-CANCER.

Eating Hints—Recipes and Tips for Better Nutrition During Cancer Treatment. NIH Publication No. 87-2079, Rev. 1986. Available free and in quantity from: Office of Cancer Communication, National Cancer Institute, Bldg. 31, Room 10A24, Bethesda, MD 20892.

Enteral Products and Literature Guide. Mead Johnson, Evansville IN 47721.

Ross Laboratories, Columbus, OH 43216.

Knowledge Deficit Related to Prevention and Early Detection of Lung Cancer

Bernadine Cimprich

Population at Risk

- Tobacco smokers over 40 years of age who have a history of long-term smoking
- Workers exposed to lung carcinogens
- arsenic (copper and cobalt smelters, arsenical pesticide manufacturers and insulators)
- asbestos (asbestos miners, textile manufacturers, and insulators)
- chloromethyl ethers (chemical workers)
- hydrocarbons in oil, soot, and tar (coal gas manufacturers, steel and iron foundry workers, roofers, aluminum refiners, asphalters)
- radioactive gases (uranium and other ore miners, atomic energy workers)
- Individuals who have familial history of lung cancer
- Individuals who have chronic vitamin A deficiency

LEVEL 1A: Prevention

EXPECTED OUTCOME

1. Patient demonstrates knowledge of prevention of lung cancer:
   - identifies personal risk based on history of tobacco smoking and/or occupational exposure to lung carcinogens.
   - develops or maintains strategies to reduce personal risk factors.

NURSING MANAGEMENT

Assessment

1. Evaluate patient's risk for developing lung cancer including:
   - tobacco use.
   - high-risk occupation.
   - past exposure to environmental carcinogens.
   - family history of lung cancer.
   - general nutritional status.

Knowledge Deficit Related to Prevention and Early Detection of Lung Cancer

2. Assess patient/family knowledge of lung cancer risk factors and measures to reduce personal risk.

Patient Teaching

1. Clarify personal risk factors as indicated:
   - cigarette smoking is the single greatest cause of lung cancer.
   - the risk of developing lung cancer is proportional to the amount and duration of tobacco use:
     - number of cigarettes smoked.
     - depth of inhalation.
     - age when smoking began.
     - number of years smoking.
     - amount of tar in cigarettes smoked.
   - for ex-smokers, the risk of lung cancer approximates that of individuals who never smoked beginning 10 to 15 years following cessation of smoking.
   - high-risk occupations involve exposure to known lung carcinogens from the products of coal combustion or the constituents of asbestos, hydrocarbons, arsenic, chromium, radiation.
   - lung carcinogens have a synergistic effect (a smoker who works with asbestos has an increased risk of developing lung cancer).
   - chronic vitamin A deficiency may increase risk of developing lung cancer, especially in heavy smokers.
2. Discuss appropriate measures for reducing risk factors:
   - provide positive reinforcement for not smoking (the best preventive measure is never to start smoking).
   - reinforce the health benefits of a smoke-free home and work environment (involuntary smoking may increase risk of lung cancer in nonsmokers).
   - provide a clear message to cigarette smokers to quit smoking:
     - determine willingness to quit smoking.
     - provide information aimed at increasing motivation to quit smoking (e.g., health risks of continued smoking and benefits of quitting).
   - advise smokers who want to quit about how to quit smoking:
     - provide positive feedback for previous efforts to quit (long-term success often involves a process of learning through repeated attempts to quit).
     - suggest possible "models" for quitting (self-help, individualized counseling, behavior modification, hypnosis, group programs, peer support).
     - identify potential barriers to quitting (e.g., weight gain, nicotine withdrawal effects); help patient formulate strategies to overcome perceived barriers.
     - provide appropriate self-help literature.
     - provide information concerning community smoking cessation programs.
   - if patient is unable to quit smoking, help identify strategies to reduce tobacco use (e.g., smoke low tar cigarettes, fewer cigarettes per day, less of each cigarette).
   - if high-risk occupation, discuss safety procedures to reduce exposure to carcinogens emphasizing:
     - compliance with work safety regulations, policies, and specific protective measures.
     - importance of not smoking.
   - offer nutritional guidance:
     - include foods rich in vitamin A or carotene in daily diet (e.g., deep green and yellow vegetables and fruits).
     - caution against unprescribed vitamin A supplements because of possible toxicity.

EXPECTED OUTCOME

1. Patient demonstrates knowledge of measures for early detection of lung cancer:
   - participates in health screening procedures.
   - recognizes signs and symptoms to report to health care team.
   - identifies health care resources.

NURSING MANAGEMENT

Assessment

1. Evaluate patient's risk for developing lung cancer. See Assessment Level 1A.
2. Obtain history of respiratory problems.
3. Assess signs and symptoms of lung cancer:
   - pulmonary signs and symptoms:
     - persistent cough or change in smoker's cough.
     - increased sputum.
     - hemoptysis.
     - prolonged or repeated respiratory infection.
     - chest pain (dull ache, or pleuritic pain).
     - unilateral wheeze, dyspnea (suggests obstruction).
     - dullness on chest percussion (suggests underlying fluid or solid mass).
   - signs and symptoms of intrathoracic invasion:
     - Horner's syndrome due to paralysis of cervical sympathetic nerves (unilateral drooping of eyelid, contraction of pupil, recession of eye within the orbit, absence of facial sweating).
     - shoulder and arm pain due to invasion of eighth cervical and first thoracic nerves (superior sulcus or Pancoast's tumor).
     - hoarseness or huskiness of voice due to recurrent laryngeal nerve paralysis.
     - superior vena cava syndrome from obstruction (edema of face, neck, and upper extremities, engorged veins on chest wall, shortness of breath).
   - signs and symptoms of paraneoplastic syndromes:
     - anorexia/cachexia.
     - hypercalcemia (ectopic parathyroid hormone).
     - hyponatremia (inappropriate secretion of antidiuretic hormone).
     - Cushing's syndrome (ectopic ACTH).
     - hypertrophic pulmonary osteoarthropathy (clubbing, painful joints).
   - signs and symptoms of metastatic lung cancer:
     - lymph node adenopathy (e.g., enlarged supraclavicular or axillary node).
     - bone pain (e.g., back, vertebral, thoracic).
     - change in mental status, headache, seizure.
     - anorexia, right upper quadrant pain, enlarged liver.
4. Determine diagnostic and laboratory test results as indicated: chest x-ray, pulmonary function studies, CBC, serum electrolytes, calcium, phosphorus, and alkaline phosphatase, and liver and renal function tests.

29

Knowledge Deficit Related to Prevention and Early Detection of Lung Cancer

Patient Teaching

1. Explain signs and symptoms to report to health care team:
   - pulmonary signs and symptoms:
     - persistent cough or change in the character of a smoker's chronic cough (common first symptom).
     - excessive sputum and/or change in sputum (e.g., blood-tinged or frothy).
     - prolonged or repeated respiratory infection or "cold."
     - chest pain (e.g., constant ache or pleuritic pain).
     - wheezing, shortness of breath.
   - extrapulmonary symptoms may be first indication of tumor presence:
     - severe pain in shoulder, axilla, arm.
     - bone pain.
     - hoarseness.
     - enlarged lymph node in the neck or axilla.
     - swelling of face and neck, engorged veins on chest wall.
     - unexplained weight loss, fatigue, and anorexia.
2. Explain lung cancer detection methods:
   - lung cancer is difficult to detect early.
   - emphasize importance of regular health check-up (American Cancer Society guidelines: annual cancer check-up and health counseling for asymptomatic persons over age 40).
   - periodic chest x-ray and sputum cytologic examination may aid early detection of lung cancer in high-risk individuals.
   - for symptomatic individuals, a series of measures may be required:
     - complete physical examination without delay to determine cause of symptoms.
     - chest radiograph and serial sputum cytologic examinations to aid detection of lung cancer.
     - further diagnostic procedures to confirm presence of lung cancer depending on tumor location: chest imaging including tomography; bronchoscopy and bronchial brushing, washings and biopsy; percutaneous fine needle aspiration biopsy guided by fluoroscopy; or occasionally thoracotomy and biopsy.
3. Provide appropriate literature concerning detection and diagnosis of lung cancer.
4. Discuss health care resources:
   - provide literature describing community screening clinics and health care clinics.
     - assist patient with health care referrals as needed.

SUGGESTED READINGS

American Cancer Society: Guidelines for the cancer-related check-up: Recommendations and rationale. CA: A Cancer Journal for Clinicians 30:193–240, 1980.

Doll, R., and Peto, R.: The causes of cancer: Quantitative estimates of avoidable risks of cancer in the United States today. Journal of the National Cancer Institute 66(6):1194–1265, 1981.

Doyle, L.A., and Aisner, J.: Clinical presentation of lung cancer. In Roth, J., Ruckdeschel, J.C., and Weisenburger, T.H. (Eds.): Thoracic Oncology. Philadelphia, W.B. Saunders, 1989, pp. 52–76.

Groenwald, S.L. (Ed.): Cancer Nursing Principles and Practices. Boston, Jones & Bartlett, 1987.

Harwood, K.V.: Non-small cell lung cancer: Issues in diagnosis, staging and treatment. Seminars in Oncology Nursing 3(3):183–193, 1987.

Minna, J.D., Higgins, G.A., and Glatstein, E.J., Cancer of the lung. In DeVita, V.T., Hillman, S.Y., and Rosenberg, S.A. (Eds.): Cancer Principles and Practice of Oncology, 2nd ed. Philadelphia, J.B. Lippincott, 1985, pp. 507–597.

National Cancer Institute Cooperative Early Lung Cancer Detection Program: Early lung cancer detection: Conclusions and summary. Annual Review of Respiratory Disease 130:565–570, 1984.

Oleske, D.: The epidemiology of lung cancer: An overview. Seminars in Oncology Nursing 3(3):165–173, 1987.

Risser, N.L.: The key to prevention of lung cancer: Stop smoking. Seminars in Oncology Nursing 3(3):228–236, 1987.

U.S. Department of Health and Human Services: Clinical opportunities for smoking intervention, 1986.

PATIENT EDUCATION MATERIALS AND COMMUNITY RESOURCES

Printed Materials

Fifty Questions (fifty most often asked questions about smoking and health and the answers) (American Cancer Society, 1982).

Lung Cancer, What You Need To Know (types, symptoms, diagnosis) (National Cancer Institute, 1987).

Occupational Lung Cancer (major causes, high-risk groups) (American Lung Association, 1985).

Smart Move, A Stop Smoking Guide (self-help) (American Cancer Society, 1987).

Smoker's Risk Test (American Cancer Society, 1984).

The Smoke Around You (risk of involuntary smoking) (American Cancer Society, 1987).

Quit For Good: How To Help Your Patients Stop Smoking (a kit containing clinician guide and patient information materials) (National Cancer Institute, 1986).

Stop Smoking Programs

Fresh Start (American Cancer Society Divisions) (group program, donation optional).

The Freedom from Smoking Clinic (American Lung Association Regional Offices) (group program, fee).

In Control (American Lung Association Regional Offices) (video program for individual or group use, fee).

Organizations

Patient and professional educational materials on prevention and detection of lung cancer can be obtained from the following organizations:

American Cancer Society
National Headquarters
1599 Clifton Road N.E.
Atlanta, GA 30329

American Lung Association
1740 Broadway
New York, NY 10019

Office of Cancer Communications
National Cancer Institute
National Institutes of Health
Bethesda, MD 20205
Telephone: 1-800-4-CANCER

Office on Smoking and Health
U.S. Department of Health and Human Services
Park Lawn Building, Room 110
5600 Fishers Lane
Rockville, MD 20857.

Knowledge Deficit Related to Prevention and Early Detection of Prostate Cancer

June P. Martin

Population at Risk

- Older men (>50 years of age) with incidence increasing rapidly with age
- Black males
- Men with a family history of prostate cancer
- Men with a high-fat diet

LEVEL 1A: Prevention

EXPECTED OUTCOME

1. Patient demonstrates knowledge related to prevention of prostate cancer:
   - identifies type of diet associated with prostate cancer.
2. Patient demonstrates behaviors for prevention of prostate cancer:
   - restricts fat content in diet.

NURSING MANAGEMENT

Assessment

1. Assess factors that influence health behaviors:
   - predisposing (desire or motivation to perform a health action, attitudes, values, beliefs, perceptions).
   - enabling (resources needed to perform a health action).
   - reinforcing (those that reward or support positive health behavior).
2. Assess present knowledge about food high in fat.
3. Assess knowledge of association between prostate cancer and a high-fat diet.
4. Conduct diet history to determine typical fat intake.

Patient Teaching

1. Evaluate diet history for evidence of high fat intake.
2. Explain and identify foods high in fat and ways to decrease fat in the diet.
3. Stress association between high-fat diet and prostate cancer.
4. Refer to dietary resources if necessary.

EXPECTED OUTCOME

1. Patient demonstrates knowledge related to early detection of prostate cancer:
   - states individual risk factors.
   - states signs and symptoms of prostate cancer.
2. Patient demonstrates behaviors related to early detection of prostate cancer:
   - states rationale for routine screening examinations.
   - visits physician yearly for routine digital rectal examination and prostate ultrasound.
   - seeks health care for symptoms of prostate cancer.

NURSING MANAGEMENT

Assessment

1. See Assessment, Level 1A.
2. Obtain history of individual risk factors:
   - race—Black.
   - age—> 50 years.
   - family history of prostate cancer.
   - history of high-fat diet.
3. Assess for signs and symptoms of prostate cancer:
   - perineal pain.
   - blood in the ejaculate.
   - urinary hesitancy.
   - decreased urinary stream.
   - urinary frequency/nocturia.
   - dysuria.
   - urinary retention.
   - continuous pain in the lower back, hips, or upper thighs.
4. Perform a digital rectal examination.

Patient Teaching

1. See Patient Teaching, Level 1A.
2. Explain rationale for routine screening examinations:
   - detect prostate abnormalities before symptoms develop.
   - decreased morbidity and mortality when prostate cancer is detected in early stages.
3. Discuss digital rectal examination as a method used for routine screening of prostate cancer:
   - explain that the posterior part of the prostate gland lies against the rectal wall.
   - stress that most prostate tumors occur on the posterior wall of the gland.
   - explain that palpation of the gland through the rectum can detect hardness, enlargement, changes in consistency, or other abnormalities before symptoms occur.
   - state that the recommended screening for prostate cancer is a yearly digital rectal examination for all men over age 40.
4. Discuss prostate ultrasound as a new, but as yet unproven, screening method for prostate cancer.
   - explain that transrectal ultrasound uses sound waves to take pictures of the prostate gland.
   - describe the preparation for prostate ultrasound: Fleet enema 30–60 minutes before; no dietary restrictions.
   - explain the ultrasound examination.
   - stress that transrectal ultrasound is showing promise in its ability to detect lesions too small to be palpated by digital rectal examination.
5. Assist patient with referral to appropriate agency for routine screening.

6. Explain importance of seeking medical attention immediately if any symptoms of prostate cancer occur.

SUGGESTED READINGS

American Cancer Society, Texas Division: Male cancer awareness speaker training manual. (Publication #809). Austin, TX, 1988.

Bruce, A.W., and Trachtenberg, J. (Eds.): Adenocarcinoma of the Prostate. New York, Springer-Verlag, 1987.

Chodak, G.W., Keller, P., and Schoenberg, H.: Routine screening for prostate cancer using digital rectal examination. Progress in Clinical and Biological Research 269:87–95, 1988.

Chodak, G.W., and Schoenberg, H.W.: Early detection of prostate cancer by routine screening. Journal of the American Medical Association 252(3):3261–3264, 1984.

Ericksen, M.P., Green, L.W., and Fultz, F.G.: Principles of changing health behaviors. Cancer 62(8):1768–1775, 1988.

Hall, F.M.: The coming of age of radiologic imaging screening. Radiology 168:579–589, 1988.

Hopkins, G.J., and Carroll, K.K.: Role of diet in cancer prevention. Journal of Environmental Pathology, Toxicology 5(6):279–298, 1985.

Lee, F., Littrup, P.J., Torp-Pedersen, S.T., et al.: Prostate cancer: Comparison of transrectal US and digital rectal examination for screening. Radiology 168:389–394, 1988.

Martin, J.P.: Male cancer awareness—Equal time for men. Family and Community Health 19(3):66–70, 1987.

Martin, J.P.: Male cancer awareness: Impact of an employee education program. Oncology Nursing Forum 17(1):59–64, 1990.

Martin, J.P.: Cancer screening: Will prostate ultrasound be the mammogram of tomorrow? Manuscript submitted for publication, 1989.

McClennan, B.L.: Transrectal US of the prostate: Is the technology leading the science? Radiology 168:571–575, 1988.

Murphy, G.P.: Screening for prostate carcinoma—Useful or not? Progress in Clinical and Biological Research 269:131–137, 1988.

Resnick, M.I.: Background for screening—Epidemiology and cost effectiveness. Progress in Clinical and Biological Research 269:111–120, 1988.

Rose, D.P.: The biochemical epidemiology of prostatic carcinoma. Progress in Clinical and Biological Research 222:43–68, 1986.

Smith, J.A., and Middleton, R.G.: Clinical Management of Prostatic Cancer. Chicago, Year Book Medical Publishers, 1987.

Thompson, I.M., Rounder, J.B., Teague, J.L., et al.: Impact of routine screening for adenocarcinoma of the prostate on stage distribution. Journal of Urology 137:424–426, 1987.

Torp-Pedersen, S.T., Littrup, P.J., Lee, F., and Mettlin, C.: Early prostate cancer: Diagnostic costs of screening transrectal US and digital rectal examination. Radiology 169:351–354, 1988.

Watanabe, H.: Screening for prostatic cancer in Japan. Progress in Clinical and Biological Research 269:99–107, 1988.

Wynder, E.L., Laakso, K., Sotarauta, M., and Rose, D.P.: Metabolic epidemiology of prostatic cancer. The Prostate 5:47–53, 1984.

PATIENT EDUCATION MATERIALS AND COMMUNITY RESOURCES

American Cancer Society: Cancer Facts for Men. (American Cancer Society Publication #2008-LE). New York, 1984.

American Cancer Society: For Men Only: What You Should Know About Prostate Cancer. (American Cancer Society Publication #2632-LE). New York, 1985.

American Cancer Society: Nutrition, Common Sense and Cancer. (American Cancer Society Publication #2096-LE). New York, 1985.

American Cancer Society: Taking Control: 10 Steps to a Healthier Life and Reduced Cancer Risk. (American Cancer Society Publication # 2019.05). New York, 1985.

Diet, Nutrition, and Cancer Prevention: The Good News. (NIH Publication #87-2878). Bethesda, MD, US Department of Health and Human Services, National Cancer Institute, September 1987.

What You Need to Know About Prostate Cancer. (NIH Publication #88-1576). Bethesda, MD, US Department of Health and Human Services, National Cancer Institute, January 1988.

Knowledge Deficit Related to Prevention and Early Detection of Skin Cancer

Mary C. Fraser and Inga Tokar

Population at Risk

Individuals with:

- history of primary melanoma or nonmelanoma skin cancer
- history of immunosuppression (e.g., renal transplant patients)
- xeroderma pigmentation
- fair skin that burns or freckles rather than tans, red or blond hair, blue or light-colored eyes, albinism
- resides in geographic areas that receive high levels of UV radiation (e.g., southwestern United States, Australia, South Africa)

Melanoma:

- dysplastic nevi; large irregular pigmented lesions; an increased number of nevi (moles); large congenital nevi (>20 cm in diameter)
- history of changing nevi

Nonmelanoma:

- a lesion that does not heal or that persists for more than 4 weeks
- a lesion that continues to itch, hurt, crust, scab, erode, or bleed
- premalignant lesions—actinic keratoses, arsenical keratoses, leukoplakia
- lymphoproliferative malignancy, xeroderma pigmentosum, nevoid basal cell carcinoma syndrome
- chronic exposure to ultraviolet radiation (UVR) from sunlight and tanning salons; exposure to ionizing radiation (from x-rays or uranium), arsenic, petroleum products including coal tars and creosotes, asphalt, pitch, soot, paraffin waxes, lubricating and cutting oil preparations; scars following skin injuries and burns; treatment with PUVA (psoralens and UV light)

LEVEL 1A: Prevention

EXPECTED OUTCOME

1. Patient demonstrates knowledge of risk factors associated with development of skin cancer.

Knowledge Deficit Related to Prevention and Early Detection of Skin Cancer

2. Patient identifies and demonstrates personal habits that help prevent skin cancer:
   - minimizes exposure to sun by following sun protection guidelines (avoids sunburns, minimizes suntanning, wears protective clothing, uses sunscreens appropriately, avoids artificial sources of ultraviolet (UV) radiation).
   - minimizes exposure to high-risk agents.
   - performs skin self-examination (SSE) routinely, monthly if high risk.

NURSING MANAGEMENT

Assessment

1. Assess present knowledge level:
   - risk factors.
   - prevention measures.
2. Evaluate readiness and intellectual capacity to learn (including motivating factors, impeding factors, attention span, and stress level).
3. Obtain history:

Melanoma:

- previous treatment of melanoma(s).
- mole(s) changing in a "suspicious" way, "funny" or atypical moles.
- sun exposure history, i.e., cumulative sun exposure over the patient's lifetime.
- intermittent sun exposure (e.g., weekend sun-worshippers; travel to areas of intense sun exposure such as southern latitudes, "sunbelt" areas near the equator, warm climates in the winter; frequent blistering sunburns especially before age 20).
- chronic sun exposures (e.g., many years of frequent and long-term sun exposure, as in farmers, sailors).

Nonmelanoma:

- previous treatment of skin lesions—actinic keratoses that are premalignant; scarring from chronic infection or repeated trauma (topical ulcers, burns, fistulas); leukoplakia is associated with squamous cell carcinoma (SCC); repeated small doses of x-ray for benign skin conditions and PUVA are associated with basal cell carcinoma (BCC) and SCC.
- occupation—outdoor workers (farmers, sailors), radiologists, uranium miners, workers exposed to polycyclic aromatic hydrocarbons (PAH) including oil workers, jute processors, tool setters who operate automatic lathes, wax pressmen.
- chronic exposure to arsenic—some orchard sprays, well water, and solutions such as Fowler's.
- history of immunosuppression.
- geographic area of residence—risk of developing cancer related to amount of sun exposure, greater UV exposure with decreasing latitude, compounded 4 per cent increase for every 100 feet above sea level.
- outdoor recreation habits resulting in chronic exposure to UV radiation.
4. Assess patient's skin type (see Table 8–1) and other risk factors for skin cancer.
5. Assess prior and current use of preventive measures that minimize exposure to UV radiation (see Patient Teaching, sun protection guidelines).

TABLE 8–1. SKIN TYPES

Type	Skin Reactions	Examples
I	Always burns easily and severely (painful burn); peels, tans little or not at all.	Individuals with fair skin. Blue, green, or even brown eyes, freckles; unexposed skin is white.
II	Usually burns easily and severely (painful burn); peels, tans minimally or lightly.	Individuals with fair skin, blond or brown hair, blue, hazel, or brown eyes; unexposed skin is white.
III	Burns moderately; tans about average.	Average Caucasian; unexposed skin is white.
IV	Burns minimally; tans easily and more than average with each exposure.	Individuals with white or light brown skin, dark brown hair, dark eyes; unexposed skin is white or light brown.
V	Rarely burns, tans easily and substantially.	Brown-skinned individuals; unexposed skin is brown.
VI	Never burns and tans easily.	Blacks, unexposed skin is black.

Developed by Pathak, M.A., Fitzpatrick, T.B. Parrish, J.A., and Mosher, D.B. Harvard Medical School, Massachusetts General Hospital, Boston, MA; and Greiter, F.J., Vienna, Austria. Reprinted with permission.

Patient Teaching

1. Define risk factors. Help patient identify personal risk factors.
2. Discuss effects of UVA and UVB exposure:
   - Ultraviolet A (UVA), long-wavelength radiation (320–400 nm), which penetrates the dermis and has been identified as causing both acute and chronic photodamage, is the principal UV ray in tanning salons, and causes the skin to be more sensitive to UVB.
   - Ultraviolet B (UVB), is shorter wavelength radiation (290 to 320 nm), is both the principal cause of sunburn reaction and is the cancer-causing component of UV light.
3. Describe rationale for minimizing exposure to UV radiation, including avoiding sunburning and minimizing suntanning:
   - Solar UV radiation is the major known environmental risk for skin cancer.
   - Nonmelanoma skin cancers: chronic overexposure.
   - Melanoma: particularly acute intermittent exposures that result in bad blistering sunburns before age 20.
   - Sun damage occurs with each unprotected sun exposure and accumulates over individual's lifetime.
4. Describe and discuss measures to minimize UV radiation to protect skin:
   - Avoid getting sunburned; do not try to get a "good" tan.
   - Limit exposure to sunlight during hours that UV radiation is most intense (e.g., between 10 AM and 2 PM, 11 AM and 3 PM during daylight savings time). Plan outdoor activities for early in the morning or late afternoon.
   - Wear protective clothing (e.g., broad-brimmed hats, long-sleeved shirts, long pants) made of tightly-woven fabrics while out in the sun. Note that UV radiation can penetrate a single layer of thin cotton (e.g., T-shirts) or loosely woven fabrics, so sunscreen may be needed in addition to lightweight clothing.
   - Apply a sunscreen to all exposed body areas 15 to 30 minutes before sun exposure. Remember to include the ears, back of the neck, and bald spots on the head.
   - Broad-spectrum sunscreens containing

benzophenones that block both UVA and UVB rays and have a sun protection factor (SPF) of 15 or more provide the best protection.

- Suntanning lotions are not protective. Adults need to apply approximately 5½ tsp of sunscreen to receive the SPF protection listed on the container: ½ tsp to face and neck, ½ tsp to each arm and shoulder, ½ tsp to the anterior torso, ½ tsp to back, 1 tsp to each leg and top of feet.
- Reapply sunscreens every 2 hours while in the sun and after swimming or perspiring heavily.
- Use a sunscreen during high-altitude activities (e.g., skiing, mountain climbing). For every 100 ft above sea level, there is a compounded 4 per cent increase in UV radiation exposure.
- Remember to use sunscreens on cloudy or hazy days. Because UV radiation penetrates clouds easily, it is as damaging on cloudy days as it is on sunny days.
- Individuals at high risk for melanoma and other skin cancers should apply sunscreens daily.
- Follow extra precautions while taking medications or treatments that cause photosensitivity reactions, an increased susceptibility to the sun (e.g., certain antibiotics, diuretics, oral contraceptives, chemotherapy agents, radiation therapy treatments).
- Change sunscreens if rash, irritation, or allergic reaction develops. Many types of commercial products are available.
- Be aware that reflective surfaces (e.g., water, sand, snow, and concrete can reflect up to 85 per cent of the sun's rays onto the skin). Staying in the shade does not guarantee protection from sunburn.
- Avoid artificial UV radiation sources including sun lamps, tanning beds, booths, and salons.
- Wear sunglasses that screen out UV radiation.

- Keep infants out of the sun. Begin using sunscreens at 6 months of age and then allow sun exposure with moderation.
- Teach children sun protection early. Preliminary studies have shown that attitudes about sun exposure are fixed by the sixth grade.

5. Discuss importance of and procedure for routine skin self-examination (SSE):
- In well-lit area, using hand mirror and full-length stationary mirror, systematically inspect and examine all accessible skin surfaces from head to toe, including scalp.
- Give attention to both preexisting and changing lesions such as nevi, freckles, warts, birthmarks, persistent sores, or new lesions.
- Obtain assistance from another individual who should systematically inspect entire scalp and hairline.
- Inspect face, lips, and neck, including posterior neck and postauricular area.
- Inspect and palpate all surfaces of upper extremities including axillae, hands, finger webs, and nail beds.
- With the back to a full-length mirror, use hand mirror to inspect the back, buttocks, and backs of legs. Pay particular attention to skin folds.
- Inspect external genitalia using a hand mirror.
- Women should separate the skin folds of the labia and perineum to adequately view surfaces.
- Men should inspect all sides of the penis and scrotal sac. Retract foreskin if present.
- Both men and women should examine the skin between the buttocks.
- Inspect the anterior surfaces of the legs including toe webs, toenail beds, and plantar surfaces.
- Inspect and palpate all hairy surfaces such as those beneath axillary, thoracic, and pubic hair.

EXPECTED OUTCOME

1. Patient demonstrates knowledge related to early detection of skin cancer:
   - states signs and symptoms of skin cancer.
   - states individual risk factors.
2. Patient demonstrates measures to promote early detection of skin cancer:
   - performs SSE routinely, monthly if at increased risk.
   - observes lesions closely, noting changes.
   - minimizes exposure to UV radiation.
   - identifies signs and symptoms to report to health care team.
3. Patient states appropriate plan for follow-up skin care:
   - identifies physician or health care provider for ongoing skin exams.
   - states frequency of exams recommended by health care provider.

NURSING MANAGEMENT

Assessment

1. See Assessment, Level 1A.
2. Obtain history:

Melanoma:

- ask patient about "suspicious" moles:
  - moles that have recently changed.
  - "ugly" moles or spots.
  - large atypical moles.

Nonmelanoma:

- recent change in lesion or spot that does not heal.
3. Systemically observe and assess entire body skin surface (including scalp) for suspicious pigmented or nonpigmented lesions.

Melanoma:

- think about the ABCD system when assessing individual lesions:
  - A = Asymmetry (shape of one half does not match the other.)
  - B = Border (edges are irregular, ragged, notched, blurred, or fade off into the surrounding skin).
  - C = Color (color is uneven. Shades of black, brown, or tan are present. Areas of white, gray, red, or blue may be seen).
  - D = Diameter (change in size, especially increase).
- usual sites for melanomas:
  - approximately half develop in pre-existing nevus, approximately half develop de novo (spontaneously arise in previously normal skin).
  - trunk (back) is most common site for melanoma in Caucasian males.
  - lower extremities is most common site for melanoma in Caucasian females.
  - head and neck are next most common sites in male and female Caucasians.
  - acral lentiginous melanoma occurs on the palms of hands, soles of feet, nail beds, and mucous membranes.
  - melanomas are rare in non-whites. They usually occur on areas of the skin with the least amount of pig-

ment (e.g., palms and soles, fingers and toes, mucous membranes).

Nonmelanoma:

- visually inspect skin for signs of chronic sunburn, actinic damage (wrinkling, varied pigment changes), freckling:
  - actinic keratoses (premalignant) are usually found on sun-exposed skin (head and neck, hands, arms). The lesions are flat or slightly elevated, irregularly shaped, reddened with a rough and scaly surface.
  - basal cell cancers (BCC) commonly present as a dome-shaped papule that has a pearly, shiny, translucent appearance (particularly the borders), and a depression or ulceration in the center. They may have telangiectases (permanently dilated capillaries) beneath the surface. They usually appear on sun-exposed skin and occasionally on the trunk, especially the upper back and chest, and legs.
  - squamous cell carcinomas (SCC) begin as a red papule or plaque with a scaly or crusted surface. They may become nodular and ulcerate. SCC confined to the epidermis is called Bowen's disease (carcinoma in situ). These lesions occur predominantly on sun-exposed skin and can occur in areas free from chronic sun damage.

4. Assess characteristics of suspicious or changing nevi or lesions including:
   - symptoms experienced (e.g., itching, bleeding).
   - location.
   - color.
   - size and shape.
   - surface texture (e.g., scaly, nodular, smooth).
   - condition of surrounding skin.
   - presence of drainage, bleeding.

Patient Teaching

1. See Patient Teaching, Level 1A.
2. Discuss signs and symptoms of early skin cancers.

Melanoma:

- change in size of a mole (sudden increase in size is of special concern; slow change is much more common).
- change in color of a mole (of special concern is the mixing of shades of red, white, and blue or a sudden darkening of brown or black shades).
- change in mole surface (scaliness, flaking, oozing, erosion, ulceration, bleeding, nodular or bulging, sudden elevation, mushrooming mass).
- change in shape or outline of a mole (irregular, notched border where it used to be regular and smooth).
- change in how a mole feels to the touch (getting hard, lumpy).
- change in skin around a mole (spread of pigment from the edge of the mole into skin that formerly appeared normal, inflammation of surrounding skin).
- satellite pigmentation.
- onset of new feelings or symptoms in a mole (itching, tenderness, pain). Early melanoma does *not* cause pain.
- sudden appearance of a new pigmented lesion in previously normal skin.
- early melanoma (e.g., change in size, color, itchiness).
- *advanced* melanoma (e.g., bleeding, ulceration).

Nonmelanoma:

- an open sore that bleeds, oozes, crusts, and remains open for 3 weeks or more.
- a reddish patch, or irritated area frequently occurring on chest, shoulder, arms, or legs.

- a smooth growth with an elevated rolled border and an induration in the center. Tiny blood vessels may develop on the surface as the growth enlarges.
- a shiny bump that is pearly or translucent and is often pink, white, or red.
- a scar-like area with a white, yellow, or waxy appearance that often has poorly defined borders. Skin appears shiny or taut. Most SCC develop on sun damaged skin or in preexisting actinic keratoses. The lesion continues to scale, scab, itch, hurt, bleed, or erode.

3. Outline characteristics of normal moles (common acquired nevi), use photographs for comparison, if available:
   - uniformly tan, brown (normal moles look very similar to each other).
   - usually less than 5 mm in diameter.
   - round or oval.
   - sharp border between mole and surrounding skin.
   - flat or elevated.
   - typical adult has 10 to 40 scattered over body, generally located on sun-exposed surfaces above waist (scalp, breasts, buttocks rarely involved).

4. For individuals affected with dysplastic nevi, outline characteristics of dysplastic nevi, using pictures:
   - contain color mixtures of tan, brown, black, red, and pink. Moles often look quite different from one another.
   - irregular borders that may include notches. May fade into surrounding skin and include a flat portion.
   - may be smooth, slightly scaly, or have a rough, irregular "pebbly" appearance.
   - often larger than 5 mm and sometimes larger than 10 mm.
   - many people do not have increased number; persons severely affected may have more than 100 nevi.
   - may occur anywhere on the body but most common on back. May also appear on scalp, buttocks, and breasts in females.

5. Emphasize the importance of reporting changes to health care team and of follow-up for suspicious lesions.

Melanoma:

- biologically early melanoma (<0.76 mm thick [Clark Level II], horizontal growth phase present, vertical growth phase absent) is readily cured by surgical excision. Survival rate decreases progressively with lesion thickness. Most patients with lesions > 1.50 mm thick (Clark Levels IV, V) have relatively poor prognoses.

Nonmelanoma:

- cure rate > 95 per cent for lesions treated early.
- actinic keratoses are premalignant lesions.
- BCCs are usually growing and metastasis is rare; however, considerable localized tissue destruction may occur and may invade vital structures such as bone, eye, or ear.
- SCCs are more rapidly growing, may also infiltrate surrounding structures, and may metastasize to lymph nodes.

6. Emphasize importance of routine follow-up examinations with health care team.

Melanoma:

- patients at high-risk should be examined at least twice yearly; during times of "increased mole activity" (e.g., pregnancy), may need to be seen more often.

Nonmelanoma.

- individuals who have already had one or more skin cancers are in a high-risk group and need to be followed on a regular basis by a qualified skin care specialist.

Knowledge Deficit Related to Prevention and Early Detection of Skin Cancer

SUGGESTED READINGS

Carter, D.M.: Basal cell carcinoma. *In* Fitzpatrick, T., Eisen, A., Wolff, K., et al. (Eds.): Dermatology in General Medicine. New York, McGraw-Hill, 1987, pp. 756–766.

Cassileth, B.R., Clark, W.H. Jr., Lusk, E.J., et al.: How well do physicians recognize melanoma and other problem lesions? Journal of the American Academy of Dermatology 14:555–560, 1986.

Cassileth, B.R., Lusk, E.J., Guerry, D., et al.: "Catalyst" symptoms in malignant melanoma. J Gen Intern Med 2:1–4, 1987.

Cassileth, B.R., Temoshok, L., Frederick, B.E., et al.: Patient and physician delay in melanoma diagnosis. Journal of the American Academy of Dermatology 18:591–698, 1988.

Coody, D.: Pediatric Nurses—Sun protection advocates and educators. The Skin Cancer Foundation Journal 5:16, 62, 1987.

DeSimone, E.M.: Sunscreens and suntan products. *In* Handbook of Non-Prescription Drugs, 8th ed. Washington, D.C., American Pharmaceutical Association, 1986, pp. 533–543.

Frank-Stromborg, M.: The role of the nurse in early detection of cancer: Population sixty-six years of age and older. Oncology Nursing Forum 13: 66–74, 1986.

Fraser, M.C.: The role of the nurse in the prevention and early detection of malignant melanoma. Cancer Nursing 5:351–360, 1982.

Friedman, R.J., Rigel, D.S., and Kopf, A.W.: Early detection of malignant melanoma: The role of physician examination and self examination of the skin. CA: A Cancer Journal for Clinicians 35:130–151, 1985.

Hill, M.: Dermatology nurses: Proponents of skin cancer awareness. The Skin Cancer Foundation Journal 4:41, 101, 1988.

Lawler, P.E.: Be sunsensible: Steps toward safety in the sun—An information handout. Oncology Nursing Forum 16:424–427, 1989.

Lawler, P.E., and Schreiber, S.: Cutaneous malignant melanoma: Nursing's role in prevention and early detection. Oncology Nursing Forum 16:345–352, 1989.

National Cancer Institute: Working Guidelines for Early Cancer Detection, 1987.

National Cancer Institute Research Report: Melanoma. NIH Publication No. 89-3020, 1988.

National Cancer Institute Research Report: Nonmelanoma Skin Cancers—Basal and Squamous Cell Carcinomas. NIH Publication No. 88-2977, 1988.

Nichol, N.H.: Actinic keratosis: Preventable and treatable like other precancerous and cancerous skin lesions. Plastic Surgical Nursing 9:49–55, 1989.

Nichol, N.H.: Early detection and prevention of skin cancer. Dermatology Nursing 1:11–20, 1989.

Nichol, N.H.: What's new with sunscreens? Choices, choices, choices. Pediatric Nursing 15:417, 1989.

Ramstack, J., White, S., Hazelkorn, K., et al.: Knowledge, attitude, and behavior (KAB) changes in pre and early adolescents exposed to a school-based cancer prevention program. Proceedings of ASCO 5:217 (Abstr # 850), 1986.

Schleper, J.R.: Cancer prevention and detection: Skin cancer. Cancer Nursing 7:67–83, 1984.

Sober, A., Rhodes, A., and Mihm, M.: Neoplasms: Malignant melanoma. *In* Fitzpatrick, T., Eisen, A., Wolff, K., et al. (Eds.): Dermatology in General Medicine. New York, McGraw-Hill, 1987, pp. 733–746.

Stewart, D.S.: Indoor tanning, the nurse's role in preventing skin damage. Cancer Nursing 10: 93–99, 1987.

Stoll, H.L., and Schwartz, R.: Epithelial precancerous lesions. *In* Fitzpatrick, T., Eisen, A., Wolff, K., et al. (Eds.): Dermatology in General Medicine. New York, McGraw-Hill, 1987, pp. 733–746.

Stoll, H.L., and Schwartz, R.: Squamous cell carcinoma. *In* Fitzpatrick, T., Eisen, A., Wolff, K., et al. (Eds.): Dermatology in General Medicine. New York, McGraw-Hill, 1987, pp. 746–759.

Tucker, M.A.: Individuals at high risk of melanoma. *In* Mackie, R.M. (Ed.): Pigment Cell. New York, Karger, 1988, pp. 95–108.

Tucker, M.A., Shields, J.A., Hartge, P., et al.: Sunlight exposure as risk factor for intraocular malignant melanoma. New England Journal of Medicine 313:789–792, 1985.

White, L.N.: Cancer Prevention and detection: From twenty to sixty-five years of age. Oncology Nursing Forum 13:59–64, 1986.

PATIENT EDUCATION MATERIALS AND COMMUNITY RESOURCES

Organizations

1. American Academy of Dermatology (AAD)
   1567 Maple Avenue
   P.O. Box 3116
   Evanston, IL 60204-3116
   312-869-3954
   Professional organization of specialists who diagnose and treat skin problems. Patient education pamphlets for general public available. Patients may receive referrals to dermatologists by calling 1-800-238-2300.

2. American Cancer Society
   Tower Place
   3340 Peachtree Road, NE
   Atlanta, GA 30026
   404-320-3333

404-320-3333
State and local offices listed in the telephone book under "American Cancer Society"

3. Cancer Information Service
1-800-4-CANCER

4. Office of Cancer Communications
National Cancer Institute
Building 31, Room 10 A24
Bethesda, MD 20892

5. The Skin Cancer Foundation
245 Fifth Avenue, Suite 2402
New York, NY 10016
212-725-5176

Nonprofit organization provides a wide variety of publications on the diagnosis and treatment of skin cancers. The Foundation also publishes *Sun and Skin News* and *The Skin Cancer Foundation Journal* that have nontechnical articles on the prevention and treatment of melanoma and non-melanoma skin cancers.

6. American Society of Plastic and Reconstructive Surgeons
444 East Algonquin Road
Arlington Heights, IL 60005
1-800-635-0635
This society offers names of board-certified plastic surgeons in a patient's area. It also sends information on various surgical procedures.

Knowledge Deficit Related to Prevention and Early Detection of Testicular Cancer

June P. Martin

Population at Risk

- White males 15 to 44 years of age
- History of cryptorchidism

LEVEL 1A: *Prevention*

EXPECTED OUTCOME

1. Patient demonstrates knowledge related to prevention of testicular cancer:
   - states definition of cryptorchidism.
   - states risk of testicular cancer.
2. Patient demonstrates behaviors for prevention of testicular cancer:
   - seeks medical treatment of cryptorchidism.

NURSING MANAGEMENT

Assessment

1. Assess present knowledge level about cryptorchidism.
2. Assess readiness and ability to learn.
3. Assess newborn and pediatric patients for the presence of cryptorchidism:
   - perform a scrotal examination to determine the presence of both testicles in the scrotum.

Patient Teaching

1. When appropriate, define cryptorchidism:
   - explain development of testicles in the fetus as occurring high in the posterior abdominal wall.
   - explain the normal descent of the testicles down the inguinal canal during the third trimester of pregnancy.
   - explain that by birth or shortly thereafter, the testicles have moved to their normal location in the scrotum.
   - explain that cryptorchidism occurs when a testis fails to descend normally into the scrotum.
2. Stress association between development of testicular cancer in a cryptorchid testis (20 to 40 times greater risk).
3. State importance of early surgical treatment of cryptorchidism by orchiopexy (recommended before age 2).
4. Refer patient to appropriate agency for treatment of cryptorchidism.

EXPECTED OUTCOME

1. Patient demonstrates knowledge related to early detection of testicular cancer:
   - states individual risk factors.
   - states signs and symptoms of testicular cancer.
2. Patient demonstrates behaviors related to early detection of testicular cancer:
   - states rationale for testicular self-examination (TSE).
   - performs testicular self-examination monthly.
   - seeks health care for symptoms of testicular cancer.

NURSING MANAGEMENT

Assessment

1. See Assessment, Level 1A.
2. Assess factors that influence health behaviors:
   - predisposing (desire or motivation to perform TSE, e.g., attitudes, values, beliefs, perceptions).
   - enabling (skill needed to perform TSE).
   - reinforcing (those that reward or support positive health behavior).
3. Obtain history of individual risk factors:
   - race–Caucasian.
   - age–15 to 44 years.
   - history of cryptorchidism.
   - history of orchipexy.
4. Assess for signs and symptoms of testicular cancer:
   - testicular lump or hardening that may be painless.
   - scrotal enlargement or swelling.
   - dull ache or dragging sensation in scrotal, inguinal, or lower abdominal area.
   - gynecomastia.
5. Perform a testicular examination.

Patient Teaching

1. See Patient Teaching, Level 1A.
2. Explain rationale for testicular self-examination:

   - most common early symptom of testicular cancer is a lump.
   - testicular lumps or abnormalities are easy to find by self-examination.
   - testicular cancer is highly curable when detected and treated early.
3. Demonstrate the procedure for testicular self-examination:
   - perform TSE monthly.
   - the best time to perform TSE is after a bath or during a shower when the scrotal skin is relaxed.
   - Gently roll the testicle, between the thumb and fingers of both hands.
   - Locate the epididymis on the posterior side of the testicle and do not confuse this with a lump. Repeat the examination on the other testicle.
   - Palpate each testicle for size, shape, consistency, tenderness, and masses.
4. Explain importance of seeking medical attention immediately if any abnormalities or changes are found.
5. Assist patient with referral to appropriate agency if necessary.

SUGGESTED READINGS

American Cancer Society, Texas Division: Male Cancer Awareness Speaker Training Manual. (American Cancer Society Publication #809). Austin, TX, 1988.

Knowledge Deficit Related to Prevention and Early Detection of Testicular Cancer

Blesch, K.S.: Health beliefs about testicular cancer and self-examination among professional men. Oncology Nursing Forum *13*(1):29–33, 1986.

Eriksen, M.P., Green, L.W., and Fultz, F.G.: Principles of changing health behaviors. Cancer *62*(8):1768–1775, 1988.

Friman, P.C., Finney, J.W., Glasscock, S.G., et al.: Testicular self-examination: Validation of a training strategy for early cancer detection. Journal of Applied Behavior Analysis *19*(1):87–92, 1986.

Javadpour, N. (Ed.): Principles and Management of Testicular Cancer. New York, Thieme Inc., 1986.

Martin, J.P.: Male cancer awareness—Equal time for men. Family and Community Health *19*(3):66–70, 1987.

Martin, J.P.: Male cancer awareness: Impact of an employee education program. Oncology Nursing Forum *17*(1): 59–64, 1990.

Ostwald, S.K., and Rothenberger, J.: Development of a testicular self-examination program for college men. Journal of American College Health *33*(6):234–239, 1985.

Rudolf, V.M., and Quinn, K.L.M: The practice of TSE among college men: Effectiveness of an educational program. Oncology Nursing Forum *15*(1):45–48, 1988.

Vaz, R.M., Best, D.L., and Davis, S.W.: Testicular cancer: Adolescent knowledge and attitudes. Journal of Adolescent Health Care *9*(6):474–479, 1988.

Vaz, R.M., Best, D.L., Davis, S.W., and Kaiser, M.: Evaluation of a testicular cancer curriculum for adolescents. Journal of Pediatrics *114*(1):150–153, 1989.

PATIENT EDUCATION MATERIALS AND COMMUNITY RESOURCES

American Cancer Society: Cancer Facts for Men. (American Cancer Society Publication #2008-LE). New York, 1984.

American Cancer Society: For Men Only: Testicular Cancer and How to Do TSE (a Self-Exam). (American Cancer Society Publication #2093-LE). New York, 1982.

American Cancer Society (Producer): Testicular Self-Examination. (American Cancer Society Film #P266V). New York, 1987.

What You Need to Know About Testicular Cancer. (NIH Publication #88-1565). Bethesda, MD, U.S. Department of Health and Human Services, National Cancer Institute, June, 1988.

Knowledge Deficit Related to Prevention and Early Detection of HIV Disease

10

James P. Halloran, Jr. and Anne M. Hughes

Population at Risk

- Individuals who are heterosexually, homosexually, or bisexually active
- Individuals who share needles or equipment to inject drugs, licit or illicit
- Sexual partners of individuals who are HIV positive
- Offspring of HIV-infected mothers
- Individuals who received blood or blood product transfusion in the United States between 1975 and 1986
- Individuals who received organ transplants prior to routine testing of donors
- Individuals with occupational exposure to potentially infectious bodily substances

LEVEL 1A: *Prevention of Viral Transmission*

EXPECTED OUTCOME

1. Patient states that a knowledge deficit exists.
2. Patient demonstrates knowledge of HIV:
   - identifies modes of transmission.
   - identifies personal risk factors and behaviors.
3. Patient demonstrates knowledge of specific techniques to reduce personal risk:
   - use of latex condoms, other safer sex techniques.
   - avoidance of sharing injection equipment.
   - avoidance of unsafe sexual activity.
   - sexual abstinence.
   - monogamy or limiting number of sex partners.
   - cleaning injection equipment.
   - pre-pregnancy counseling.
4. Patient identifies personal strategies to apply risk reduction techniques, acknowledging potential or actual barriers to personal change.

NURSING MANAGEMENT

Assessment

1. Evaluate readiness to learn: motivation to change health behavior, barriers to learning (language, culture, anxiety, sensory deficits), perceived learning needs, present knowledge base.
2. Acknowledge anxiety generated by discus-

sion of topics relating to sexuality, drug use, or potentially life-threatening disease.

3. Assess history of risk factors:
   - Sexual:
     - multiple sex partners.
     - anonymous sex partners.
     - homosexual activity.
     - sexual activity with high-risk individuals.
   - Parenteral
     - IV drug use.
     - needle and equipment sharing.
     - transfusion(s) or organ transplantation between 1979 and 1986.
     - occupational exposure.
4. Assess personal behaviors to decrease risk:
   - limiting number of sex partners.
   - avoiding unsafe sexual practices.
   - use of safer sex techniques.
   - avoidance of sharing injection equipment.
   - potential testing for antibody to HIV.
   - appropriate infection control techniques in occupational setting.

Patient Teaching

1. Help patient identify personal risk factors through education regarding:
   - modes of HIV transmission (e.g., sexual, parenteral, perinatal).
   - high-risk sexual activities:
     - anal intercourse without a condom.
     - manual-anal intercourse (fisting).
     - unprotected oral-anal contact.
     - blood contact.
     - vaginal intercourse without condom.
   - moderate-risk sexual activities:
     - anal intercourse with a condom.
     - vaginal intercourse with a condom.
     - fellatio with a condom (Note: risk due to possibility of breakage or improper use of condom).
     - cunnilingus (oral-vaginal contact).
     - urine contact (water sports).
   - low-risk sexual activities:
     - mutual masturbation.
     - social kissing.
     - body massage, hugging.
     - body to body rubbing (frottage).
     - using one's own sex toys.
     - fantasy, voyeurism.
     - light S&M activities (without bleeding).
2. Assist patient to identify alternative sexual behaviors to reduce risk:
   - avoid practices that include exchange of semen, blood, vaginal secretions.
   - promote practices that prevent exchange of these bodily fluids.
   - acknowledge importance of sexuality, foster establishment of realistic goals and strategies to reduce risk of viral transmission.
   - proper use of condoms:
     - use of latex rather than natural skin condoms.
     - application of condom prior to penetration.
     - use of condom-compatible water-based lubricant.
     - disposal of condom after single use.
   - use of other techniques:
     - latex dental dams for oral-vaginal, oral-rectal contact.
     - use of lubricants containing viricidal spermicide (nonoxynol-9).
3. Teach patient to identify alternative parenteral behaviors to reduce risk:
   - avoidance of equipment-sharing offers the best protection against transmission.
   - clean equipment ("rig" or "works") with sodium hypochlorite (household bleach) in a 1-to-10 dilution, flushed through the syringe and needle twice, follow by two flushes with clean water.
   - avoid equipment obtained through illicit means as it may be misrepresented as sterile when in fact it has been previously used.
   - use formal needle exchange programs, which are illegal in most areas, but may be available through drug treatment or AIDS community service agencies.
   - state that transmission risk is through potential viral exposure regardless of

the substance injected (e.g., illicit recreational drugs, steroids, insulin).
- state that transmission may occur without venous penetration (i.e., subcutaneous injection or "skin popping").
- recognize that substance use may inhibit clear thinking, leading to high-risk behaviors.
- potential referral for drug and alcohol treatment.
- never recap, bend, or break used needles or sharps, as accidental needlestick injury presents the greatest risk for nurses. Impervious needle disposal containers should be kept as close as possible to site of needle use.
4. Teach patient alternative perinatal behaviors to reduce risk:

- refer females considering pregnancy for counseling regarding risk of perinatal transmission.
- refer females as appropriate for HIV antibody testing.
- explore with the patient alternatives such as adoption or foster parenting.
5. Explore with the patient resources available to facilitate and support behavior changes. Make referral(s) as appropriate to:
- support groups/persons.
- treatment programs, aftercare.
- counseling.
- informational resources.
6. Acknowledge that behavior changes may be difficult; encourage continued commitment to change despite occasional lapses or "slips."

LEVEL 1B: Early Detection of HIV Infection

EXPECTED OUTCOME

1. Patient acknowledges personal risk for HIV exposure.
2. Patient recognizes signs and symptoms that require professional evaluation.
3. Patient seeks health care for chronic constitutional signs and symptoms associated with HIV infection or opportunistic disease.
4. Patient describes diagnostic measures used to determine HIV infection, immune function, and HIV viral activity.
5. Patient demonstrates knowledge of self-care strategies that promote health and reduce risk of viral transmission:
   - uses skills to negotiate the health care system.
   - practices good personal hygiene.
   - manages stress.
   - seeks early detection and treatment of any symptoms of illness whether or not believed to be related to HIV.

NURSING MANAGEMENT

Assessment

1. See Assessment, Level 1A.
2. Assess patient fear and concerns regarding potential HIV seropositivity, risk of AIDS.

3. Determine patient knowledge level, personal experience with, attitudes and beliefs about HIV disease.
4. Ascertain if patient has been tested for HIV. If so, gently inquire as to date(s), method(s), and result(s). If not, assess

willingness to be tested, concerns regarding testing, knowledge of testing methods, and reasons for reluctance to test.

5. Assess patient's perception of what a positive/negative test result means regarding HIV infectivity and development of AIDS.

6. Obtain health history.

7. Perform physical examination to assess for chronic constitutional signs and symptoms not attributable to other cause(s) and associated with HIV infection or immune dysfunction:
   - symptoms: fevers, night sweats, fatigue, unexplained persistent diarrhea, skin problems.
   - signs: lymphadenopathy, chronic vaginitis, unexplained weight loss, oral thrush, oral hairy leukoplakia: viral, fungal, or bacterial skin infections and/or allergic skin reactions.

8. Determine whether patient has had laboratory monitoring of immune function and/or HIV viral activity such as T4 counts and percentages, T4/T8 ratio, p24 antigen, or beta-2-microglobulin, and the results.

9. Evaluate for signs and symptoms of *Pneumocystis carinii* pneumonia (PCP), the most prevalent opportunistic infection (OI) associated with HIV disease (signs and symptoms listed in number 7), plus dry cough, shortness of breath, $+/-$ rales on auscultation.

10. Assess for signs and symptoms of neurologic impairment associated with opportunistic disease or primary HIV disease: headache, stiff neck, visual changes or symptoms, motor and/or sensory deficits, seizure activity, cognitive impairment.

11. Clarify patient knowledge of: hopes and expectations of standard medical treatment (i.e., cure vs. control vs. palliation vs. prophylaxis); optimism or hopefulness regarding standard medical treatment. Is patient investigating alternative or unproven treatment methods? If so, what methods? interest in or eligibility for participation in clinical trials.

12. Evaluate patient's previous experience with the health care system. How satisfied is patient with relationship with health care providers? What is patient's preference regarding his or her role in decision-making regarding care? What are patient's hopes and expectations of interactions with health care providers?

13. Assess patient's available resources, encouraging patient to identify his or her own resources:
   - intrapersonal—include appraisal of patient's self-esteem, coping strategies, stress management, substance use patterns, emotional response to illness, perceived meaning of illness.
   - interpersonal—evaluate composition, size, and adequacy of patient support system, including relationships with partner or spouse, family (as defined by patient), friends, neighbors, coworkers; explore communication patterns.
   - community—availability and accessibility of resources, identification of services provided and eligibility requirements.
   - financial—health insurance coverage, disability benefits, other financial assets and resources.

Nursing Interventions

1. Establish trusting, supportive, nonjudgmental, therapeutic relationship.

2. Advocate for full health insurance coverage, other entitlement program.

3. Encourage patient to mobilize personal support system.

4. Provide supportive counseling regarding coping with uncertainty, potential loss of health, stigma, death and dying.

5. Support and maintain a sense of hope.

6. Explore long-term planning options such as durable power of attorney for health care and finances, patient preferences for treatment.

Patient Teaching

1. See Patient Teaching, Level 1A.
2. Establish realistic goals based on patient's identified needs and essential basic information regarding early detection of HIV, transmission prevention, disease progression.
3. Provide information that can be applied directly to patient's life situation based on patient's life experiences (e.g., how to negotiate safer sex with potential sex partners).
4. Describe spectrum of HIV disease from initial infection to asymptomatic carrier state to development of symptoms to diagnosis of AIDS:
   - outline pathophysiology.
   - identify signs and symptoms.
   - state self-care activities for each stage.
   - relate that no reliable predictor of disease progression has been identified.
5. Discuss specifically and reinforce with written materials how to prevent transmission of HIV:
   - safer sex techniques.
   - if continued injectable drug use seems likely, discourage sharing of equipment; explain methods for cleaning "works" (Level 1A, Patient Teaching).
   - counsel females considering pregnancy regarding risk of HIV transmission to offspring.
   - identify general household hygiene practices.
6. Review signs and symptoms to report to health care provider, stress those that require immediate attention, and review mechanism(s) for contacting health care provider(s).
   - explain that many of the signs and symptoms of HIV infection are nonspecific and may relate to other conditions; however, they do require evaluation.
7. Describe various methods of HIV testing (ELISA, antibody test, Western blot, assay polymerase chain reaction), differences in sensitivity and specificity.
8. Describe various methods for testing immune function and HIV viral activity:
   - absolute T4/CD4 lymphocyte count.
   - percentage T4/CD4 lymphocytes.
   - T-cell helper/suppressor ratio.
   - p24 antigen.
   - beta-2-microglobulin.
9. Discuss meaning of test result (positive or negative) and necessary health practices; emphasize that a negative test result does not negate the need to modify behavior to reduce risk.
10. Provide time for discussion of risks/benefits of HIV testing and early detecting; if testing is to be conducted elsewhere, ensure referral to be qualified, reliable agency that will provide appropriate pre- and post-test counseling.
11. Review current health maintenance activities, including regular primary health care and importance of adequate exercise, rest, nutrition, and stress management.
12. For HIV seropositive patients:
    - describe rationale for antiviral therapy and opportunistic infection prophylaxis.
    - discuss management of side effects of medical therapies, and side effects to report to health care provider.
13. Teach negotiation and problem-solving skills to be used in managing day-to-day realities of being seropositive.
14. Discuss strategies for managing demands of chronic illness: value of peer support, importance of nonillness-related activities.
15. Provide written information about available health care, legal and social support resources and agencies. Make referral as appropriate or explain mechanism to access resource providers.
16. Facilitate meeting for patient and members of support system to provide basic information about HIV and its transmission, to demonstrate appropriate infection control techniques and methods of discussing sensitive topics.

Knowledge Deficit Related to Prevention and Early Detection of HIV Disease

SUGGESTED READINGS

American Nurses Association: Nursing and the human immunodeficiency virus. Kansas City, MO, American Nurses Association, 1988.

Bennet, J.: AIDS: What precautions do you take in the hospital? American Journal of Nursing 86:952–953, 1986.

Brown, M.L.: AIDS and ethics: Concerns and considerations. Oncology Nursing Forum 14(1):69–73, 1987.

Centers for Disease Control: Condoms for prevention of sexually transmitted disease. MMWR 37(9):133–137, March 11, 1988.

Centers for Disease Control: AIDS and human immunodeficiency virus infection in the United States: 1988 update. MMWR 38(S-4), (suppl): 1–38, May 12, 1989.

Centers for Disease Control: Update: Serologic testing for antibody to human immunodeficiency virus. MMWR 36:52, 833–839, 845, January 8, 1988.

AIDS etiology, diagnoses, treatment and prevention. In Devita, V., Hellman, S., and Rosenberg, S. (Eds.): Cancer Medicine. Philadelphia, J.B. Lippincott, 1985.

Flaskerud, J.H.: AIDS/HIV Infection: A Reference Guide for Nursing Professionals. Philadelphia, W.B. Saunders, 1989.

Gee, G., and Moran, T.A.: AIDS: Concepts in Nursing Practice. Baltimore, Williams & Wilkins, 1988.

Grady, C.: Acquired immune deficiency syndrome: The impact on professional nursing practice. Cancer Nursing 12(1):1–9, 1989.

Holloran, J., Hughes, A., and Mayer, D.: Oncology Nursing Society position paper on HIV-related issues. Oncology Nursing Forum 15(2):206–217, 1988.

Hollander, H., Greenspan, D., Stringari, S., et al.: "Hairy" leukoplakia and the acquired immunodeficiency syndrome. Annals of Internal Medicine 104(6):892, 1985.

Lewis, A.: Nursing care of the person with AIDS/ARC. Rockville, MD, Aspen, 1988.

Lovejoy, N.: The pathophysiology of AIDS. Oncology Nursing Forum 15(5): 563–571, 1988.

Marion S.A., Schecter, M.T., Weaver, M.S., et al.: Evidence that prior immune dysfunction predisposes to human immunodeficiency virus infection in homosexual men. Journal of Acquired Immune Deficiency Syndrome 2(2):178–186, 1989.

Meisenhelder, J.B., and LaCharite, C.L.: Comfort in caring: Nursing the person with HIV infection. Boston, Scott Foresman, 1989.

Moran, T.A., Lovejoy, N., Viele, C.S., et al.: Informational needs of homosexual men diagnosed with AIDS or AIDS-related complex. Oncology Nursing Forum 15(3):311–314, 1988.

Moss, A.R., Bacchetti, P., Osmond, D., et al.: Seropositivity for HIV and the development of AIDS or AIDS-related condition: Three year followup of the San Francisco General Hospital cohort. British Medical Journal 296:745–750, 1988.

Sande, M.A., and Volberding, P.A. (Eds.): The Medical Management of AIDS. Philadelphia, W.B. Saunders, 1988.

Taylor, J.M., Fahey, J.L., Detils, R., and Giorgi, J.V.: CD4 percentage, CD4 number and CD4:CD8 ratio in HIV infection: Which to choose and how to use. Journal of Acquired Immune Deficiency Syndrome 2(2):114–124, 1989.

Ungvarski, P.: Demystifying AIDS: Educating nurses for care. Nursing and Health Care 8(10):571–573, 1987.

PATIENT EDUCATION MATERIALS AND COMMUNITY RESOURCES

The following list includes organizations that the San Francisco AIDS Home Care and Hospice Program have found particularly helpful in providing educational resources. These organizations produce many excellent written and audiovisual materials. We encourage you to call or write them to obtain information about their educational materials. You also should consult local listings for additional organizations in your area that might provide materials and other assistance for staff and patient education.

Educational Materials Specific for AIDS

1. AIDS Information
   U.S. Public Health Service
   Hubert Humphrey Building
   Room 721-H
   200 Independence Avenue, SW
   Washington, DC 20201
   (202) 245-6867

   AIDS Hotline (Taped message)
   1-800-342-AIDS

   AZT Information Hotline (Physicians only)
   1-800-843-9388

2. AIDS Project Los Angeles, Inc.
   (Write for "Living with AIDS: A Self-Care Manual")
   7362 Santa Monica Boulevard
   West Hollywood, CA 90046
   (213) 876-8951

3. Centers for Disease Control (CDC)
   1599 Clifton Road, NE
   Atlanta, GA 30333
   (404) 329-3472 (For statistics regarding epidemiology)
   (404) 329-3406 (Needlestick study)
   (404) 329-2891 (Information office for educational materials)

4. Gay Men's Health Crisis
   Box 274
   132 W. 24th Street
   New York, NY 10011
   (212) 807-6655

5. National AIDS Network
   (Clearinghouse for Information regarding
   AIDS)
   729 8th Street SE, Suite 300
   Washington, DC 20003
   (202) 546-2424

6. National Gay Task Force Crisis Line
   1-800-221-7044
   In New York: (212) 807-6016
   In San Francisco: 1-800-FOR-AIDS
   In Los Angeles: 1-800-922-AIDS

7. National Institute for Arthritis and Infectious
   Disease
   Bethesda, MD 20205
   (301) 496-5717 (Information regarding the immune system)

8. National Institute of Mental Health
   (Write for booklet, "Coping With AIDS," for
   health care professionals)
   Public Inquiries
   Park Lawn Building
   Room 15C-15
   5600 Fishers Lane
   Rockville, MD 20857

9. San Francisco AIDS Foundation
   (Write for catalog of educational materials)
   333 Valencia Street
   San Francisco, CA 94103

10. The Shanti Project
    (Write for list of training materials)
    890 Hayes Street
    San Francisco, CA 94117
    (415) 558-9644

11. U.S. Department of Health and Human Ser-
    vices Information Office
    Washington, DC 20201
    (202) 245-6867

12. VNA of San Francisco
    AIDS Home Care and Hospice Program
    410 Duboce Street
    San Francisco, CA 94117
    (415) 861-8705

Additional Resources with Related Information

1. American Cancer Society National Office
   4 West 35th Street
   New York, NY 10001
   (212) 371-2900

2. American Red Cross
   17th and D Street, NW
   Washington, DC 20006
   (202) 737-8300

3. Hemophilia Foundation
   19 West 34th Street, Suite 1204
   New York, NY 10001
   (212) 563-0211

4. Hospice Association of America
   214 Massachusetts Ave, NE
   Washington, DC 20002
   (202) 547-5263

5. National Association for Home Care
   519 C Street, NE
   Washington, DC 20002
   (202) 547-5277

6. National Cancer Institute
   Cancer Information Service
   1-800-422-6237

7. National Hospice Organization
   Suite 307
   1901 North Fort Meyer Drive
   Arlington, VA 22209

State and Local Resources

1. National Directory of AIDS-Related Services
   The Fund for Human Dignity
   80 Fifth Avenue, Suite 1601
   New York, NY 10011

2. For AIDS-related services in your area:
   - Check with local home health agencies and hospice programs.
   - Check with your local Department of Public Health.
   - Check with your local mental health agencies for available services.
   - Check for local community resource guides (such as guides published by the United Way).
   - Check with National AIDS Network for local and state specific AIDS organizations and gay community organizations.
   - Check with your state Department of Social Services.

53

Knowledge Deficit Related to Prevention and Early Detection of HIV Disease

- Check with your children's service programs and agencies.

Other Supportive Services:

- Alcoholics Anonymous (Check phone book for local telephone number).

- Narcotics Anonymous (Check phone book for local telephone number).
- Church councils.

Reprinted with permission from Hughes, A.M., Martin, J.P. and Franks, P.: AIDS Home Care and Hospice Manual. VNA of San Francisco, 1987.

INFORMATION

The nurse assesses the patient's current knowledge of diagnosis, treatment, resources, predictable problems, and participation in care (e.g., financial matters, spiritual concerns, and hospice) to formulate actual or potential nursing diagnoses.

Appropriate patient outcomes to consider in planning nursing interventions will specify the patient's ability to:

1. describe the state of the disease and therapy at a level consistent with patient's educational and emotional status.
2. participate in the decision-making process pertaining to the plan of care and life activities.
3. identify appropriate community and personal resources that provide information and services.
4. describe appropriate actions for highly predictable problems, oncologic emergencies, and major side effects of the disease or therapy.
5. describe the schedule when ongoing therapy is predicted.

Evaluation of the patient's responses to nursing care is based on whether the patient understands enough about the disease process and therapy to attain self-management and to participate in treatment.

Excerpted from the ANA/ONS Standards of Oncology Nursing Practice.

Knowledge Deficit Related to Chemotherapy

Eileen T. Somerville

Eileen T. Somerville

Population at Risk

- Individuals with a diagnosis of cancer potentially responsive to antineoplastic chemotherapy agents

EXPECTED OUTCOME

1. Patient demonstrates knowledge related to diagnosis and disease process:
   - states the diagnosis and explains the disease process.
   - describes previous experience with cancer and cancer treatment.
   - acknowledges need for treatment.
   - states alternatives to prescribed treatment.
2. Patient demonstrates knowledge related to rationale for treatment with chemotherapy:
   - verbalizes need for chemotherapy.
   - verbalizes attitude toward and expectations of cancer treatment.
   - states understanding of use of chemotherapy alone or in conjunction with other treatment modalities if applicable.
   - identifies treatment protocol.
3. Patient demonstrates knowledge related to potential therapeutic effects of chemotherapy:
   - states diagnosis and expected response to treatment.
   - identifies specific effects of treatment with chemotherapy drugs.
4. Patient demonstrates knowledge of treatment plan and schedule:
   - identifies drugs to be given.
   - states frequency and duration of administration.
   - identifies studies and procedures that will be done prior to administration of chemotherapy.
   - identifies follow-up studies and procedures needed to evaluate treatment effect.
5. Patient demonstrates knowledge of potential side effects of drugs:
   - states mechanism of action of drugs.
   - states reason for side effects.
   - identifies specific side effects that may occur with each drug.
   - states self-management interventions to control side effects.
   - states signs and symptoms to report to health care professionals.
   - identifies procedures for reporting signs and symptoms.

6. Patient demonstrates knowledge to manage treatment with chemotherapy:
   - maintains nutritional status to best of ability.
   - follows oral, body, and environmental hygiene measures.
   - maintains optimal rest/activity pattern.
   - uses safety precautions to prevent injury.
   - seeks and uses resources as necessary.
   - verbalizes reduced anxiety related to treatment with chemotherapy.
   - states intention to comply with treatment plan.
7. Patient demonstrates knowledge related to various access devices if applicable.

NURSING MANAGEMENT

Assessment

1. Assess educational level, ability and desire to learn, memory retention, barriers to learning (e.g., excessive fatigue, anxiety, use of denial as coping mechanism).
2. Assess knowledge level relative to cancer, previous experience with the diagnosis of cancer, and cancer treatment.
3. Evaluate knowledge relative to the individual's specific cancer diagnosis and cancer treatment.
4. Ascertain understanding of anatomy and physiology related to specific disease and treatment.
5. Ascertain attitudes and expectations related to outcome of cancer treatment.
6. Assess understanding of:
   - chemotherapy as treatment modality for disease.
   - alternatives to prescribed treatment with chemotherapy.
   - short-term/long-term process and outcome, should treatment be postponed or declined.
   - side effects and adverse effects (both immediate and long-term) of treatment with chemotherapy.
   - terminology related to disease.
7. Note previous experience with chemotherapy as a treatment modality for cancer.
8. Assess need for venous access device.
9. Determine availability of a caregiver willing to learn and participate in patient's care.
10. Assess degree of potential family/social disruption caused by compliance with chemotherapy protocol.
11. Evaluate resources needed and available to assist in compliance with treatment schedule.
12. Determine medical history; evaluate for contraindications for specific chemotherapy agents or dosage adjustments.
13. Obtain medication history, including nonprescription medications routinely or intermittently taken by patient. Review for contraindications (e.g., aspirin-containing medications, anticoagulants).
14. Note allergy history.

Patient Teaching

1. Develop a teaching plan at an appropriate level of understanding.
2. Review, clarify, and reinforce information previously given relevant to diagnosis, disease, treatment.
3. Explain informed consent and need for signed consent if applicable.
4. Explain expected therapeutic effect of chemotherapy treatment (e.g., cure, control, palliation, adjuvant).
5. Teach anatomy and physiology pertinent to disease and treatment. Explain how drugs work to kill cancer cells.

6. Provide patient/caregiver with oral and written information regarding:
   - name of each drug to be given.
   - route of administration of each drug.
   - anticipated schedule of administration of each drug.
   - frequency and duration of administration of each drug (e.g., continuous infusion, short-term infusion, bolus infusion, or daily, weekly, monthly).
7. When appropriate, discuss venous access devices, advantages, and potential.
8. Explain that time space between administration of drugs allows time for normal cells to recover.
9. Explain rationale for follow-up procedures and studies to evaluate effectiveness and side effects to therapy:
   - routine blood counts and chemistries.
   - testing of urine and stool.
   - x-ray and scans.
   - bone marrow studies.
10. Define relevant terminology.
11. Explain mode of action of antineoplastic drugs and reasons for side effects:
    - anticancer drugs act on rapidly dividing cells.
    - anticancer drugs affect normal cells as well as malignant cells.
    - normal cells can recover from the damage caused by these drugs while cancer cells cannot.
12. Identify known side effects of each drug patient will receive.
13. Teach which side effects will occur immediately (e.g., nausea and vomiting; red urine with Adriamycin).
14. Teach which side effects will be delayed (e.g., decreased blood counts approximately 7 to 10 days, hair loss approximately 3 weeks).
15. Explain that some side effects are reversible (e.g., blood counts will recover, hair will regrow).
16. Provide information regarding medical and nursing interventions available for adverse side effects.
17. Provide printed material related to chemotherapy side effects, interventions for self-management.
18. Give verbal and written instructions for self-management of anticipated side effects:
    - nausea and vomiting:
      - antiemetics.
      - carbonated beverages.
      - cold and bland foods.
      - small and frequent intake.
      - high-protein and carbohydrate diet.
      - avoidance of foods with strong or unpleasant aromas.
    - diarrhea:
      - antidiarrheal medications.
      - replacement fluids.
      - avoidance of highly seasoned/greasy foods and stimulants such as coffee.
    - constipation:
      - cathartics/stool softeners.
      - high-fiber/fluid diet.
    - hair loss: use of wigs, scarfs, and hats.
    - decreased white blood cells (WBC):
      - avoidance of others with infectious/contagious disease.
      - daily bath.
      - hand-washing routine.
    - decreased red blood cells (RBC): alter activity and increase rest.
    - decreased platelets:
      - avoid contact sports, trauma, injury.
      - use electric razor only.
    - stomatitis:
      - routine mouth care AM, after eating, bedtime.
      - rinse with salt water or salt and baking soda.
      - use soft toothbrush.
      - use of high-protein liquid supplements.
      - avoid alcohol-containing mouthwashes, foods that irritate oral mucosa, citrus, spices, alcohol, smoking.
19. Review medications and foods to be avoided:

- aspirin-containing medications.
- all medications not approved by the oncology treatment team.
- high-tyramine diet if taking procarbazine.

20. Discuss literature and resources available to patient.
21. Teach signs and symptoms to observe and report to the health care team:
    - blood in urine, stool, emesis.
    - bleeding gums, nose.
    - rash, jaundice.
    - fever.
    - fatigue, shortness of breath.
    - sore mouth, pain or difficulty in swallowing.
    - change in mental status.
    - numbness or tingling in fingers or toes.
    - change in bowel habits.
    - change in urinary output, edema, dehydration.
22. Teach where and how to reach appropriate health care persons if necessary.
23. Reassure patient about continued availability of health care service should adverse or side effects develop beyond self-care/family management.
24. Discuss possibility of treatment as outpatient or need for hospital admission for future treatment.
25. Discuss contraception, potential for infertility (see Chapters 17 and 54).
26. Assure healthy family members/friends that cancer is noncontagious and noninfectious.
27. Instruct family and care providers to use caution when handling patient's emesis and excreta for 48 hrs after drug treatment, and to use good handwashing regimen.

Calabresi, P., and Parks, R.E.: Chemotherapy of neoplastic disease. *In* Gilman, A.G., Goodman, L.S., Rally, T.W., and Murad, F. (Eds.): The Pharmacological Basis of Therapeutics (7th ed). New York, Macmillan, pp. 1240–1306, 1985.
Cancer Chemotherapy Guidelines. Modules I–V. Pittsburgh, PA, Oncology Nursing Society, 1988.
Dodd, M.J.: Cancer patients' knowledge of chemotherapy: Assessment and information interventions. Oncology Nursing Forum 9:39–44, 1982.
Donovan M.I., and Pierce, S.: Cancer Care: A Guide for Patient Education. New York, Appleton-Century Crofts, 1981.
Dorr, R.T., & Fritz W.L.: Cancer Chemotherapy Handbook. New York, Elsevier, 1980.
Fisher, D.S., and Knobf, M.T.: The Cancer Chemotherapy Handbook (3rd ed). Chicago, Year Book Medical Publishers, 1989.
Krakoff, I.H.: Cancer Chemotherapeutic Agents. Atlanta, American Cancer Society Professional Education Publication, 1987.
Maxwell, M.B.: Reexamining the dietary restrictions with procarbazine (an MAOI). Cancer Nursing 3:451–457, 1980.
Oncology: Programmed Modules for Nurses, Volume 1: The Basics of Cancer. Syracuse, NY, Bristol-Myers Oncology Division, 1985.
Oncology: Programmed Modules for Nurses, Volume 2: The Basics of Cancer Treatment. New York, L.P. Communications, 1988.
Oncology: Programmed Modules for Nurses, Volume 3: Types of Cancer. New York, L.P. Communications: 1990.
Oncology Nursing Society: Access Device Guidelines: Module I—Catheters. Pittsburgh, PA, 1989.
Oncology Nursing Society: Access Device Guidelines: Module II—Ports and Reservoirs. Pittsburgh, PA, 1989.
Oncology Nursing Society: Access Device Guidelines: Module III—Pumps. Pittsburgh, PA, 1990.
Oncology Nursing Society and American Nurses' Association. Standards of Oncology Nursing Practice. Kansas City, MO, American Nurses' Association, 1987.
Tenebaum, L.: Cancer Chemotherapy: A Reference Guide. Philadelphia, W.B. Saunders, 1989.
Wittes, R.E. (Ed.): Manual of Oncologic Therapeutics 1989/1990. Philadelphia, J.B. Lippincott, 1989.

SUGGESTED READINGS

Becker, T.: Cancer Chemotherapy Manual for Nurses. Boston, Little, Brown & Co., 1987.
Brager, B.L. and Yasko, J.M.: Care of the Client Receiving Chemotherapy. Reston, VA, Reston Publishing Co., 1984.

PATIENT EDUCATION MATERIALS AND COMMUNITY RESOURCES

Baker, L.S.: You and Leukemia: A Day at a Time. Philadelphia, W.B. Saunders, 1978.
Chemotherapy and You. Columbus, OH, Adria Laboratories, 1980.

Chemotherapy and You. A Guide to Self-Help During Treatment. (N.I.H. Publication No. 82-1136). Bethesda, MD, National Institutes of Health, 1982.

Diet and Nutrition: A Resource for Parents of Children with Cancer. (N.I.H. Publication No. 80-2038). Bethesda, MD, National Institutes of Health, 1979.

Eating Hints: Recipes and Tips for Better Nutrition During Treatment. (N.I.H. Publication No. 80-2079). Bethesda, MD, National Institutes of Health, 1980.

Leukemia: Looking Toward Tomorrow: A Patient's Handbook. New York, American Cancer Society, 1977.

12

Knowledge Deficit Related to Radiation Therapy

Judith A. Shell

Population at Risk

- Individuals with cancer who are to receive external radiation therapy

1. Patient demonstrates knowledge of radiation therapy:
   - identifies radiation therapy as one of the treatment modalities for curing, controlling, or relieving symptoms of cancer.
   - identifies rationale for use of radiation therapy for patient's particular disease.
   - identifies principles of radiation therapy and methods of action.
   - states purpose and procedures for use of radiation therapy.
   - identifies different types of machines used for radiation therapy relative to patient's treatment plan.
2. Patient demonstrates knowledge related to treatment plan and procedures prior to and during treatment with radiation therapy:
   - identifies that treatment planning includes disease evaluation, immobilization devices, simulation, and cast blocks.
   - identifies that treatment course involves length of daily treatment, actual number of treatments given; understands importance of completion of prescribed treatment schedule.
   - identifies need and rationale for assessment during treatment.
3. Patient demonstrates knowledge related to measures to manage general side effects of radiation therapy:
   - prevent/minimize fatigue.
   - promote adequate nutritional and fluid intake.
   - promote healing of skin.
   - promote adequate hematopoietic function.
   - promote coping mechanisms.
4. Patient identifies when and what side effects to report to health care team.

NURSING MANAGEMENT

Assessment

1. Assess patient/family awareness and understanding of the cancer diagnosis. Note verbal and nonverbal communication. If illness is denied, learning is minimized.

2. Evaluate patient's/family's current knowledge of diagnosis, disease, and radiation therapy:

- has patient had previous instruction/treatment?
- what has patient been told by physician, nurse, others?
- what, if any, are patient's misconceptions?

3. Determine patient's ability to read and comprehend new information.
4. Gauge patient's readiness to learn (emotional state, level of anxiety) and intellectual capability.
5. Assess patient's current knowledge of treatment planning and the purpose of treatment. (Has the patient had previous instruction/treatment? What has the patient been told by the physician? What, if any, are the patient's misconceptions? What are the expectations of treatment?)
6. Assess patient's readiness to learn about treatment planning and the treatment course.
7. Assess patient's current knowledge of general side effects:
   - has patient had previous instruction/treatment?
   - what has patient been told by physician, nurse, others?
   - what, if any, are patient's misconceptions?
8. Assess patient's general physical status (e.g., nutritional, hematopoietic, skin and mucous membrane integrity, ADL performance) and concept of self.
9. Assess patient's method of coping with diagnosis and treatment with radiation therapy.
10. Obtain history of any previous radiation therapy, including dose, length of therapy, type of radiation equipment, treatment port.
11. Obtain history of previous chemotherapy since drugs (e.g., Adriamycin) may increase response or side effects.

Patient Teaching

1. Discuss principles of radiation therapy and the method of action.

2. Explain that radiation therapy may be used alone, combined with chemotherapy, used preoperatively or postoperatively or intraoperatively for cure, control of tumor growth, or palliation of symptoms.
3. Describe (and possibly illustrate) according to individual patient treatment, different modes of radiation therapy and their functions (e.g., x-rays, gamma rays, electrons, neutrons, types of hyperthermia).
4. Discuss (possibly illustrate) according to individual patient treatment, different types of machines used for radiation therapy and their functions.
5. Provide patient with current literature concerning treatment with radiation therapy.
6. Teach radiation safety precautions for certain types of radiation therapy if appropriate (see Chapter 13).
7. Assure patient/family that patient is not radioactive and that no special precautions are required during external treatment.
8. Explain basis for treatment planning, including evaluation of:
   - type of cancer.
   - stage of disease.
   - patient's age and concomitant disease.
   - area of body being treated and vital organs to be protected.
   - body size.
   - tumor response.
   - tests (x-rays, blood test, biopsy, scans).
   - Karnofsky Scale status.
9. Describe the schedules for treatment. Identify length of time required for each treatment and number of treatments planned. Emphasize the importance of adhering to the prescribed schedule and completing the course of treatments.
10. Treatment may require the use of immobilization devices (e.g. alpha cradle and/or light cast, bite block, sand bags, foam cushions.). Explain rationale for use of these devices:
   - helps keep patient more comfortable on table during radiation treatment.

- helps keep patient from moving during treatment.
- provides more accurate treatment since the patient is in the same position each day.

11. Treatment planning includes simulation:
   - special x-rays called "port films" are made of area to be treated.
   - marks are drawn, usually with magic marker, around the treatment area for exact treatment location. These are removed after entire treatment course is completed.
   - tattoos may also be placed at this time or later during treatment. These are small permanent pinpoint marks that indicate the treatment area.
   - simulation may need to be repeated during the course of treatment.

12. Treatment planning may include cast block production. Describe this device and its purpose:
   - a shield made of lead-like substance, to be placed in beam pathway during treatment.
   - one block made for each treatment port.
   - purpose is to spare normal tissue surrounding tumor area.

13. Describe radiation treatment:
   - usually consists of treatment 5 days per week (patient may be treated only twice a week or up to twice a day); number of treatments will depend on disease, treatment goal (cure versus palliation), total dose needed.
   - actual treatment is short, but preparation and positioning on treatment table can take up to 10 to 15 minutes per port.
   - patient will be alone in room but will be under constant observation via window or TV screen.
   - machine often makes a whirring noise or a noise like a vacuum.
   - the patient will not experience any pain during treatment itself, but if the patient is already in pain, the hard table may cause discomfort. Tell patient to use pain medications 1 hour before radiation therapy.

14. Describe possible physical assessment measures during treatment:
   - hematologic lab tests.
   - nutritional status (weight, calorie intake).
   - ability of patient to perform ADL.
   - side effects (depend on treatment field, daily and total dosage, elapsed time of therapy, type of cancer, pretreatment condition, concurrent therapy).
   - tumor status and response (tests done, assessment made regarding increase or decrease in number of treatments, port size, and/or possible boost to the tumor area with regular beam or with electrons).

15. Explain rationale and measures to limit, as necessary, patient's activities during treatment and 6 to 8 weeks after treatment:
   - activity must be limited due to increased fatigue.
   - help plan a daily schedule including rest periods according to patient's life style, occupation, and hobbies.
   - discuss assistive devices for saving energy (e.g., wheelchair, bedside commode).

16. Discuss rationale and measures to maintain adequate nutritional intake:
   - instruct in planning meals within high-protein/high-carbohydrate diet.
   - obtain dietary consultation if necessary.
   - explain need for small frequent meals, finger foods, dietary supplements.
   - record patient's weight once per week.
   - provide copy of *Eating Hints* from NCI for menus.

17. Explain rationale and measures to control radiodermatitis (see Chapter 37).

18. Describe rationale and measures to take following a decrease in hematopoietic function:
   - if WBC is low (below 3000):

- treatment may be temporarily discontinued until WBC climbs to 3000.
  - ○ Refer to Chapter 31, Potential for Infection.
- if hemoglobin is low (under 10 gm):
  - ○ packed cells may be transfused to elevate hemoglobin so radiation treatment will be effective.
  - ○ Refer to Chapter 33, Injury, Potential for, Related to Anemia.
- if platelet count is low:
  - ○ patient's treatment may be tempo-

rarily discontinued until platelet count is above 40,000.
  - ○ Refer to Chapter 32, Injury, Potential for, Related to Thrombocytopenia.

19. Explain potential problems regarding sexual identity and function and identify alternate methods of sexual expression and satisfaction (see Chapter 53).

20. Encourage and support patient's coping mechanisms regarding treatment with radiation therapy (see Chapter 19).

Specific Side Effects Related to Site of Treatment with Radiation Therapy: Head and Neck, Chest and Back, Abdomen and Pelvis

EXPECTED OUTCOME

1. Patient demonstrates knowledge of side effects of head and neck radiation therapy:
   - identifies specific potential side effects.
   - verbalizes appropriate self-care behaviors to prevent or manage side effects.
   - states side effects to report to health care team.
2. Patient demonstrates knowledge of side effects of radiation to chest and back:
   - identifies specific potential side effects.
   - verbalizes appropriate self-care behaviors to prevent or manage side effects.
   - states side effects to report to health care team.
3. Patient demonstrates knowledge of side effects of radiation to abdomen and pelvis:
   - identifies specific potential side effects.
   - verbalizes appropriate self-care behaviors to prevent or manage side effects.
   - states side effects to report to health care team.

NURSING MANAGEMENT

Assessment

1. Assess patient's current knowledge of side effects of treatment.

2. Assess patient's readiness and ability to learn.
3. Assess patient's physical condition, with specific emphasis on area of treatment.

4. Ascertain whether dental consult has been arranged prior to head and neck radiation therapy.

Patient Teaching

1. Teach procedures to avoid/ameliorate side effects of radiation to head and neck:
   - describe signs and symptoms of side effects of radiation therapy to head and neck (mucositis, xerostomia, altered tastes, dental caries, sore throat, hoarseness, dysphagia, decreased sense of smell, alopecia in treated area only, headache, nausea and vomiting).
   - discuss need for dental consultation *before* radiation therapy begins and regularly during and following radiation therapy.
   - explain rationale and measures for clean mouth (brushing teeth or dentures, fluoride application, saline rinse, artificial saliva):
     ○ advise patient to brush teeth after each meal and to floss at least once per day (if platelets are low, clean with moist gauze or toothette).
     ○ if patient has dentures, they should be cleaned each day with a denture cleaner or salt and soda.
     ○ mouth should be irrigated with soda, salt (1 tsp of each), and water (1 quart), at least qid and more often if possible.
     ○ if mucositis is present, the soda-salt solution can be chilled and used in a gavage fashion. (An enema bag is an excellent device for gavage).
   - explain signs and symptoms of mucositis, stomatitis, and xerostomia, indicating those that should be reported to health care team (see Chapter 38).
   - explain possible formation of pseudomembrane (white or tan glistening membrane). Membrane should not be removed because ulceration and bleeding will occur.
   - teach measures to prevent tooth decay including use of artificial saliva and topical fluoride.
     ○ explain need for application of topical fluoride to the teeth for remainder of patient's life. Fluoride is available in mouthwashes, toothpaste, topical solution and gels, and in tablet form.
   - teach measures to control sore mouth and throat:
     ○ use of Xylocaine Viscous mixed with Mylanta or Maalox (1 to 3).
     ○ Carafate 1 tablet dissolved in 30 ml water may be used one-half hour before meals and at bedtime for discomfort in swallowing.
     ○ zinc sulfate 110 mg every day, may be used to help minimize taste loss.
     ○ Refer to Chapter 38, Mucous Membrane Integrity, Impairment of, Related to Stomatitis.
   - for radiation to head, instruct patient regarding:
     ○ whether hair loss is likely to be temporary or permanent. (In adults treated with whole-brain radiation therapy, with doses greater than 5000 rad, hair loss is usually permanent. If temporary, hair usually grows back approximately 6 months after completion of treatment).
     ○ not to shampoo hair if marks are placed on head for treatment guidelines, since marks may wash off of head.
     ○ avoiding excessive brushing and using wide-toothed comb.
     ○ purchasing a wig or hairpiece before radiation begins.
     ○ wearing a cover for head (turban, sports cap) when not using wig.
     ○ avoiding hair dyes and hot rollers during radiation treatments.
   - explain possible alterations and interventions during sexual relations (see Chapter 53).
   - explain different stages of skin reaction and treatment (see Chapter 37).

- explain importance of follow-up exams to watch for soft tissue necrosis/osteoradionecrosis.
- provide information related to availability of local services and patient information booklets.

2. Teach procedures to avoid/ameliorate side effects of radiation to chest and back:
   - describe signs and symptoms of pneumonitis (dyspnea, dry cough, fever, night sweats, hemoptysis) and esophagitis (sore throat, difficulty swallowing).
   - explain possibility of late effect fibrosis in the lung, and that this may cause infection, fever, chills, dyspnea, clubbing, and abscess formation.
   - discuss rationale and measures to maintain adequate oxygenation:
     ○ oxygen or steroids may be administered if there is shortness of breath from pneumonitis.
     ○ positioning and breathing through pursed lips may help decrease anxiety from shortness of breath.
     ○ cough suppressant may be used for dry cough.
     ○ an increase in fluid intake and use of a humidifier will help loosen secretions.
   - discuss rationale and measures to maintain hydration and nutritional status (Refer to Chapter 27, Nutrition, Alteration in, Related to Disease Process and Treatment).
     ○ provide patient information booklet.

3. Teach procedures to avoid/ameliorate side effects of radiation to abdomen and pelvis:
   - describe signs and symptoms of bladder/bowel and vaginal/penal irritation to report to the health care team (diarrhea, cramping, hematuria, tenesmus, urinary frequency, urinary urgency, nausea, vomiting, and dyspareunia).
   - fluids should be forced to prevent cystitis.
   - to reduce symptoms of cystitis and urethritis, anticholinergics such as Ditropan (oxybutynin chloride) and antispasmodics such as Pyridium (phena-

zopyridine) or Urispas (flavoxate HCl) may be used.
- Lomotil or Immodium, not to exceed 8 tablets per day may be used for cramping and diarrhea. If patient experiences *severe* diarrhea and cramping, paregoric or tincture of opium may be used.
- describe hygienic measures to prevent undue perineal irritation and infection:
  ○ perineum should be carefully cleansed after bowel movement or urination (cotton balls and warm water, wash front to back).
- explain rationale and measures to maintain hydration and nutritional status (low-residue diet, force fluids, antiemetics).
- explain effects of radiation therapy if patient has a stoma:
  ○ stoma may become inflamed, prolapsed, retracted, or narrowed if in the treatment field.
  ○ if moist desquamation occurs, a steroid cream or a skin barrier such as Stomahesive or Hollihesive may be used.
  ○ patient should avoid taking medication such as bismuth subgallate, an oral ostomy deodorant, as this contains metal and causes increased reactions around the stoma.
- explain possible alterations in vaginal mucous membrane and effect during sexual activity:
  ○ vaginal intercourse may be painful due to narrowed vaginal opening, fissured mucous membrane, and burning sensation from semen on tender tissue, but may be continued during treatment as long as pain is tolerable.
  ○ after radiation therapy is completed, vaginal dilators inserted for 5 to 10 minutes daily or qod or vaginal intercourse performed weekly will maintain the vaginal opening.
  ○ during sexual intercourse or vaginal dilator use, an estrogen cream and water based lubricant (KY Jelly) must be used.

- men may experience painful redness of the penis and scrotum, decreased ejaculate, or may have difficulty with attaining/maintaining an erection.
- for further discussion of male and female sexual concerns, please see Chapters 39, 53, and 54.
- explain importance of follow-up for late complications of small bowel injury and fistula formation.
- provide patient information booklets.

SUGGESTED READINGS

Conkey, C.: Intraoperative radiation therapy: Procedures protocols. AORN Journal 46(2):226–227, 229–232, 1987.

Dolinger, D.: How radiation complicates stoma care. RN 49(9):32–34, 1986.

Doyle, M.A.: Whole body hyperthermia: Making things too hot for cancer. RN 50(8):39–40, 1987.

Dudjak, L.A.: Mouth care for mucositis due to radiation therapy. Cancer Nursing 10(3):131–140, 1987.

Eardley, A.: Planning nutritional support. Nursing Times 82(16):26–29, 1986.

Gardner, M.E.: Notes from a waiting room. American Journal of Nursing 80(1):86–89, 1980.

Gunderson, L.L., Martin, J.K., Beart, W., et al.: Intraoperative and external beam irradiation for locally advanced colorectal cancer. Annals of Surgery 207(1):52–60, 1988.

Hassey, K.M.: Radiation therapy for rectal cancer and the implications for nursing. Cancer Nursing 10(6):311–318, 1987.

Hassey, K.M.: Skin care for patients receiving radiation therapy for rectal cancer. Journal of Enterostomal Therapy 14(5):197–200, 1987.

Hellman, S.: Principles of radiation therapy. In DeVita, V.T., Hellman, S., and Rosenberg, S.A. (Eds.): Cancer: Principles and Practice of Oncology (Vol. 1). Philadelphia, J.B. Lippincott, 1985, pp. 227–256.

Hilderly, L.: Clinical reviews: Skin care in radiation therapy: A review of the literature. Oncology Nursing Forum 10(1):51–58, 1983.

Hilderly, L.: Radiotherapy. In Groenwald, S.L. (Ed.): Cancer Nursing: Principles and Practices. Boston, Jones & Bartlett, 1987, pp. 320–344.

King, K.B., Nail, L.M., Kreamer, K., et al.: Patients' description of the experience of receiving radiation therapy. Oncology Nursing Forum 12(4):55–61, 1985.

Klein, F.A., Ali, M.M., Marks, S., et al.: Bilateral pelvic lymphadenectomy, iridium 192 template, and external beam therapy for localized prostate carcinoma: Complications and results. Southern Medical Journal 81(1):27–31, 1988.

Lewis, F., and Levita, M.: Understanding radiotherapy. Cancer Nursing 11(3):174–185, 1988.

McNaull, F.W.: Radiation therapy. In McIntire, S.N., and Cioppa, A.L. (Eds.): Cancer Nursing: A Developmental Approach. New York, John Wiley & Sons, 1984, pp. 91–114.

Mossman, K., Shatzman, A., Chencharick, J., et al.: Long-term effects of radiotherapy on taste and salivary function in men. International Journal of Radiation, Oncology, Biology and Physics 8: 991–997, 1982.

Phillips, T.: Principles of radiobiology and radiation therapy. In Carter, S., Glatstein, E., and Livingston, R. (Eds.): Principles of Cancer Treatment. New York, McGraw-Hill, 1982, pp. 58–88.

Richards, S., and Hiratzka, S.: Vaginal dilatation post-pelvic irradiation: A patient educational tool. Oncology Nursing Forum 13(4):89–91, 1986.

Saver, S., and McCune, K.: An introduction to fast neutron therapy for the radiation therapy technologist. Radiologic Technology 58(6):517–522, 1987.

Schwade, J., and Lichter, A.: Management of acute effects of radiation therapy. In Cater, S., Glatstein, E., and Livingston, R. (Eds.): Principles of Cancer Treatment. New York, McGraw-Hill, 1982.

Snyder, C.C.: Nursing care of the client receiving radiotherapy. In Snyder, C.C. (Ed.): Oncology Nursing. Boston, Little, Brown and Co., 1986, pp. 116–135.

Strohl, R.A.: The nursing role in radiation oncology: Symptom management of acute and chronic reactions. Oncology Nursing Forum 15(4):429–434, 1988.

Welch, O.: Radiation-related nausea and vomiting. Oncology Nursing Forum 6(4):8–11, 1979.

Wickham, R.: Pulmonary toxicity secondary to cancer treatment. Oncology Nursing Forum 13(5):69–76, 1986.

PATIENT EDUCATION MATERIALS AND COMMUNITY RESOURCES

Radiation Therapy and You: A Guide to Self-Help During Treatment. NIH Publication, National Cancer Institute, Bethesda, MD 20892.

Radiation Therapy: A Treatment For Early Stage Breast Cancer. NIH Publication, National Cancer Institute, Bethesda, MD 20892.

Gurganus, E.: Cesium Implants for Gynecologic Cancer.

University of Texas Health Sciences Center at San Antonio, Department of Obstetrics/Gynecology.

Video

"Understanding Radiation Therapy." Grandview Hospital and Medical Center, c/o Mediatech, 110 E. Hubbard Street, Chicago, IL 60610.

Examples of Artificial Saliva

Orex—Young Dental, 2418 Northline Industrial Blvd., Maryland Heights, MO 64043.

Sal-Eze—North Pacific Dental, Inc., P.O. Box 522, Kirkland, WA 98033.

Moi-stir—Kingswood Laboratories, Inc., 336 Heather Drive, P.O. Box 744, Carmel, IN 46032.

13

Knowledge Deficit Related to Brachytherapy (Implants)

Roberta A. Strohl

Population at Risk

- Individuals with cancer who are to receive radiation therapy implants

EXPECTED OUTCOME

1. Patient demonstrates knowledge of radiation therapy implants:
   - states effect of radiation therapy implants.
   - states precautions that will be taken by health care personnel and visitors with sealed and unsealed sources.
   - identifies procedure for implantation.

NURSING MANAGEMENT

Assessment

1. Assess patient's current knowledge of and misconceptions about radiation implant therapy:
   - information learned from physician and health care providers.
   - information learned from family and friends.
2. Obtain history of previous external or implant radiation therapy: assess patient's feelings and concerns regarding radiation therapy implants.
3. Ascertain patient's willingness and ability to learn about radiation therapy implants.
4. Determine whether radiation implant is a sealed or unsealed source.
5. Evaluate patient's nutritional, cardiovascular, and pulmonary status.

Patient Teaching

1. Explain types of implant procedures:
   - afterloading (carrier is inserted in operating room and radioactive source is inserted later).
   - preloading (radioactive source is inserted with carrier).
2. Explain that implant is used to give high dose of radiation therapy to one area, sparing surrounding normal tissue.
3. Radioactivity is produced by the implanted source and thus the patient is radioactive. Precautions are required to protect health care staff and visitors.
4. Discuss principles of safety with patient and family.
5. Reassure patient that safe nursing care will be provided.
6. Sealed Sources:
   - time spent with patient by nurses and visitors will be limited.
   - nearness to the radioactive source lessens the amount of time visitors and nurses may stay.
   - staff caring for patient must wear film badge or type of dosimeter.
   - a shield may be placed at the bedside to protect visitors and health care personnel.
   - excreta (urine, sweat, feces) are not radioactive.

- linen and tray precautions are not needed.
- post phone number of radiation safety office and radiation oncology department on patient's door.
- procedure to follow if implant becomes dislodged:
  ○ notify Radiation Therapy and Radiation Safety Departments immediately. Use long-handled tongs to pick up implant and place in lead container in patient's room.
  ○ do not touch implant with hands. Gloves offer no protection.
7. Unsealed Source ^{32}P, ^{131}I, ^{198}Au:
   - determine type of sources; select appropriate precautions.
   - avoid contamination when administering injections.
   - post "Caution Radioactive Materials" sign on door.
   - label patient's chart with "radioactive" tag.
   - patient should be in private room.
   - health care providers must wear film badges or dosimeters.
   - visitors (no pregnant women or children) should remain 6 ft away and stay a maximum of 30/min per day.
   - patient should remain in bed unless other orders given.
   - cover mattress and pillow with plastic or rubber material.
   - prepare a plastic-lined waste basket and linen hamper and label with radiation warning signs.
   - use disposable tray and utensils and dispose of items in radioactive waste container. Patient is not to share food with anyone.
   - wear gloves to prevent contamination when handling waste and all items patient has touched.
   - patient should wear hospital pajamas or gowns.
   - if doctor requests, have patient collect urine.
   - keep all items that patient has had contact with in room.
   - samples (blood, urine, and the like) are sent only when nuclear medicine, radiation oncologist, or patient's physician gives authorization and should be labeled "radioactive."
   - room must be monitored by radiation safety after discharge before it can be released.
   - if spill occurs, contact nuclear medicine or radiation safety immediately to monitor and clean. Personnel involved must also be monitored. Be careful, as a spill may render a room unusable until source decays.
   - bandages must be monitored before they are discarded.
8. Encourage patients to ask for teaching tools in radiation oncology department, as many departments have developed instructions for patients.

Gynecologic Implants

EXPECTED OUTCOME

1. Patient demonstrates knowledge of implant procedure:
   - states placement will occur in operating room or treatment room.
   - identifies need for bedrest while implant is in body.
   - identifies measures to prevent movement of radioactive source.

71

2. Patient demonstrates knowledge of measures to prevent or manage complications of gynecologic implants:
   - states measures to dilate cervix.
   - states measures to prevent emboli.

NURSING MANAGEMENT

Assessment

1. See General Information, Assessment.
2. Do vaginal exam for drainage, bleeding, tenderness.
3. Assess bowel function.
4. Assess for phlebitis.
5. Evaluate urinary elimination.

Patient Teaching

1. See General Information, Patient Teaching.
2. Explain rationale and measures for implant placement:
   - cervical implants require anesthesia and operating room for insertion.
   - vaginal implants may not require anesthesia and operating room for insertion.
3. Radioactive source may be radium, or more commonly, cesium.
4. Discuss rationale and measures to prevent movement of radioactive source:
   - bowel cleansing before insertion of source is usually required before implantation to prevent bowel movement.

Enemas or colonic lavage (e.g., Golytely) are usually required.
   - placement of urinary Foley catheter while source is implanted.
   - bedrest while source is implanted.
5. Review measures to prevent complications of implant therapy and procedures.
   - patient should do isometric exercises while on bedrest.
   - patient should wear antiembolic hose while on bedrest.
   - patient may receive prophylactic heparin therapy to prevent emboli.
   - Foley catheter care should be provided to prevent infection.
   - gradual ambulation with assistance will be begun after source is removed.
   - after source is removed, patient should dilate vagina by vaginal sexual intercourse or vaginal dilator to avoid fibrosis/stenosis.
   - bowel program should be followed after implantation to prevent further constipation.
   - patient should be taught to report signs and symptoms of infection (e.g., fever, discharge, local pain).

Head and Neck

EXPECTED OUTCOME

1. Patient demonstrates knowledge of implant procedure.
2. Patient demonstrates knowledge of methods to prevent/manage complications:
   - states use of oral hygiene to prevent infection.

- states use of steroids to control edema.
- describes alternative communication methods if speaking will be difficult to understand.
- states measures to control pain.

NURSING MANAGEMENT

Assessment

1. See General Information, Assessment.
2. Assess nutritional status (e.g., weight and height, anthropometric measurements, serum albumin, total protein and albumin/globulin [A/G] ratio).
3. Check for fever (elevated temperature, redness at insertion site).
4. Observe oral pharyngeal area.

Patient Teaching

1. See General Information, Patient Teaching.
2. Explain types of implants and methods of placement:
   - sources used may be iridium or ^{125}I seeds.
   - catheters or permanent seeds are implanted at time of surgery.
3. Discuss measures for nutritional support during implant:
   - soft or liquid high-protein diet.
   - IV therapy often needed for hydration.

4. Teach signs and symptoms of infection (usually does not occur with seeds):
   - fever.
   - redness at insertion site.
   - drainage at insertion site.
   - pain at insertion site.
5. Describe measures to prevent infection:
   - oral hygiene 4 to 6 times daily with saline, water, baking soda, during and 1 week after implant therapy.
   - teach patient to perform suctioning procedures.
6. Discuss measures to control edema (e.g., steroids may be administered).
7. Identify alternate communication systems if patient's speech deteriorates (e.g., use of magic slate, cards).
8. Describe rationale and measures to control pain (e.g., use of analgesics around the clock).
9. Teach rationale and measures for radiation safety.
10. Describe measures to control pain:
    - topical applications of Xylocaine Viscous (lidocaine).
    - analgesics.

Breast

EXPECTED OUTCOME

1. Patient demonstrates knowledge of breast implant procedures.
2. Patient identifies measures to prevent complications:
   - describes appropriate skin care.
   - identifies signs and symptoms to report to health care team.

Knowledge Deficit Related to Brachytherapy (Implants)

NURSING MANAGEMENT

Assessment

1. See General Information, Assessment.
2. Assess skin over breast for redness, lesions, drainage.

Patient Teaching

1. See General Information, Patient Teaching.
2. Discuss implant procedures:
   - implants may be preloaded or, more commonly, afterloaded.
   - iridium is usual source.
3. Explain measures for providing comfort (analgesics as needed).
4. Teach signs and symptoms of infection (redness, fever, pain, drainage at site of insertion).
5. Describe measures for skin care during and after implant:
   - avoid trauma to implant area.
   - keep skin clean and dry.

Prostate

EXPECTED OUTCOME

Patient demonstrates knowledge of prostate implant procedures.

NURSING MANAGEMENT

Assessment

1. See General Information, Assessment.
2. Assess urine output.
3. Inspect all voided urine for presence of radiation seeds.

Patient Teaching

1. See General Information, Patient Teaching.
2. Discuss prostate implant therapy:
   - implants are inserted in operating room during surgery.
   - removable catheters may also be used.
   - permanent ^{125}I seeds are the usual source.
   - implanted ^{125}I seeds produce a low level of radioactive energy on skin surface.
3. Teach measures to promote safety with prostate-implanted ^{125}I seeds:
   - patient may be in semiprivate room.
   - urine and linens will be examined for seeds.
   - caregivers will limit time at dressing site.
4. Teach measures to promote safety with removable catheters:
   - antiembolism stockings must be worn.
   - anticoagulants may be given to prevent emboli.
   - urine should be monitored for bleeding.

SUGGESTED READINGS

Battles, C.S.E.: Nursing Management of the Radiation Therapy Client. *In* Marino L.B. (Ed.): Cancer Nursing. St. Louis, MO, C.V. Mosby, 1981, pp 260–286.

Hassey, K.: Principles of radiation safety and protechia. Seminars in Oncology Nursing *3*(1):23–30, 1987.

Instructor's Guide: Nursing Care of Radionuclide Therapy Patients (Vol. 19). Columbia, MD, Training Resources Division, Nuclear Support Services, 1982.

McCarthy, C.: The role of interstitial implantation in the treatment of primary breast cancer. Seminars in Oncology Nursing *3*(1):47–54, 1987.

Shell, J., and Carter, J.: The gynecological implant patient. Seminars in Oncology Nursing *3*(1):54–67, 1987.

Strohl, R.: Head and neck implants. Seminars in Oncology Nursing *3*(1):30–47, 1987.

PATIENT EDUCATION MATERIALS AND COMMUNITY RESOURCES

Radiation Therapy and You.—Available from NCI.

14

Knowledge Deficit Related to Biotherapy

Patricia F. Jassak

Population at Risk

- Patients who are eligible to receive biologic response modifier (BRM) agents
- Family members of patients who are to receive BRMs

EXPECTED OUTCOME

1. Patient/family demonstrate knowledge of disease process and available treatment modalities:
   - verbalize disease process.
   - state available treatment options.
   - acknowledge willingness to participate in clinical trial if appropriate.
   - verbalize attitude toward and expectations of therapy to be undertaken.
2. Patient/family demonstrate knowledge related to biotherapy treatment:
   - state rationale for treatment with BRM agent.
   - identify action of BRM agent in relation to immune system.
3. Patient/family demonstrate knowledge of specific biotherapy protocol and treatment plan to be administered:
   - state name of BRM agent(s) to be administered.
   - identify route and sites of administration of BRM agent.
   - state frequency and duration of administration.
   - identify studies and procedures that will be done prior to and during administration of BRM agent.
   - identify follow-up studies and procedures to be performed.
4. Patient/family demonstrate knowledge related to potential side effects of biotherapy treatments:
   - identify frequency and duration of potential side effects.
   - state signs and symptoms of potential side effects.
   - describe self-care strategies to manage side effects.
   - identify signs and symptoms of local and systemic side effects that must be reported to the health care team.
   - state procedures to follow for reporting signs and symptoms.
5. Patient/family demonstrate knowledge to manage biotherapy treatment:
   - maintain optimal rest and activity patterns.
   - request clarification and assistance as necessary.
   - verbalize intent to actively participate in treatment plan.

NURSING MANAGEMENT

Assessment

1. Assess educational level, ability, and desire to acquire knowledge related to biotherapy treatment.
2. Determine barriers to learning.
3. Identify attitude and expectations related to outcome of biotherapy.
4. Gauge understanding of:
   - biotherapy as a treatment modality for disease.
   - choice of participation in clinical trial and treatment plan.
   - potential side effects and adverse effects of treatment.
   - self-care strategies for management of side effects.
   - specific protocol and treatment plan to be implemented.
5. Obtain baseline psychologic and physiologic parameters.
6. Evaluate resources needed and available to assist patient/family during treatment course.

Patient Teaching

1. Review patient's/family's current knowledge of disease state and treatment plan.
2. Explain that the function of the immune system is to protect the body from invasion by bacteria, viruses, and foreign materials. Cancer is thought to develop from a dysfunction in the immune system, where the cancer (abnormal) cells are not recognized as abnormal by the immune system, and thus allowed to reproduce or are not adequately destroyed.
3. Explain that the goal of biotherapy as a treatment modality is to promote the immune system's ability to control and destroy malignant disease by modulating, restoring, or augmenting immune function.
4. Review knowledge of rationale and expected outcomes of specific clinical trial, if appropriate.

5. Explain rationale of informed consent process and requirement of written consent form if appropriate.
6. Determine if patient's/family's outcome expectations are in congruence with the purpose of the clinical trial, if appropriate.
7. Explain expected therapeutic effect of biotherapy.
8. Instruct and provide written information on the specific treatment plan to be implemented including:
   - name of each BRM agent to be administered (e.g., interferon, interleukin, colony-stimulating factor, monoclonal antibodies, and tumor necrosis factor).
   - route of administration of each agent (e.g., intramuscular, subcutaneous, intravenous, intracavitary, intralesional).
   - setting of BRM administration (e.g., inpatient, clinic/outpatient, home/self-administration).
   - frequency and duration of administration of each agent (e.g., daily, once daily for 5 days for 2 weeks, monthly).
   - administration of any other medications or agent required by the treatment plan.
   - patient/family role in the treatment plan.
9. Identify the frequency and rationale for studies and procedures prior to and during biotherapy and follow-up studies post-administration to evaluate immune function and therapeutic effectiveness of biotherapy:
   - blood counts and chemistries.
   - pharmacokinetics and immune parameters.
   - urine analysis: diagnostic studies (e.g., CT scan, x-rays).
10. Instruct patient/family that most side effects directly related to biotherapy usually will disappear within 72 to 96 hours after treatment is discontinued.
11. Teach patient/family signs and symp-

Knowledge Deficit Related to Biotherapy

toms of potential side effects of the BRM agent and self-care strategies to manage symptoms:

Flu-like syndrome
- signs and symptoms:
  - acute: fever, chills/rigors, myalgia, headaches.
  - chronic: malaise, fatigue, anorexia.
- management strategies:
  - check temperature at onset of chills and when warm.
  - use guided imaging and relaxation techniques.
  - use layers of blankets and extra clothing to promote warmth during periods of chilling.
  - use acetaminophen and Benadryl as prescribed.
  - avoid use of aspirin and aspirin-containing products.
  - arrange for a quiet environment.
  - maintain record of each symptom occurrence.
  - seek assistance with activities as needed.
  - rest when tired, attempt to develop progressively increased activities over time.
  - notify health care team if profound fatigue occurs (e.g., patient is confined to bed or couch more than 12 hours per day.

Integumentary
- signs and symptoms: rash, pruritus, irritation at injection site, skin desquamation.
- management strategies:
  - use fragance-free, high-fat, or oil lotions.
  - avoid scratching red and irritated areas.
  - apply cool compresses to irritated injection sites.
  - report any continued redness, swelling to health care team immediately.
  - use Benadryl as prescribed for pruritus.

Central Nervous System
- signs and symptoms: changes in cerebral function, mood alteration, confusion, agitation, anxiety.
- management strategies:
  - avoid alcoholic beverages.
  - report occurrence of any difficulty in concentration, confusion, or somnolence to health care personnel immediately.

Pulmonary
- signs and symptoms: dry cough, stridor, wheezing, dyspnea, rales.
- management strategies: report any symptoms to health care personnel immediately.

Cardiovascular
- signs and symptoms: peripheral edema, weight gain, chest pain, orthostatic hypotension.
- management strategies:
  - obtain daily weight; slowly change positions, lying-to-sitting-to-standing, to avoid dizziness.
  - report any symptoms to health care personnel immediately.

Renal
- signs and symptoms: decreased urine output, inability to take oral fluids.
- management strategies: maintain adequate oral fluid intake; report to health care personnel immediately if urine output is decreased or if color of urine becomes dark yellow.

Hepatic
- signs and symptoms: increased liver enzymes as evidenced by jaundice, increased abdominal girth.
- management strategies: report any signs of jaundice or abdominal swelling to health care personnel immediately.

Hematopoietic
- signs and symptoms: bleeding, dyspnea, bruising, temperature > 38°C or 101°F, or other signs of infection.
- management strategies: report any

signs and symptoms immediately to health care team.

Gastrointestinal

- signs and symptoms: nausea and vomiting, diarrhea, anorexia, taste alterations, stomatitis.
- management strategies:
  - avoid foods with strong or unpleasant odors.
  - eat small frequent meals.
  - if nausea persists, use antiemetics as prescribed.
  - use high-caloric food supplements instead of routine meals.
  - use antidiarrheal medications as prescribed.
  - monitor fluid intake to prevent dehydration.
  - maintain good oral hygiene.
  - avoid oral irritants (e.g., alcohol, spicy foods, commercial mouthwashes).
  - report weight loss and oral discomfort to health care personnel.

12. Instruct patient/family in techniques of drug administration (e.g., subcutaneous injection, ambulatory pump manipulation).
13. Instruct patient/family in procedure to use to contact health care personnel when appropriate.
14. Instruct patient to check with health care personnel prior to taking any unprescribed medication.
15. Review written patient education materials and available resources with patient/family.
16. Reinforce continued availability of health care services should adverse side effects occur.

SUGGESTED READINGS

Abernathy, E.: Biotherapy: An introductory overview. Oncology Nursing Forum *14*(6) Supplement: 13–15, 1987.

Biological Response Modifier Guidelines and Recommendations for Nursing Education and Practice. Pittsburgh, Oncology Nursing Society, 1989.

Bucholtz, J.: Radiolabeled antibody therapy. Seminars in Oncology Nursing *3*(1):67–73, 1987.

Chamoro, T., and Appelbaum, J.: Informed consent: Nursing issues and ethical dilemmas. Oncology Nursing Forum *15*(6):803–808, 1988.

Dewey, D.: Role of the nurse in the use of biological response modifiers. American Association of Occupational Health Nurses Journal *35*(4):163–167, 1987.

Dillman, J.B.: New antineoplastic therapies and inherent risks: Monoclonal antibodies, biologic response modifiers and interleukin-2. Journal of Intravenous Nursing *12*(2):103–113, 1989.

Dillman, J.B.: Toxicity of monoclonal antibodies in the treatment of cancer. Seminars in Oncology Nursing *2*(4):107–111, 1988.

Haeuber, D.: Recent advances in the management of biotherapy-related side effects: Flu-like syndrome. Oncology Nursing Forum *16*(6):35–41, 1989.

Haeuber, D., and DiJulio, J.E.: Hematopoietic colony stimulating factors: An overview. Oncology Nursing Forum *16*(2):247–255, 1989.

Hahn, M.B., and Jassak, P.F.: Nursing management of patients receiving interferon. Seminars in Oncology Nursing *4*(2):95–101, 1988.

Irwin, M.M.: Patients receiving biological response modifiers: Overview of nursing care. Oncology Nursing Forum *14*(6) Supplement:32–37, 1987.

Jassak, P.F., and Sticklin, L.A.: Interleukin-2: An overview. Oncology Nursing Forum *13*(6):17–22, 1987.

Moldawer, N.P., and Figlin, R.A.: Tumor necrosis factor: Current clinical status and implications for nursing management. Seminars in Oncology Nursing *4*(2):120–125, 1988.

PATIENT EDUCATION MATERIALS AND COMMUNITY RESOURCES

At home with Roferon[R]-A therapy. (Videotape). Nutley, NJ, Roche Laboratories, 1989.

Intron[R]A: Five steps to subcutaneous self-injection. (Videotape). Kenilworth, NJ, Schering, 1986.

Managing interleukin-2 therapy. (N.I.H. Publication No. 89-3071). Bethesda, MD, National Institutes of Health, 1989.

Schindler, L.W.: Understanding the immune system. (N.I.H. Publication No. 88-529. Bethesda, MD, National Institutes of Health, 1988.

Tips on Teaching Self-Administration Techniques to the Cancer Patient. (Pamphlet). Nutley, NJ, Roche Laboratories, 1987.

Knowledge Deficit Related to Surgery

Christine Miaskowski

Population at Risk

- Individuals with an actual or potential diagnosis of cancer who will undergo surgery as a diagnostic procedure, as a therapeutic intervention, or as a palliative procedure

Preoperative

EXPECTED OUTCOME

1. Patient demonstrates knowledge of preoperative routines:
   - states routine preoperative procedures.
   - relates information related to scheduling.
   - describes the surgical environment (holding area, OR, post-anesthesia care unit).
   - identifies rationale for and type of anesthesia.
2. Patient demonstrates knowledge of the planned surgical procedure:
   - states name or description of planned surgical procedure.
   - states reason for the surgical procedure and the expected outcome.
   - uses common surgical terminology appropriately.
   - states expectations of intraoperative care.
   - identifies immediate preoperative and postoperative care routines.
   - identifies expectations regarding immediate postoperative condition and care.
3. Patient provides an acceptable return demonstration of the following procedures:
   - coughing and deep breathing exercises.
   - use of an incentive spirometer
   - leg exercises.

NURSING MANAGEMENT

Assessment

1. Assess prior experience with surgery.
2. Determine present knowledge base and major concerns regarding surgery.
3. Note prior experience with anesthesia, including knowledge and fears.
4. Ascertain familiarity with common surgical terminology.
5. Assess readiness to learn.

6. Assess barriers to learning.
7. Assess patient's knowledge of potential sequelae of surgery:
   - changes in body functions.
   - limitations in mobility.
   - loss of body organs.
   - changes in appearance.

Patient Teaching

1. Review purpose of the surgical procedure:
   - diagnostic/evaluative (sometimes done to stage the cancer or to evaluate the effects of adjuvant treatment [e.g., chemotherapy, radiation therapy, or biotherapy]).
   - curative (usually done in cancers that are localized to a primary region and have not spread beyond regional lymph nodes).
   - debulking (done to decrease tumor size).
   - palliative (used to treat cancer that has spread beyond the primary site). The goals are to promote comfort, relieve clinical symptoms, and prevent further deterioration.
2. Describe the type of surgical procedure:
   - incisional biopsy (used to determine the presence of tumor and may indicate a need for further surgery).
   - local excision of tumor (removal of a localized lesion).
   - excision with wide margin (sometimes done in order to excise any tumors that have spread beyond the primary site).
   - block dissection (includes the tumor itself, all of the surrounding tissue, and the primary nodes surrounding the tumor).
   - radical surgery (removal of the tumor, surrounding tissue, regional lymph nodes, as well as muscle and sometimes major organs. This type of surgery often involves physical disfigurement and psychologic sequelae).

- resection of metastases (done after treatment of a primary tumor. If a solitary metastasis appears with no clinical evidence of other metastases, a resection of the lesion may be performed).
- cytoreductive surgery (done on inoperable cancer in conjunction with chemotherapy, radiation therapy, or biotherapy, usually to devascularize the tumor).
3. Describe special surgical techniques that attempt to conserve normal tissue:
   - electrosurgery—performed by needle, blade, or disk electrode using the cutting and coagulating effects of high current (e.g., used in some skin, oral, and rectal malignancies).
   - cryosurgery—performed by a probe containing liquid nitrogen that is inserted into the tumor (e.g., used in some cancers of the oral cavity, brain, prostate, and chronic cervicitis).
   - chemosurgery—performed by applying escharotic paste to the tumor; requires multiple frozen sections to determine surgical margins.
   - laser surgery—performed by laser therapy to resect delicate areas.
4. Explain common terms and procedures regarding pathology specimen.
5. Discuss potential sequelae of surgery:
   - changes in bodily appearance.
   - changes in bodily functions.
   - limitations in mobility.
   - loss of body organs.
6. Explain that various nursing and medical personnel will be visiting and the purpose of these visits.
7. Inform the patient that a consent must be signed for the procedure.
8. Inform the patient of place on the OR schedule and approximate time patient will spend in the holding area, OR, and post-anesthesia care unit.
9. Describe preoperative surgical preparations and procedures and their purposes:
   - area to be operated on may be shaved.
   - enema may be given.

- nothing should be eaten or drunk after midnight to prevent reflux and possible aspiration of abdominal contents.
- nail polish and makeup are removed to facilitate assessment of oxygenation and circulatory status via nail beds and mucous membranes.
- hair pins, glasses, contact lenses, dentures are removed to prevent trauma to the patient.
- prostheses and jewelry are removed to prevent loss.
- immediately prior to transfer to the holding area, the following will be done:
  - voiding (to maintain comfort and prevent postoperative retention).
  - hospital gown will be worn (to prevent loss or damage to patient's clothing).
  - thromboembolic stockings (if ordered) will be put on (to promote venous return and prevent thrombus formation).
  - preoperative medications will be given. (A narcotic is ordered to promote comfort, and an agent is given to decrease secretions, thereby lessening respiratory difficulties. Emphasize that the patient will become drowsy and probably experience a dry mouth).

9. Describe the procedures and routine completed in the holding area:
   - there will be a waiting period prior to being taken into the OR.
   - the patient's chart is checked to ensure that all necessary information is present.
   - an IV line may be started to maintain and provide easy access for medications.
10. Describe the atmosphere of the operating room.
11. Review what anesthesiologist/surgeon have told the patient regarding anesthesia and describe the specific anesthetic technique to be employed.

12. Describe the immediate postoperative routine and the environment of the post-anesthesia care unit:
    - length of time in the post-anesthesia care unit is variable. Minimum time is approximately 1 hour. The time is usually half the operating room time or until the patient's condition is stable.
    - patient will awaken with some type of oxygen device (usually a face mask). This is a routine procedure for patients who receive general anesthesia.
    - patient may be on a cardiac monitor.
    - post-anesthesia care unit nurse will check vital signs, dressings, breath sounds, temperature, drainage at least every 15 minutes. Explain that this is a routine procedure.
    - explain that there may be a great deal of noise in the post-anesthesia care unit.
    - explain to the patient that pain medication is readily available.
    - explain that the patient may experience unusual sensations while recovering from anesthesia.
13. Explain routine postoperative care when the patient is returned to the nursing unit:
    - vital signs, temperature, dressings, tubes will be checked frequently.
    - pain medication is available, and there is a true physical need for such medication, usually every 3 to 6 hours for 24 to 48 hours postoperatively. Patients should be told to ask for pain medication *before* pain becomes severe. If patient controlled analgesia (PCA) is to be used postoperatively, patient should be taught the rationale for this type of administration and how to use the device.
14. Demonstrate deep breathing and coughing exercises and obtain a return demonstration. Explain that breathing exercises will begin in the post-anesthesia care unit and should be done every 4 hours for 24 to 48 hours. If ordered, explain the im-

portance of an incentive spirometer to prevent postoperative complications, demonstrate its use, and obtain a return demonstration.
15. Explain that the patient will be helped to turn from side to side every 2 hours for 24 hours to prevent pulmonary and circulatory complications:
    • explain the importance of leg exercises/thromboembolic stockings (if ordered) to prevent circulatory complications, demonstrate leg exercises, and obtain a return demonstration when appropriate.
16. Explain that the patient will be helped out of bed as soon as possible after surgery to

prevent pulmonary and circulatory problems.
17. Describe the specific devices that may be employed after the surgical procedure (e.g., Foley catheter, chest tubes, nasogastric tubes, drains, dressings, and so on).
18. Explain to the patient that the family will be kept informed about the patient's progress.
19. Explain the importance of the patient's participation in the postoperative recovery period.
20. Utilize other resource persons (e.g., physical therapist, respiratory therapist, social worker, chaplain).

Postoperative

EXPECTED OUTCOME

Patient demonstrates knowledge of postoperative course:
• identifies surgical findings.
• demonstrates ability to perform self-care activities.
• states plans for long-term follow-up.
• identifies appropriate community resources.
• describes/demonstrates discharge plans and care.
• identifies emergency procedures and persons to contact.

NURSING MANAGEMENT

Assessment

1. Assess patient's response to outcome of surgery.
2. Assess knowledge of postoperative routines.
3. Evaluate knowledge and understanding of results of surgery including pathology report.
4. Determine knowledge of planned post-surgical resources.

Patient Teaching

1. Review results of surgery and reinforce physician's teaching and explanations.
2. Reinforce teaching regarding postoperative care and routines.
3. Explain plans for follow-up treatment as indicated.
4. Teach emergency procedures and appropriate persons to contact after discharge.

Knowledge Deficit Related to Surgery

5. Describe/demonstrate techniques for self-care after discharge from the hospital.
6. Initiate appropriate referrals for home care and instruct patient on available community resources.

SUGGESTED READINGS

Brunner, L.S., and Suddarth, D.S.: The Lippincott Manual of Nursing Practice, 4th ed. Philadelphia, J.B. Lippincott, 1986.

Goulart, A.E.: Preoperative teaching for surgical patients. Perioperative Nursing Quarterly *3*:8–12, 1987.

Johnson, S.: Preoperative teaching: A need for change. Nursing Management *10*:80B, 80F, 80H, 1989.

Kozier, B., and Erb, G.: Techniques in Clinical Nursing: A Comprehensive Approach. Menlo Park, CA, Addison-Wesley, 1982.

Lewis, S.M., and Collier, I.C.: Medical-Surgical Nursing Assessment and Management of Clinical Problems, 2nd ed. New York, McGraw-Hill, 1987, pp. 259–309.

Lindeman, C.A.: Patient education. Annual Review of Nursing Research *6*:29–60, 1988.

Smith, S., and Duell, D.: Clinical Nursing Skills: Nursing Process Model—Basic to Advanced Skills. Los Altos, CA, National Nursing Review, Inc., 1988.

Knowledge Deficit Related to Bone Marrow Transplant

Eileen T. Somerville

16

Population at Risk

- Adults with a malignant disease potentially responsive to bone marrow transplantation
- Adults with aplastic anemia

EXPECTED OUTCOME

1. Patient demonstrates knowledge related to diagnosis and disease process:
   - states diagnosis and explains disease process.
   - relates previous treatment for disease.
2. Patient demonstrates knowledge related to bone marrow and its function; dysfunctional bone marrow and outcome:
   - describes location of bone marrow.
   - states that bone marrow is responsible for blood cell production.
   - states importance of sufficient healthy red cell, white cell, platelet production and function.
   - verbalizes outcome of dysfunctional bone marrow.
3. Patient demonstrates knowledge related to bone marrow transplant:
   - discusses knowledge or experience related to bone marrow transplants.
   - identifies type of bone marrow transplant being considered.
   - discusses rationale for bone marrow transplant as potential treatment modality.
   - acknowledges potential therapeutic and adverse effects of bone marrow transplant.
   - identifies varied outcome possibilities of bone marrow transplant.
   - discusses alternatives to treatment with bone marrow transplant.
   - acknowledges financial commitment and ability to meet that commitment.
4. Patient demonstrates knowledge related to treatment plan:
   - acknowledges need for hospitalization for protracted period of time.
   - identifies pretransplant conditioning regimen.
   - states time involved from admission to transplant.
   - identifies time from transplant to bone marrow recovery.
   - describes medical and nursing interventions available and required during treatment program.

Note: This guideline does not address pediatric bone marrow transplants.

- acknowledges need for placement of venous access device.
- acknowledges need for blood product replacement infusions.
- discusses post-transplant follow-up studies, procedures, and time commitment.
- identifies resources available.
- identifies constraints to commitment to treatment program.
- identifies needs requiring assistance and willingness to explore availability of assistance.
- states desire and commitment to comply with treatment program.

5. Donor (self or other) demonstrates knowledge related to bone marrow harvest:
   - discusses potential self-donation of blood for replacement during bone marrow harvest.
   - describes anesthesia, operating room, and post-recovery unit and procedures.
   - describes multiple bone marrow aspiration procedure.
   - states postdischarge plan.
   - relates situations to report to health care personnel.
   - states procedure to contact health care personnel if needed.
   - identifies time between bone marrow harvest and bone marrow transplantation.

6. Patient and family demonstrates knowledge related to allogeneic bone marrow transplantation:
   - identifies immediate family members, relationship, and availability as donors.
   - verbalizes willingness to participate in testing.
   - verbalizes commitment to participate as bone marrow donors/blood product donors in supportive role.
   - states willingness to participate in treatment program.
   - verbalizes long-term availability and commitment.
   - states willingness to identify resources needed and to use resources available.
   - discusses potential complications of treatment.
   - acknowledges possible inability of treatment to cure patient.

NURSING MANAGEMENT

Assessment

1. Assess educational level, ability and desire to learn, barriers to learning, learning style.
2. Assess anxiety level, retention/memory ability, comprehension.
3. Evaluate knowledge level relative to disease and treatment.
4. Assess knowledge level relative to anatomy and physiology of specific disease.
5. Assess knowledge level relative to:
   - bone marrow and its function.
   - bone marrow transplantation as a treatment modality.
6. Explore previous experience with or knowledge of bone marrow transplantation.
7. Ascertain attitude and expectations related to outcome of treatment with bone marrow transplantation.
8. Evaluate knowledge of:
   - potential therapeutic effect of bone marrow transplantation.

- potential complications/adverse effects of bone marrow transplantation, both immediate and long-term.
9. Assess understanding of alternative treatment modalities for specific disease.
10. Assess extent of knowledge of pretreatment work-up, preparation for transplant, and long-term follow-up.
11. Determine psychosocial and emotional ability to comply with long-term treatment plan; utilize resource persons to contribute to evaluation.
12. Determine family structure, relationships, support, availability, commitment to involvement in treatment plan.
13. Determine family understanding of involvement in treatment program: as potential bone marrow donors if appropriate; as potential donors of blood products.
14. Evaluate degree of family disruption caused by commitment to treatment program, resources available and those needed; utilize resource persons to contribute to evaluation and availability of assistance.
15. Assess relevant medical/surgical history; previous medical treatment.
16. Assess history of allergies, adverse reactions to medications/transfusion therapy.
17. Assess financial resources.

Patient Teaching

1. Develop a teaching plan appropriate for the patient/family level of understanding and learning style.
2. Review information patient/family have been given; clarify, reinforce; allow for questions and discussion.
3. Explain investigational nature of bone marrow transplantation if appropriate.
4. Discuss informed consent and need for signed consent.
5. Explain that bone marrow transplantation is the replacement of damaged, insufficient, incompetent, or diseased bone

marrow with normal, healthy bone marrow cells.
6. Explain the anatomic location and distribution of bone marrow.
7. Explain bone marrow function
   - review red cell, white cell, and platelet production and function.
8. Discuss the results of inadequate or abnormal bone marrow function.
9. Explain that there are two primary types of bone marrow transplants
   - autologous bone marrow transplants—from self—using individual's own bone marrow cells for transplantation.
   - allogeneic bone marrow transplants—from a donor—using bone marrow cells from another individual for transplantation. If the other individual (donor) is an identical twin, the term syngeneic transplant is used.
10. Discuss the difference between:
   - replacing abnormal or inadequate bone marrow with normal, healthy bone marrow cells from another individual.
   - the use of an individual's own bone marrow cells as a replacement (rescue) following the bone marrow depleting effects of treatment with chemotherapy/radiation therapy.
11. Explain that an allogeneic bone marrow transplant requires the donor and the recipient (the patient) to be genetically matched; they must have the same human leukocyte antigens (HLA match):
   - usually limits the donor to a brother or a sister.
   - in rare instances an unrelated HLA-matched donor may be found.
   - donor and patient should be under 45 years of age or as specified in protocol.
   - risks increase with unmatched donors.
   - increased risks of complications over age 40.
12. Identify the type of bone marrow transplant being considered and the rationale for the treatment choice.

13. Provide full explanation of:
    - bone marrow harvest
    - transplantation procedure and process
    - pretransplant regimen.
    - potential therapeutic outcome.
    - potential adverse complications/side effects, both immediate and long-term.

(See Patient Teaching: Bone Marrow Harvest; Autologous Transplant; Allogeneic Transplant; Autologous Peripheral Stem Cell Harvest and Transplant.

Patient Teaching

Bone Marrow Harvest—Self or Other Donor

1. Provide written and verbal instructions relative to bone marrow harvest.
2. Explain process and procedure for bone marrow harvest:
    - a preharvest bone marrow aspiration will be done using local anesthesia to ensure that the donor marrow is healthy, normal, appropriate for transplantation
    - greatest and most accessible source of bone marrow is the hip bones, posterior and anterior iliac crest.
    - bone marrow to be harvested is in the center of these bones.
    - bone marrow harvested is liquid and full of healthy young cells that can reproduce themselves when transplanted.
    - approximately one quart of liquid marrow is required to obtain sufficient cells for transplantation.
    - bone marrow is obtained by inserting a special needle into the center of the hip bones and aspirating the liquid marrow into syringes.
    - to obtain sufficient numbers of bone marrow cells, multiple needle insertions and aspirations are required.
    - the procedure must be done using sterile technique.
    - the bone marrow harvest is done in the operating room.
    - to prevent pain and discomfort the

donor is put to sleep using general anesthesia.
- the procedure usually takes 1½ to 2 hours.
- the donor must have a preoperative work-up that generally includes: interview with the anesthetist, history and physical, chest x-ray, ECG, urinalysis, blood counts and chemistries.
- preoperative instructions will be provided.
- the risk to the donor is limited to the risk of anesthesia since bone marrow can replenish itself within 2 to 3 weeks.
- replacement blood transfusion(s) may be given to the donor during the procedure.
- the bone marrow donor may give a unit of blood prior to the procedure to be used as the replacement transfusion during the harvest.
- the donor may be admitted to the hospital or to a one-day surgery unit.
- at the completion of the procedure the donor will be transferred from the operating room to a recovery room until fully recovered from the effects of anesthesia.
- the donor may be discharged the same day or kept in the hospital for observation.
- the bone marrow donor sites will be tender, sore, and stiff.
- pain medication will be provided and ambulation will be encouraged for relief of discomfort.
- the bone marrow harvest sites will be covered with a pressure dressing that must be left in place for 24 to 72 hours.
- tub or shower bathing is contraindicated until the pressure dressings are removed.
- specific instructions as to site care and follow-up may vary and will be provided per institutional policy.
- vitamins or iron supplements may be prescribed after bone marrow harvest.
- instructions will be provided regarding observations for signs and symptoms of

bleeding and infection and for increased or unrelieved discomfort.

- instructions for contacting the appropriate health care professionals if problems arise will be provided.

Patient Teaching

Autologous Bone Marrow Transplant

1. Explain that auto refers to self; autologous bone marrow transplantation utilizes the individual's own bone marrow cells.
2. Explain that cancer chemotherapy is dose-limited by bone marrow toxicity; that autologous bone marrow transplantation allows for treatment with higher doses of chemotherapy, alone or in conjunction with radiation therapy.
3. Explain that bone marrow may be:
   - harvested in conjunction with an immediate treatment plan.
   - harvested and stored for future use if needed.
   - harvested and purged to remove abnormal or malignant cells for immediate or future use.
4. Explain that autologous bone marrow transplantation may be considered:
   - when a malignant disease is unresponsive to conventional therapy.
   - for treatment of resistant or residual disease following conventional therapy.
   - for treatment of relapsed disease following initial successful treatment.
   - when prognosis for long-term disease-free state is limited with conventional therapy.
   - when high-dose chemotherapy/radiation therapy provide a greater potential for cure than conventional therapy.
5. Explain that:
   - bone marrow may be harvested and stored prior to treatment if the disease does not involve the bone marrow.

- if the disease involves the bone marrow, the bone marrow is harvested following treatment when the disease is in clinical remission.
6. Explain that the overall treatment protocol requires approximately 3 to 4 weeks of hospitalization and long-term follow-up.
7. Discuss the pretransplant conditioning regimen: chemotherapy drugs to be used, schedule and timing; radiation therapy if appropriate.
8. Discuss the bone marrow transplant procedure:
   - following treatment with chemotherapy alone or with radiation therapy, the stored bone marrow is thawed and returned to the patient.
   - thawed bone marrow cells are given back to the patient as an intravenous infusion, much like a blood transfusion.
   - cells circulate and return to the bone marrow, reproduce, and repopulate the damaged bone marrow with red cells, white cells, and platelets.
   - the patient will be monitored throughout the transfusion for potential adverse effects such as:
     ○ nausea, vomiting, chest pain, dyspnea, allergic reactions.
     ○ patient will be premedicated to avoid these adverse effects.
     ○ patient can expect an unpleasant taste and odor from the dimethyl sulfoxide that the cells have been stored in.
     ○ Pink to red tinge to urine is not unusual following infusion of cells.
     ○ time between transplant and sufficient circulating blood cells is approximately 3 weeks.
9. Discuss the side effects the patient will experience as a result of the pretransplant conditioning regimen; chemotherapy/radiation therapy that may include:
   - nausea, vomiting, anorexia, diarrhea, stomatitis, esophagitis, gastritis.
   - fluid imbalance.

- hair loss.
- potential pulmonary, cardiac, renal, liver, or CNS effects.
- bone marrow depletion.

10. Provide information regarding medical and nursing interventions available for adverse side effects.

11. Discuss the potential need for nutritional support, either intravenously or with dietary supplements.

12. Discuss the need for a venous access device (VAD) and the placement procedure.

13. Explain that bone marrow depletion causes:
    - decreased white blood cells, increased risk of infection that may require treatment with antibiotics.
    - decreased red blood cells, increased risk of anemia that may require replacement red cell transfusions.
    - decreased platelet cells, increased risk of bleeding that may require replacement platelet transfusions.

14. Explain that the increased risk of infection may require some protective precautions. Depending on institutional protocol these may or may not include:
    - private room, protective environment, sterile environment, laminar air flow environment.
    - visitor restrictions.
    - diet restrictions (sterile food, low-bacterial diet, or cooked foods only).
    - no live plants or flowers in room.
    - use of gowns, gloves, masks, by health care personnel.
    - various oral, personal and environmental regimens.

15. Discuss:
    - need for post-transplant procedures to evaluate effect of treatment.
    - postdischarge follow-up per institutional protocol.
    - procedure for contacting medical or nursing personnel following discharge.

16. Provide written and verbal instructions for postdischarge requirements and regimen.

Patient Teaching

Allogeneic Bone Marrow Transplant

1. Explain that allogeneic bone marrow transplants usually require a genetically matched donor, most often a sibling:
   - unrelated genetically matched donors may be found, but the occurrence is rare.
   - mismatched donors may be used in specific instances.

2. Explain that:
   - preparation for an allogeneic transplant requires a pretransplant evaluation of both patient and donor.
   - if available, all siblings will be tested as potential bone marrow donors/blood product donors.
   - allogeneic transplant requires a long-term commitment for both donor and recipient.
   - to determine a matched donor two blood tests are done using blood taken intravenously from both the potential donor and the patient:
     - the first blood test determines if the patient and donor have the same cell surface antigens, human leukocyte antigens (HLA) match.
     - once an HLA match is established a second blood test is done, a mixed lymphocyte culture assay (MLC) to determine if the donor and patient cells are compatible.
   - if a match is established a bone marrow aspiration is done on the donor to assure the donor that bone marrow is suitable for transplantation.

3. Discuss potential outcomes of allogeneic bone marrow transplant, therapeutic and adverse:
   - total engraftment, ablated bone marrow replaced with new healthy bone marrow.
   - no engraftment of new marrow, rejection by patient that may require a second transplant; may be lethal.

- possible recurrent disease following bone marrow transplant.
- graft-versus-host disease (GVHD); acute/chronic: Donor marrow reacts against the patient's tissues and organs; may require intensive therapy, long-term therapy; may cause long-term disabilities; and may be lethal. (See Potential for Injury Related to Graft-Versus-Host Disease, Chapter 35).

4. Discuss the bone marrow harvest procedure with potential bone marrow donor. (See Patient Teaching, Bone Marrow Harvest):
   - discuss with donor the need of post-transplant availability.

5. Provide patient with outline of overall treatment plan:
   - may require 6 to 8 weeks of hospitalization if no complications are encountered.
   - pretransplant conditioning regimen may take 10 days to 2 weeks.
   - bone marrow harvest from the donor and transplant to the patient are done on the same day.
   - time from transplant to engraftment may be 3 to 4 weeks.
   - post-transplant follow-up will be intensive and long-term usually requiring 90 to 100 days in transplant center area.
   - complete immunologic recovery will take approximately 1 year.
   - continuous monitoring will be required during the first year and intermittently therafter.

6. Discuss pretransplant conditioning regimen with patient as appropriate:
   - chemotherapy drugs to be used, schedule and route of administration.
   - total body irradiation (TBI) schedule and procedure.
   - limited site-specific irradiation.

7. Discuss the side effects of the pretransplant regimen, both immediate and long-term, which may include:
   - nausea, vomiting, anorexia, diarrhea, stomatitis, esophagitis, gastritis.
   - fluid imbalance.
   - hair loss.
   - potential pulmonary, cardiac, renal, liver, or CNS effects.
   - bone marrow ablation.
   - dry mouth and parotitis may result from TBI.
   - long-term complications may include infertility, cataracts, chronic pulmonary disease, secondary malignancies, GVHD.

8. Provide information regarding medical and nursing interventions available for adverse side effects.

9. Describe bone marrow transplant procedure:
   - the bone marrow harvested from the donor in the OR is processed and brought immediately to the patient's room.
   - the donor's marrow cells are given to the patient as an intravenous infusion, much like a blood transfusion.
   - the patient will be given premedications to prevent adverse reactions to the transplanted cells.
   - the patient will be monitored throughout the transfusion for potential adverse effects (e.g., nausea, vomiting, chest pain, dyspnea, allergic reactions).
   - red to pink urine is not unusual following infusion of bone marrow.

10. Explain that bone marrow depletion causes:
    - decreased white blood cells, increased risk of infection that may require treatment with antibiotics.
    - decreased red blood cells, increased risk of anemia that may require replacement red cell transfusions.
    - decreased platelets, increased risk of bleeding that may require replacement platelet transfusions.

11. Explain that the increased risk of infection may require some protective precau-

tions; depending on institutional protocol these may or may not include:
- private room/protective environment/ sterile environment, laminar air flow environment.
- visitor restrictions.
- diet restrictions (sterile diet, low-bacterial diet, or cooked food only).
- no live plants or flowers in room.
- use of gowns, gloves, masks by health care personnel.
- various oral, personal, and environmental regimens.

12. Discuss the potential need for nutritional support, either intravenously or with dietary supplements.
13. Provide information regarding
    - post-transplant procedures and the need for these procedures to evaluate effect of treatment
    - postdischarge follow-up per institutional protocol.
    - procedure for contacting medical or nursing personnel following discharge from the hospital.
14. Provide written and verbal instructions for postdischarge requirement and regimen.

Patient Teaching

Autologous Peripheral Blood Stem Cell Harvest and Transplant

1. Discuss with patient that in selected instances peripheral stem cell harvest may be used:
   - in addition to bone marrow harvest if the number of cells from the bone marrow is insufficient for bone marrow recovery.
   - as an alternative to bone marrow harvest if:
     - the bone marrow is hypocellular.
       - the bone marrow harvest sites have been previously irradiated.
       - the bone marrow is known to contain tumor cells.

2. Instruct patient that peripheral stem cells are collected from the circulating blood via apheresis. Peripheral stem cell harvest:
   - is generally done as an out-patient procedure.
   - is not an operating room procedure and does not require general anesthesia.
   - requires insertion of a venous access catheter.
   - involves attaching the venous access catheter to an apheresis machine that removes venous blood, separates and collects stem cells, returns all remaining blood to the patient.

3. Explain that peripheral circulating stem cells are the same as bone marrow stem cells:
   - number of peripheral stem cells in the circulating blood is less than in the bone marrow.
   - to harvest enough peripheral stem cells for transplantation requires numerous apheresis procedures.
   - the number of apheresis procedures depends on the number of peripheral stem cells collected from each procedure.
   - peripheral stem cell harvest may require 1 to 2 weeks of daily or every other day apheresis to obtain sufficient numbers of cells for transplantation.
   - peripheral stem cells are frozen and stored after each apheresis, the same process as harvested bone marrow cells.

4. Explain that peripheral stem cells are thawed and administered intravenously similar to bone marrow harvested cells.
5. Discuss the pretransplant conditioning regimen, side effects, and outcome, which are the same as for autologous bone marrow transplantation.
6. Discuss the pre- and post-transplant procedures, evaluation and follow-up that are the same for autologous bone marrow

transplantation (See Patient Teaching, Autologous Bone Marrow Transplant).

SUGGESTED READINGS

Bell, A.J., Hamblin, T.J., and Oscier, D.G.: Peripheral blood stem cell autografting. Hematological Oncology 5:45–52, 1987.

Coglians-Shutta, N.A., Broda, E.J., and Gress, J.S.: Bone marrow transplantation: An overview and comparison of autologous, syngeneic and allogeneic treatment modalities. Nursing Clinics of North America 20(1):49–66, 1985.

Collins, C., Upright, C., and Aleksick, J.: Reverse isolation: What patients perceive. Oncology Nursing Forum 16: 675–679, 1989.

Corcoran-Buchsel, P.: Long-term complications of allogeneic bone marrow transplantation: Nursing implications. Oncology Nursing Forum 13: 61–69, 1986.

Corcoran-Buchsel, P., and Porchem, C.: Ambulatory care of the bone marrow transplant patient. Seminars in Oncology Nursing 4(1):41–46, 1988.

Dicke, K.A., Jagannath, S., Spitzer, G., et al.: The role of autologous bone marrow transplantation in various malignancies. Seminars in Hematology 29:109–119, 1984.

Ford, R., and Ballard, B.: Acute complications after bone marrow transplantation. Seminars in Oncology Nursing 4(1):15–24, 1988.

Freedman, S.: An overview of bone marrow transplantation. Seminars in Oncology Nursing 4:3–8, 1988.

Groenwald, S., Hanson, M., Varbro, C.H., and Stuart, M.: Cancer Nursing: Principles and Practice. Boston, Jones & Bartlett, 1990.

Haberman, M.R.: Psychosocial aspects of bone marrow transplantation. Seminars in Oncology Nursing 4(1):55–59, 1988.

Holland, J., Plumb, M., Yates, J., et al.: Psychological response of patients with acute leukemia to germ-free environments. Cancer 40:871–879, 1977.

Jett, M.F., and Lancaster, L.E.: The inflammatory immune response: The body's defense against invasion. Critical Care Nurse 3:64–86, 1983.

Kellerman, J., Rigler, D., and Siegel, S.E.: Psychological effects of isolation in protected environments. American Journal of Psychiatry 134:563–565, 1977.

Kessinger, A.: Autologous transplantation with peripheral blood stem cells: A review of clinical results. Journal of Clinical Apheresis 5:97–99, 1990.

Kessinger, A., Armitage, J.O., Smith, D.M., et al.: High-dose therapy and autologous peripheral blood stem cell transplantation for patients with lymphoma. Blood 74:1260–1265, 1989.

Mueller, S.K.: Bone marrow teaching and documentation tool. Oncology Nursing Forum 9:57–64, 1982.

Nims, J.W., and Strom, S.: Late complications of bone marrow transplant recipients: Nursing care issues. Seminars in Oncology Nursing 4(1):47–54, 1988.

O'Quin, T., and Moranic, C.: The critically ill bone marrow transplant patient. Seminars in Oncology Nursing 4(1):25–30, 1988.

Pizzo, P.A., Purvis, D.S., and Waters, C.: For patients undergoing gastrointestinal decontamination and protected isolation: Microbiological evaluation of food items. Journal of the American Dietetic Association 81:272–279, 1982.

Reheis, C.E.: Neutropenia: Causes, complication, treatment, and resulting nursing care. Nursing Clinics of North America 20(1):219–225, 1985.

Ruggiero, M.R.: The donor in bone marrow transplantation. Seminars in Oncology Nursing 4(1):9–14, 1988.

Schryber, S., La Casse, C.R., and Barton-Burke, M.: Autologous bone marrow transplantation. Oncology Nursing Forum 14:74–80, 1987.

Siena, S., Bregni, M., Brando, B., et al.: Circulation of CD34+ hematopoietic stem cells in the peripheral blood of high-dose cyclophosphamide treated patients: Enhancement by intravenous recombinant human granulocyte-macrophage colony-stimulating factor. Blood 74:1905–1914, 1989.

Somerville, E.T.: Special diets for neutropenic patients: Do they make a difference? Seminars in Oncology Nursing 4(1):55–58, 1988.

Stewart, F.M., Thomas, R.M., Somerville, E.T., and Stewart, K.J.: Bone marrow transplantation: Three treatments for disease. AORN Journal 42:196–205, 1985.

Sullivan, K.M., Deeg, G., Sanders, J.E., et al.: Late complications after marrow transplantation. Seminars in Hematology 21:53–63, 1984.

Zander, A.R., and Cockerill, K.J.: Autologous transplantation with circulating hemopoietic stem cells. Journal of Clinical Apheresis 3:191–201, 1987.

PATIENT EDUCATION MATERIALS AND COMMUNITY RESOURCES

Audio Tapes

Bone Marrow Transplantation: Basic Concepts. (#8, A & B). Oncology Nursing Society Congress, Washington, DC, 1990. Available from Oncology Nursing Society, 1016 Greentree Road, Pittsburgh, PA 15220.

New Strategies for Continuing Issues in Bone Marrow Transplantation. (#36, A & B). Oncology Nursing Society Congress, Washington, DC, 1990. Available from Oncology Nursing Society, 1016 Greentree Road, Pittsburgh, PA 15220.

Knowledge Deficit Related to Bone Marrow Transplant

Advanced Topics Related to Bone Marrow Transplantation: BMT in the 90s. (#47, A & B). Oncology Nursing Society Congress, Washington, DC, 1990. Available from Oncology Nursing Society, 1016 Greentree Road, Pittsburgh, PA, 15220.

Bone Marrow Transplantation: Questions and Answers. Leukemia Society of America. New York, NY, 1989.

Holcombe, A.: Bone marrow harvest. Oncology Nursing Forum *14*:63–65, 1987.

Knowledge Deficit Related to Contraception

Susan Gelbard

17

Population at Risk

- Cancer patients with functional reproductive capabilities who are undergoing chemotherapy or receiving radiation therapy to pelvic area

EXPECTED OUTCOME

Patient demonstrates knowledge related to contraception:
- states information relevant to disease process and treatment and contraception as it applies to individual situation.
- identifies available contraceptive methods.
- describes implementation of various methods.
- lists advantages and disadvantages of each method.

NURSING MANAGEMENT

Assessment

1. Assess patient and scheduled cancer treatment.
2. Note reproductive history and desire to have children.
3. Determine impact of disease and treatment on sexual functioning.
4. Ascertain current and previous use of contraceptives (effectiveness, patient satisfaction, wish to continue or initiate).
5. Gauge knowledge level of alternative contraceptive methods.

Patient Teaching

1. Discuss with patient and partner information relevant to disease process and treatment and contraceptives as it applies to their situation:

- teratogenic effects of treatment.
- Many patients receiving chemotherapy/radiation therapy will experience temporary or permanent sterility. Since occurrence of sterility resulting from disease or treatment is not always predictable as to duration, contraception should continue to be practiced (see Chapter 54).
- Patient's life expectancy, as well as effect of pregnancy upon course of disease (if female), should be considered when couple is choosing whether or not to use contraception. Some relevant factors are:
  - If patient dies, *can* partner care for child alone?
  - If patient dies, would partner *want* to care for child alone?
  - Does couple have other children?

95

○ Would pregnancy preclude treatment of disease? Would this be harmful?

○ Are there any genetic concerns such as familial cancers?

2. Provide patient and partner with information regarding methods of contraception, implementation, advantages, and disadvantages. Available pamphlets include *A Guide to the Methods of Contraception* from Ortho Pharmaceutical Corporation, Raritan, NJ 08869. Other information is as follows:

• Rhythm and coitus interruptus have high failure rates usually associated with noncompliance. If pregnancy is not desired, a more reliable method should be recommended.

• Chemical barriers have varying effectiveness; may be used in combination with rhythm, coitus interruptus, diaphragm, or condom to increase reliability. If patient has impaired mucous membrane, may be vaginal irritant.

• Diaphragm used with spermicidal substance is very effective—have fit checked if patient has lost weight.

• Condoms are moderately effective. If preventing vaginal irritation or if infection is of concern, advise patient and partner to purchase prelubricated condoms or to use generous amounts of water-soluble lubricant (e.g., Lubafax, Burroughs Wellcome).

• Vaginal contraceptive sponges may be unfamiliar to patients and partners but are very effective. Fit is not affected by weight loss.

• IUDs are best inserted prior to treatment to minimize risks related to bleeding and infection:

○ Tell patient to monitor for complications (bleeding, vaginal discharge, signs and symptoms of infection).

○ Progesterone-releasing IUDs may decrease bleeding risk.

• Oral contraceptives should not be used by patients with hormonal-dependent tumors. Side effects from oral contraceptives should not be confused with treatment side effects (and vice versa).

SUGGESTED READINGS

Accola, K.M., and Sommerfeld, D.P.: Helping people with cancer consider parenthood. American Journal of Nursing 79:1580–1583, 1979.

Blatt, J., Mulvihill, J.J., and Ziegler, J.L.: Pregnancy outcome following chemotherapy. American Journal of Medicine 69:828–832, 1980.

Hassey, K.M.: Pregnancy and parenthood after treatment for breast cancer. Oncology Nursing Forum 15:439–444, 1988.

Itri, L.M.: The effects of chemotherapy on gonadal function. Your Patient and Cancer 3:45–49, 1983.

Jochinson, P.R., Spaight, M.E., and Urdaneta, L.F.: Pregnancy during adjuvant chemotherapy for breast cancer. Journal of the American Medical Association 245:1660–1661, 1981.

Kaempfer, S.H.: The effects of cancer chemotherapy on reproduction: A review of the literature. Oncology Nursing Forum 8:11–18, 1981.

Kaempfer, S.H., Wiley, F.M., Hoffman, D., and Rhodes, E.A.: Fertility considerations and procreative alternatives in cancer care. Seminars in Oncology Nursing 1:25–34, 1985.

Krebs, L.U.: Pregnancy and cancer. Seminars in Oncology Nursing 1:35–41, 1985.

MacElveen-Hoehn, P.: Sexual assessment and counseling. Seminars in Oncology Nursing 1:69–75, 1985.

Mulvihill, J.J., and Byrne, J.: Genetic counseling of the cancer survivor. Seminars in Oncology Nursing 5:29–35, 1989.

Peters, R.M.: Overview of contraception. Oncology Nursing Forum 8:38–39, 1981.

Schilsky, R.L., Lewis, B.J., and Sherins, R.J.: Gonadal dysfunction in patients receiving chemotherapy for cancer. Annals of Internal Medicine 93:109–114, 1980.

Smith, D.B.: Sexual rehabilitation of the cancer patient. Cancer Nursing 12:10–15, 1989.

Tarpy, C.C.: Birth control considerations during chemotherapy. Oncology Nursing Forum 12:75–78, 1985.

Whitehead, E., Shalate, S.N., and Blackledge, D.: The effects of Hodgkin's disease and combination chemotherapy on gonadal function in the adult male. Cancer 49:418–422, 1982.

PATIENT EDUCATION MATERIALS AND COMMUNITY RESOURCES

A Guide to the Methods of Contraception. Ortho Pharmaceutical Corporation, Raritan, NJ 08869.

Knowledge Deficit Related to Unproven Methods of Cancer Treatment

18

Karen Wojtalewicz-Friedberg, Barbara A. Flynn, Mary Beth Riley, Catherine M. Kelley, and Ellen L. Roth

Population at Risk

- Any patient/family with a diagnosis of cancer

EXPECTED OUTCOME

1. Patient verbalizes an understanding of conventional therapy:
   - describes goals of treatment.
   - verbalizes both conventional and investigational therapy options available.
   - identifies possible side effects of therapy.
2. Patient verbalizes concerns related to conventional treatment:
   - acknowledges insufficient knowledge.
   - expresses misconceptions of treatment modalities.
   - expresses fear of side effects.
3. Patient identifies resources available during conventional therapy.
4. Patient identifies motivating factors for choosing unproven treatment methods.
5. Patient demonstrates knowledge of unproven treatment methods:
   - identifies types of unproven treatment methods.
   - states the characteristics of a "quack promoter."
   - develops means to evaluate health promoters.
   - explores ways to utilize available resources/exercise options.
6. Patient verbalizes known risks and adverse reactions related to unproven treatment methods under consideration.
7. Patient recognizes the ability to continue involvement with the conventional health care system while receiving unproven methods.
   - continued contact with physician and nurse.
   - compliance with follow-up appointments.
8. Patient exhibits resolution of conflict regarding reentry into the health care system after treatment with unproven methods:
   - utilizes effective coping patterns.
   - complies with conventional therapy.
   - participates in health care system.
   - identifies reasons for pursuing unproven method of treatment.

97

Knowledge Deficit Related to Unproven Methods of Cancer Treatment

- verbalizes feelings regarding use of unproven treatment methods.
- develops and maintains nonjudgmental attitudes about treatment.

NURSING MANAGEMENT

Assessment

1. Identify population at risk:
   - those in whom conventional treatment has failed.
   - those who have not attained or maintained effective communication with the health care team.
   - those who react with fear or anger to their illness.
2. Assess:
   - patient's readiness to learn.
   - patient's previous experience/familiarity with cancer.
   - patient's level of understanding of current or planned conventional therapy.
   - patient's past and present psychologic patterns of coping with stress.
   - patient's reasons for noncompliance with conventional therapy.
   - needs of patient/family for resources (financial, dietary, psychologic).
3. Explore attitudes, experiences, feelings about conventional and unconventional treatment with patient/family.

Nursing Interventions

1. Establish therapeutic relationship with patient/family.
2. Facilitate communication between patient/family and members of health care team.
3. Maintain nonjudgmental environment.
4. Promote effective coping patterns.
5. Provide ongoing support for patient/family while decisions regarding treatment are being made, during any subsequent therapies, and while decisions to enter or learn about conventional treatment are being made:
   - provide opportunities for individual counseling as needed.

- encourage patient/family to utilize the various supportive resources available, arranging contact with the appropriate persons or organizations if requested.
- provide information to patient/family to facilitate follow-up care (phone numbers of physicians, nurse, or other health care professionals).

Patient Teaching

1. Discuss conventional therapy as it relates to:
   - treatment program (goals, logistics).
   - management of possible side effects.
   - means of evaluating effectiveness of therapy.
   - community resources.
2. Define unproven treatment methods as those that do not have scientific proof of efficacy, that conflict with conventional therapy, or that have risk for injury.
3. Identify possible types of unproven treatment methods:
   - drugs and chemical preparations (e.g., Hoxey treatment, Krebiozen, laetrile, topical applications).
   - nutritional approaches (laetrile, megadose vitamins, macrobiotic diets, coffee ground enemas, herbal diets).
   - occult psychic techniques.
4. Identify the characteristics of a quack promoter as one who:
   - promotes unusual theories.
   - has unreliable records.
   - has questionable credentials.
   - fights against the "medical monopoly."
   - exists in isolation from other health care professionals.
   - maintains secrecy of method.
   - exhibits "cult" status.
   - refuses to collaborate with health care professionals.

5. Discuss with patient possible questions to ask about product/promoters of unconventional methods:
   - does the promoter promise quick-and-easy cures?
   - is the product being paid for by a self-styled health adviser, crusader, or faith healing group, or promoted in popular advertisements?
   - is the product advertised as being good for a wide variety of ailments?
   - is the product advertised to treat condition(s) for which medical science has not yet found successful therapy?
   - does the sponsor/promoter claim persecution by the medical community/government?
   - is the product available only from the promoter or by mail order with payment in advance?
   - does the promoter use many case histories or testimonies from grateful ex-patients?
6. Identify potential sequelae/complications of unproven treatment methods:
   - direct (depending on type of method chosen, may cause dehydration, physical injury, death).
   - indirect (possible delay/inconsistency with conventional therapy may decrease chance for cure/palliation, loss of revenue/savings, psychologic disequilibrium).
7. Identify steps patient/family should take if and when a complication related to unconventional therapy occurs (identify contact person, as applicable).
8. If patient/family makes inquiries related to reporting unproven methods of treatment, provide with following information:
   - if product was received via mail, complain to U.S. Postal Service, Federal Trade Commission, and State Attorney's Office. Send written complaints to the Better Business Bureau and State Consumer Protection Agency.
   - if the complaint involves vitamins, drugs, or foods, consult Food and Drug Administration.
   - identify the following as points to include when filing a complaint:
     - explanation of problem.
     - product information.
     - where and how purchased, administered, obtained.
     - support for due process of law.
   - identify use of the legislative process in regulating unproven treatment methods:
     - send letter to legislators.
     - support formation of state and federal programs to prevent exploitation of the public and set standards for scientific investigation of all treatments.
     - provide testimony at selected hearings if applicable.

SUGGESTED READINGS

Brown, H.: Cancer quackery: What can you do about it? Nursing 5:24–26, 1975.

Burkhalter, P.: Cancer quackery. American Journal of Nursing 77:451–453, 1977.

Cameron, C.: The cancer quacks. Washington DC, Government Printing Office, 1956 (revised 1968).

Cassileth, B.: After laetrile, what? New England Journal of Medicine 306:1482–1484, 1982.

Cassileth, B.: The social implications of questionable cancer therapies. Cancer 63:1247–1250, 1989.

Cassileth, B., and Brown, H.: Unorthodox cancer medicine. CA: A Cancer Journal for Clinicians 38:176–186, 1988.

Cramp, A.: Nostrums quackery and pseudomedium. Chicago, AMA Press, 1936.

Grant, R., and Bartlett, I.: Unproven cancer remedies—A primer. New York, American Cancer Society, 1971.

Griffiths, W.: Can human behavior be modified? Cancer 47:1221–1225, 1981.

Herbert, V., and Yarbro, C.H.: Nutrition quackery. Seminars in Oncology Nursing 2(1):63–69, 1986.

Holland, J.: Why patients seek unproven cancer remedies: A psychological perspective. CA: A Cancer Journal for Clinicians 32:10–14, 1982.

Howard-Ruben, J., and Miller, N.: Unproven methods of cancer management, Part II: Current trends and implications for patient care. Oncology Nursing Forum 11: 67–73, 1984.

Isler, C.: The fatal choice: Cancer quackery. RN 37:55–59, 1974.

Janssen, W.: Cancer quackery—The past in the present. Seminars in Oncology 6:526–535, 1975.

Miller, N., and Howard-Ruben, J.: Unproven methods of cancer management, Part I: Backgrounds and historical perspectives. Oncology Nursing Forum 10:46–52, 1983.

Young, V., and Richardson, D.: Nutrients, vitamins and minerals in cancer prevention: Facts and fallacies. Cancer 43:2125–2136, 1979.

PATIENT EDUCATION MATERIALS AND COMMUNITY RESOURCES

American Cancer Society State Division/Local Unit
National Cancer Institute Toll Free Information Line 1-800-4-CANCER
National Coalition for Cancer Survivors

COPING

The nurse assesses the patient's past and present coping mechanisms, current ability and availability to mobilize resources, and alternative coping strategies during all phases of care to formulate actual or potential nursing diagnoses.

Appropriate patient outcomes to consider in planning nursing interventions will specify the patient's ability within a level consistent with physical, psychosocial, and spiritual capacities and value systems to:

1. use appropriate resources for support in coping.
2. communicate feelings about living with cancer.
3. participate in care and ongoing decision-making.
4. identify alternative resources when present coping strategies do not meet needs.
5. set accomplishable goals.

Evaluation of the patient's responses to nursing care is based on whether the patient, while living with cancer, manages stress within physical, psychological, and spiritual capacities and value systems.

Excerpted from the ANA/ONS Standards of Oncology Nursing Practice.

Ineffective Individual Coping

Joanne Doublsky

19

Population at Risk

- Individuals undergoing initial diagnostic work-up for a malignancy
- Individuals receiving a positive diagnosis for a malignancy
- Individuals undergoing initial treatment
- Individuals following relapse or those unresponsive to further treatment
- Individuals perceiving personal stress related to their perceived vulnerability (disturbance in body image, life style, roles, self-esteem, and self-concept)
- Individuals perceiving personal stress resulting from changes imposed by another's disease process, treatment and/or their responses to treatment or disease process
- Individuals who have limited resources, small social networks, few interests, lack of spiritual beliefs, or a sense of helplessness/hopelessness
- Individuals successfully completing treatment and reorienting to concept of "long-term" future

LEVEL 1: At Risk for Ineffective Coping

EXPECTED OUTCOME

1. Patient begins adaptive process to psychoemotional stressors:
   - identifies potential stressors.
   - relates how potential stressors affect the patient's behavior.
   - seeks relevant information for problem-solving.
   - identifies resources to support and enhance effective coping.
   - alters perception of stressors and stressor events (redefines thinking patterns and sets goals to meet present situation; takes action).
2. Patient demonstrates functional adaptive behaviors and problem-solving capacity:
   - maintains personal appearance.
   - meets or redefines role expectations.
   - participates in decision-making with regard to health care.
   - makes decision with regard to activities of daily living, personal plans, work, and family.
   - maintains open channels of communication with family, significant others, and health care team.

NURSING MANAGEMENT

Assessment

1. Assess specific stressors.
2. Determine patient's perception of stressors, events, and beliefs about their causes.
3. Assess patient's perceived control and "expectation of controllability" to disease, treatment options, life style, work load and environment (see Stoner, 1985).
4. Evaluate patient's/significant other's available resources and support system.
5. Assess patient's perception of hope, meaning of the cancer experience, and impact on life through diagnosis, treatment, and cure.
6. Determine patient's usual and preferred coping style.
7. Assess usefulness of patient's preferred coping style.
8. Note patient's pattern of communication and affiliative need-response patterns.
9. Ascertain patient's ability to solve problems.
10. Evaluate patient's mental status.
11. Assess patient's physiologic status.
12. Observe patient's degree of stress.
13. Assess impact of treatment outcome on patient's life style, personal and interpersonal relationships, as well as ability to function at work.
14. Assess survivor's ability to reorient to concept of future (re-establishing long-term goals, hopes, and dreams).

Nursing Interventions

1. Develop rapport; utilize active listening skills.
2. Provide consistent, empathetic, and positive regard.
3. Support patient in expression of feelings over actual and potential losses and limitations imposed by disease and treatment, and in the expression of uncertainty surrounding completion of treatment and actual/potential cure.
4. Assist patient/family in formulating and clarifying goals to meet present demands of stressors.
5. Assist and encourage individual to identify and act upon those factors and events over which the individual has control.
6. Encourage and support patient's search for information with regard to disease, treatment, life after treatment and its effect on personal plans, family, friends, and work (e.g., what is known and what needs to be taught in order to plan for the future).
7. Identify and reinforce positive self-care behaviors that are performed regularly.
8. Identify and encourage use of available community agencies fostering supportive care (e.g., ACS programs such as: I Can Cope; Look Good–Feel Better; Reach for Recovery; other community resources such as National Coalition for Cancer Survivors; National Hospice Organization; Make Today Count; United Ostomy Association).

Patient Teaching

1. Teach relationship between coping and perception of stressors.
2. Teach relationship among hope, coping, and problem-solving.
3. Note importance of developing and participating in hobbies and physical activities for developing, sustaining, and enhancing a sense of accomplishment and "healthy" body image.
4. Discuss methods to identify problems and generate options for handling stress.
5. Describe importance and benefit of emotional release of tension (crying, exercise, play, talk, humor, and so on).
6. Teach problem-solving behavior:
   - List all problems; identify the most important.

- Discern patient's thoughts, feelings, and behaviors in response to a particular problem (e.g., help patient to recognize thoughts, feelings, and behavior in response to identified problem).
- Teach importance of relaxing before tackling problem (e.g., deep breathing, exercise, play, and so on).
- Have patient fantasize how others might respond.

- List potential responses and solutions to problem.
- Teach patient to identify positives and negatives of fantasized potential responses and solutions.
- Have patient prioritize potential solutions from most possible and desirable to least.
- Encourage choice of best solution. (Sobel and Worden, 1981)

LEVEL 2: *Ineffective Coping*

EXPECTED OUTCOME

1. Patient demonstrates successful positive coping and adaptation:
   - recognizes when present coping mechanisms are not working.
   - asks for assistance.
   - initiates and utilizes self-care tasks to minimize tension.
   - identifies, cultivates, and utilizes available resources.
   - exhibits absence of or decrease in number of verbalized somatic complaints.
   - shows absence of or decrease in frequency of "sick role" behaviors (e.g., performs tasks, makes decisions, "shows up for life" when within ability to do so).
   - displays absence of or decrease in number of verbalized helpless and self-defeating statements.

NURSING MANAGEMENT

Assessment

1. See Nursing Assessment, Level 1.
2. Assess ability to use divergent thinking patterns.
3. Determine effect of any drug regimen on ability to solve problems and cope positively (e.g., inappropriate use of and potential drug interactions among analgesics, antidepressants, sedatives, hypnotics, and antianxiety drugs.

Nursing Interventions

1. See Nursing Interventions, Level 1, steps 1 through 7.

2. Respond to patient's questions with pertinent and specific information.
3. Assist patient in formulating and learning specific procedures, tasks, and strategies for enhancing positive coping:
   - "thought stopping" (Ross, 1984).
   - divergent thinking.
   - reassessment, and clarification of life values.
   - focusing on realistic projects and possible goals.
   - relaxation training.
4. Reward attempts and success of patient's development and implementation of actions to decrease tension.
5. Redefine with patient the mastery level as each new action is successfully achieved.

6. Refer patient to appropriate and qualified professional for further intervention as indicated (e.g., mental health professional, clergy, social worker, attorney, career counselor, and the like).
7. Guide patient to specific resources (e.g., support groups—see list under Nursing Interventions, Level 1, step 8).

Patient Teaching

1. See Patient Teaching, Level 1.
2. Instruct patient in keeping a journal for identification of events and feelings and strategies utilized during particular problem events.
3. Teach assertiveness strategies.
4. Teach importance of social networks and community resources for support.
5. Discuss goal setting and follow-up action plans.
6. Develop an emergency plan for handling "out of control" behavior (e.g., crisis line, physician listing, primary oncology nurse, or clinical nurse specialist).

LEVEL 3: Severely Impaired Coping with Incapacitating Psychoemotional Covert and Overt Behaviors

EXPECTED OUTCOME

1. Caregiver demonstrates awareness of patient's unsuccessful coping and impact on life:
   - identifies unhealthy behaviors to report to health care team.
   - reports signs and symptoms of unhealthy behaviors.
   - identifies consequences of continued ineffective coping.
2. Caregiver/patient accept professional help:
   - participate with a professional mental health counselor.
   - keep appointments.
3. Caregiver/patient demonstrate consistent cognitive processes and behaviors aimed at de-escalation of maladaptive coping:
   - completes thoughts and speaks in complete sentences.
   - verbalizes specific "how to" steps in resolving problems.

NURSING MANAGEMENT

Assessment

1. Assess inadequate behaviors and the degree of physical and emotional destructiveness on individual and caregiver (e.g., inappropriate medication dosing, noncompliance, failure to keep appointments, substance abuse, "failure to show up for life").
2. Determine caregiver's level of knowledge of patient's maladaptive behaviors and effects on the caregiver and others.
3. Note desire and willingness to seek and utilize intensive professional help and resources.
4. Evaluate patient's physical status for physiologic problems that may affect behavior (e.g., hormonal imbalance, electrolyte imbalance, hypoxemia, brain metastasis, drugs).

Nursing Interventions

1. See Nursing Interventions, Level 2.
2. Maintain positive regard for patient and family while setting limits.
3. Collaborate with professional mental health worker to develop therapeutic plan (including emergency plan).
4. Reenforce emergency plan with caregiver.
5. Provide support for caregiver when patient exhibits destructive behaviors/rejects caregiver.

Patient Teaching

1. Direct teaching at caregiver.
2. Teach signs and symptoms of severe incapacitation or escalation of destructive behaviors requiring immediate attention of mental health professional.
3. Explain crisis intervention techniques.
4. Discuss medication regimen (if used) to control behavior.
5. Emphasize importance of keeping appointments with mental health professional.

SUGGESTED READINGS

Burns, D.D.: Feeling Good: The New Mood Therapy. New York, The New American Library, 1981.

Friedman, B.D.: Coping with cancer: A guide for health care professionals. Cancer Nursing 3: 105–110, 1980.

Garfield, C.A.: Psychosocial Care of the Dying Patient. New York, McGraw-Hill, 1978.

Garfield, C.A.: Three Lives: Counseling the Terminally Ill. Santa Monica, CA, Pelican Films, 1981.

Hickey, S.S.: Enabling hope. Cancer Nursing 9: 133–137, 1986.

Hinds, P.S., and Martin, J.: Hopefulness and the self-sustaining process in adolescents with cancer. Nursing Research 37: 336–340, 1988.

Hoffman, B.: Cancer survivors at work: Job problems and illegal discrimination. Oncology Nursing Forum 16(1): 39–43, 1989.

Holmes, T., and Rahe, R.H.: Social readjustment rating scale. Journal of Psychosomatic Research 11(2): 213–218, 1967.

Martocchio, B.: Authenticity, belonging, emotional closeness and self-representation. Oncology Nursing Forum 14(1): 23–27, 1987.

Maxwell, M.B.: The use of social networks to help cancer patients maximize support. Cancer Nursing 5(4): 275–281, 1982.

Nowotny, M.L.: Assessment of hope in patients with cancer: Development of an instrument. Oncology Nursing Forum 16(1): 57–61, 1989.

Perls, F.S.: In and Out of the Garbage Pail. New York, Bantam Books, 1969.

Pollock, S.E.: Human responses to chronic illness: Physiologic and psychosocial adaptation. Nursing Research 35(2): 90–95, 1986.

Ross, D.M.: Thought-stopping: A coping strategy for impending feared events. Issues in Comprehensive Pediatric Nursing 7(2–3): 83–89, 1984.

Saunders, J.M., and Valente, S.M.: Career and suicide. Oncology Nursing Forum 15(5): 575–580, 1988.

Shepard, M.: Someone You Love is Dying: A Guide for Helping and Coping. New York, Harmony Press, 1985.

Sobel, H.J., and Worden, J.W.: Helping Cancer Patients Cope: A Problem-Solving Intervention for Health Care Professionals. New York, B.M.A. Audio Cassettes, Div-Guilford Publishers, 1981.

Sodestrom, K.E., and Martenson, J.M.: Patient's spiritual coping strategies: A study of nurse and patient perspectives. Oncology Nursing Forum 14(2): 41–46, 1987.

Spiegel, D.: Psychosocial interventions with cancer patients. Journal of Psychosocial Oncology 3, 83–95, Winter 1985/1986.

Stewart, G.W., and Sundeen, S.J.: Principles and Practices of Psychiatric Nursing. St. Louis, C.V. Mosby, 1979.

Stoner, C.: Learned helplessness: Analysis and application. Oncology Nursing Forum 12(1): 31–35, 1985.

Taking Time (Publication No. 80–2059). Bethesda, MD, National Institute of Health, 1980.

Tedesco-Carreras, P.: Maintaining Mental Wellness. NSNA/Imprint. pp. 38–39, Feb/March 1988.

Warr, P., and Jackson, P.: Adapting to the unemployed role: A longitudinal investigation. Social Science Medicine 25: 1219–1224, 1987.

Weisman, C.: Coping with Cancer. New York, McGraw-Hill, 1979.

Ineffective Family Coping

20

Sr. Karin DuFault, Sharon Cannell Firsich, Anne Gardner,
Margaret B. Jones, Jean R. Moseley, and Sandra Stone

Population at Risk

Individuals who significantly interact with patient throughout the course of illness, especially those with:
- Family role changes resulting from disease
- Families at crucial developmental stages (e.g., new marriages, young children, retired people)
- Preexisting patterns of dependency within relationship
- Preexisting interpersonal problems
- Inadequate financial resources
- Preexisting health problems
- Negative past experience with cancer
- History of long-term problems in adjusting to life changes

LEVEL 1: At Risk for Ineffective Family Coping

EXPECTED OUTCOME

1. Family copes effectively at a level consistent with physical, psychosocial, and spiritual capacities and value system:
    - identifies internal and external resources.
    - identifies potential and actual stressors.
    - demonstrates resourceful use of multiple positive coping strategies.
    - is productive and flexible with regard to change.
    - resolves conflicts and lives with differences.
    - recognizes and deals with realities of the situation, regulates emotional reactions, integrates the experience of illness with rest of life.
    - acknowledges and communicates changed attitudes, needs, and limitations in a way that permits new balance with the environment.

NURSING MANAGEMENT

Assessment

1. Assess family constellation (family of origin):
    - parents' and siblings' present ages.
    - geographic locations.
    - description and relationship to patient.
    - description of roles in family (evaluation of role shifts resulting from illness).
    - alliances and friction.

- developmental level of family.
- health status of family members.
- cause of death of deceased members; cancer history.
- major stressors in family of origin.
2. Evaluate present living group:
   - socioeconomic level, life style.
   - marital status.
   - if married, history and circumstances of marriage, pregnancies, children.
   - description and history of family relationships.
   - amount and kind of communication (past and present) in family.
   - comparision between present family and family of origin.
   - family strengths and liabilities.
   - decision-making processes and problem-solving skills.
   - roles of family members (e.g., financial provider, primary homemaker).
   - shared and unshared family values and beliefs.
   - important events and rituals.
   - special concerns.
   - cultural/ethnic influences on life style.
   - usual daily living pattern.
   - role of illness in family history.
   - recent crises or changes in life pattern (e.g., hospitalization, change of residence, job, income, school).
   - steps taken in adjustment to illness.
   - changes expected in life style as a result of illness.
3. Evaluate community/environment:
   - description of neighborhood (e.g., length of time at that residence, type of community, relationship to neighbors, transportation facilities available, needed, and used).
   - suitability of home to life style and needs (e.g., type of housing, living conditions, arrangements of available space).
   - availability and pattern of utilization of health care facilities.
4. Note occupation/finances:
   - present occupation and length of employment, job satisfaction.
- adequacy of income.
- identification of financial problems.
- adequacy of insurance.
- effect of illness on work dependability and productivity.
- health hazards and stressors of work environment.
5. Determine religious practices:
   - membership in religious group.
   - level of activity and satisfaction with level.
   - spiritual beliefs of client/family and their effect on client's physical and emotional health.
   - supportive individuals/clergy connected with religion and ways in which support is offered.
   - ways in which spiritual needs are met presently; anticipated changes related to illness.
6. Assess membership in other groups and organizations (role, quality of relationships, satisfaction).
7. Ascertain recreational interests:
   - individual/family leisure activities and time devoted to them.
   - opportunities for self-expression.
   - social orientation in activities.
   - friendship network.
8. Evaluate stressors:
   - sources of concern or anxiety.
   - physical and emotional disabilities.
   - problems with memory, sleep, mood, substance abuse.
   - attitudes toward illness and interpretation of present situation.
   - understanding of disease, prognosis, treatment plan.
   - present and anticipated impact on family.
   - level of confidence in coping abilities.
9. Note factors with high risk for distress:
   - marital problems.
   - living alone.
   - economic marginality.
   - alcohol abuse.
   - dysfunctional family of origin.
   - lack of church affiliation.
   - psychiatric history.

- suicidal ideation.
- low ego strength.
- high anxiety level.
- pessimistic attitude.
- advanced stage of cancer.
- multiple reported symptoms.
- multiple current concerns and problems of all types with poor resolution.
- little help or support expected or received.
- health professionals seen as unhelpful or unconcerned.
- coping strategies of suppression and passivity, fatalistic submission, isolation and withdrawal, blaming others, blaming self.

10. Ascertain usual manner of coping with stress and actions taken during crisis:
- rational inquiry (seeks additional information regarding disease, treatment, and prognosis).
- mutuality (shares concern and talks with others; note that silence and trust may provide nonverbal mutuality).
- affect reversal (makes light of a serious situation).
- suppression (attempts to forget or put out of mind).
- displacement/redirection (engages in other activities for purpose of distraction).
- confrontation of reality and appropriate action (takes firm action based on present understanding).
- redefinition/revision (accepts situation, puts it in a more favorable light).
- passive acceptance (submits to the inevitable; fatalism).
- impulsivity ("acts out" reckless, impractical, socially unacceptable behavior).
- negotiation of feasible alternatives (weighs one choice, possibility, or decision against another).
- life-threatening behavior (reduces tension through excessive drinking, drugs, other dangers).
- disengagement (withdraws into isolation).

- externalization/projection (blames someone or something).
- cooperative compliance (seeks direction; attempts to follow instructions).
- self-blame (victimizes self; sacrifices or atones for behavior).

11. Gauge effectiveness of strategies.

Nursing Actions

1. Listen supportively.
2. Determine temporary and long-term demands of the situation that must be coped with in some ways.
3. Review past coping styles and determine relevance to present situation.
4. Assist with formulation of goals to maintain effective coping.
5. Assist with identification of methods to achieve goals and reduce stress to manageable level.
6. Identify appropriate physical, social, economic resources.

Patient Teaching

1. Appropriate content of teaching includes:
   - impact of changes related to diagnosis on life style and family relationships.
   - styles of communication (passive, assertive, aggressive).
   - active listening skills (attending, tracking, questioning, focusing).
   - ways of viewing stress (harm, loss, threat, challenge).
   - identification and strengthening of coping resources (health, energy, morale, problem-solving skills, social networks, utilitarian resources).
   - coping strategies focused on efforts to regulate emotional stress and distress (e.g., use of humor).
2. Appropriate methods of teaching:
   - family unit/individual member instruction.
   - group educational opportunities (e.g., I Can Cope).
   - modeling and role playing.

EXPECTED OUTCOME

1. Family copes effectively at a level consistent with physical, psychosocial, and spiritual capacities and value system:
   - states realistic goals derived from changing situation.
   - seeks opportunities to participate in care and decision-making.
   - communicates openly feelings related to disease, treatment, prognosis.
   - develops new patterns and techniques of communication to cope with present situation.
   - expands utilization of appropriate resources to meet needs of present situation.

NURSING MANAGEMENT

Assessment

1. See Assessment, Level 1.
2. Assess family's ability to set realistic goals:
   - obtain statement of long-term/short-term goals.
   - elicit expression of realistic rather than global or idealistic goals.
3. Gauge family's participation in care and decision-making:
   - family's background and expertise in care and decision-making.
   - level of participation in care (Does family actively seek out opportunities to participate in care?).
   - expressed desire for participation in decision-making.
4. Observe communication patterns between family members:
   - understanding by family members of patient's disease, prognosis, and treatment plan.
   - feelings about changes in the patient.
   - perception of cancer, death.
5. Evaluate family/community support resources:
   - availability of support.
   - understanding of resources available.
   - actual use of support services.
   - effectiveness of resources currently used.
6. Determine family's willingness and ability to learn and accept alternative coping strategies:
   - past use of coping strategies.
   - expressed dissatisfaction with present coping strategy.

Nursing Actions

1. Assist patient/family in setting goals to regain effective coping.
2. Involve family in areas of care and decision-making through the use of contracts, support, praise.
3. Demonstrate communication techniques (use of touch, humor).
4. Model family problem-solving and expression of feelings.
5. Explore alternative coping methods and skills that could be developed to meet the demands or to manage problems consistent with intellectual capacities, goals, age, grief.
6. Share information about disease, prognosis, and treatment.
7. Identify ineffective resources and explore alternatives.
8. Make referral to appropriate resources.

Patient Teaching

1. See Patient Teaching, Level 1.
2. Appropriate family teaching includes:
   - available community/family resources, referral systems, information systems.
   - individual/family growth and developmental patterns.
   - exploration of alternative roles (e.g., husband taking on housekeeping, wife becoming wage earner, child becoming caregiver).
   - the right of patients to be informed about disease, treatment, and related issues.
   - skills, techniques, rationale, medications, for providing care.
   - problem identification, problem-solving.
   - assertiveness skills.
   - improved communication skills (how to remove barriers, use of touch, active listening, responding, humor, giving permission to communicate).
   - new skills required for role changes.

LEVEL 3: Severely Impaired Family Coping

EXPECTED OUTCOME

1. Family copes effectively at a level consistent with physical, psychosocial, and spiritual capacities and value system:
   - demonstrates ability, resources, stamina to handle physical, mental, emotional work required by the present situation.
   - recognizes, obtains, uses, maintains supports (equipment, people, systems).
   - demonstrates desire and motivation to participate in present situation.
   - states attainable goals.
   - communicates feeling about living with cancer.
   - participates in care and ongoing decision-making.
   - uses appropriate resources for support in coping.
   - identifies alternative resources when present coping strategies do not provide support.
   - maintains adequate and satisfying sensory environment.

NURSING MANAGEMENT

Assessment

1. See Assessment, Levels 1 and 2.
2. Assess present level of strength, endurance, sensory input, knowledge, desire, courage, skills, and support systems of family members.
3. Observe physiologic and behavioral coping mechanisms being used by family (e.g., use of past coping strategies, use of physical tension-reducing techniques, use of job, social activities).
4. Determine family's willingness and ability to change coping mechanisms.
5. Evaluate current status of problem-solving, emotional regulation.
6. Examine level of interaction of family/patient, family/environment.

Nursing Actions

1. See Nursing Actions, Levels 1 and 2.
2. Assist family to identify reasonable goals for physical, mental, and emotional work required by present situation.
3. Assist family to identify personally satisfying means of participating in patient care.
4. Support family as they choose to take risks in coping with changing situation.
5. Assist family to identify crucial elements in sensory environment and reasonable goals for maintaining comfortable, peaceful environment.
6. Assist family to participate in care.
7. Encourage family to express feelings about the impact of cancer on their lives in order to identify possible resources, potential risks, and environmental effects.
8. Assist family to recognize when present resources are not sufficient and to identify and use alternative resources.

Patient Teaching

1. See Patient Teaching, Levels 1 and 2.
2. Appropriate family teaching includes:
   - information relevant to present situation.
   - alternative coping strategies, problem-solving and decision-making, time management, organizational skills.
   - normal and pathologic emotional responses.
   - identification of resources.
   - interpersonal and communication skills.
   - relevant manual skills.

SUGGESTED READINGS

Anderson, S.V., and Bauwens, E.E.: Chronic health problems: Concepts and applications. St. Louis, C.V. Mosby, 1978.

Bean, F., Cooper, S., Renee, A., et al.: Coping mechanisms of cancer patients: A study of 33 patients receiving che-motherapy. CA: A Cancer Journal for Clinicians 30:2516–2519, 1980.

Carnevali, D.L.: Nursing care planning: Diagnosis and management. Philadelphia, J.B. Lippincott, 1983.

Cohen, F., and Lazarus, R.S.: Coping with the stresses of illness. In Stone, G.C., Cohen, F., and Adler, N.E. (Eds.): Health Psychology—A Handbook: Theories, Applications, and Challenges for Psychological Approach to the Health Care System. San Francisco, Jossey-Bass, 1979, pp. 217–254.

Folkman, S., Schaefer, C., and Lazarus, R.S.: Cognitive processes as mediators of stress and coping. In Hamiton, V., and Warbutor, D.M. (Eds.): Human Stress and Cognition: An Information Processing Approach. New York, John Wiley & Sons, 1979, pp. 265–298.

Forsyth, D.M.: The hardest job of all. Nursing 12(4):86–90, 1982.

Garland, L.M., and Bush, C.T.: Coping Behaviors and Nursing. Reston, VA, Reston, 1982.

George, J.B.: Nursing Theories Conference Group: Nursing Theories: The Base for Professional Nursing Practice. Englewood Cliffs, NJ, Prentice-Hall, 1980.

Grobe, M.E., Ahmann, D.L. and Ilstrup, D.L.: Needs assessment for advanced cancer patients and their families. Oncology Nursing Forum 9:26–30, 1982.

Hackett, T.P., and Cassem, N.J.: Massachusetts General Hospital Handbook of General Hospital Psychiatry. St. Louis, C.V. Mosby, 1978.

Hansen, D.A., and Hill, R.: Families under stress. In Christensen, H.T. (Ed.): Handbook of Marriage and the Family. Chicago, Rand McNally, 1964, pp. 782–823.

Hickey, M.: What are the needs of families of critically ill patients? Focus on Critical Care 12:41–43, 1985.

Holmes, B.C.: Psychological evaluation and preparation of the patient and family. Cancer 60:2021–2024, 1987.

Kaempler, S.H.: Family coping: Assessment and family coping: Strategies. In Baird, S.B. (Ed.): Decision Making in Oncology Nursing. Toronto, B.C. Decker, 1988, pp. 50–53.

Kirschling, J.M.: The experience of terminal illness on adult family members. The Hospice Journal 2:121–138, 1986.

Lazarus, E.S., and Launier, R.: Stress-related transactions between person and environment. In Pervin, L.A., and Lewis, M. (Eds.): Perspectives in International Psychology. New York, Plenum, 1987, pp. 287–322.

Lewis, F.M.: Family level services for the cancer patient: Critical distinctions, fallacies, and assessment. Cancer Nursing 6:193–200, 1983.

Luce, J.K.: Selecting patients for supportive therapy. In Stoll, BA (Ed.): Mind and Cancer Prognosis. Chichester, NY, John Wiley & Sons, 1979, pp. 127–138.

Mages, N.L., and Mendelsohn, G.A.: Effects of cancer on patients' lives: A personological approach. In Stone, G.C., Choen, F., and Adler, N.E. (Eds.): Health Psychology—A Handbook: Theories, Applications, and Challenges for a Psychological Approach to the Health Care System. San Francisco, Jossey-Bass, 1979, pp. 255–284.

Marino, L.B., and Kooser, J.A.: The psychosocial care of cancer clients and their families: Periods of high risk. *In* Marino, L. (Ed.): Cancer Nursing. St. Louis, C.V. Mosby, 1981, pp. 53–65.

NCI: Coping with cancer: A resource for health professionals. Bethesda, MD: National Institutes of Health, 1980.

Olsen, E.: The impact of serious illness on the family system. Postgraduate Medicine *46:*169–174, 1970.

ONS and ANA: Standards of Nursing Practice. Kansas City, MO: American Nurses' Association, 1987.

Riehal, J.D., and Roy, C., Sr.: Conceptual Models for Nursing Practice. New York, Appleton-Century-Crofts, 1980.

Robinson, V.M.: Humor and the Health Professional. Thorofare, NJ: Charles B. Slack, 1977.

Roskies, E., and Lazarus, R.S.: Coping theory and the teaching of coping skills. *In* Davidson, P. (Ed.): Behavioral Medicine: Changing Health Styles. New York, Brunner/Mazel, 1979, pp. 36–69.

Stetz, K.M.: Caregiving demands during advanced cancer—The spouse's needs. Cancer Nursing *10*(5):260–268, 1987.

Thomas, S.G.: Breast cancer: The psychosocial issues. Cancer Nursing *1:*53–60, 1978.

Tringali, C.A.: The needs of family members of cancer patients. Oncology Nursing Forum *13*(4):65–69, 1986.

Vess, J.D. Moreland, J.R., and Schwebel, A.I.: An empirical assessment of the effects of cancer on family role functioning. Journal of Psychosocial Oncology *3:*1–16, 1985.

Vess, J.D., Moreland, J.R., and Schwebel, A.I.: A follow-up study of role functioning and the psychological environment of families of cancer patients. Journal of Psychosocial Oncology *3*(2):1–14, 1985.

Weisman, A.D.: Coping with Cancer. New York, McGraw-Hill, 1979.

Weisman, A.D., and Worden, J.W.: The existential plight in cancer: Significance of first 100 days. International Journal of Psychiatry in Medicine *7:*1–15, 1976–1977.

Whitman, H.H., and Gustafson, J.P.: Group therapy for families facing a cancer crisis. Oncology Nursing Forum *16:*539–543, 1989.

Woods, N.F., Lewis, F.M., and Ellison, E.S.: Living with cancer: Family experiences. Cancer Nursing *12:*28–33, 1989.

PATIENT EDUCATION MATERIALS AND COMMUNITY RESOURCES

Organizations

Association for Brain Tumor Research, 3725 N. Talman Avenue, Chicago, IL 60618, 312–286–5571.

Cancer Care, Inc., 1180 Avenue of the Americas, New York, NY 10036, 212–302–2400.

Contact the social work department of your local hospital.

Coping with Survival—Support for People Living with Adult Leukemia and Lymphoma, Leukemia Society of America, Inc., 733 Third Avenue, New York, NY 10017, 212–573–8484.

I Can Cope, Contact your local unit of the American Cancer Society.

National Hospice Organization, 1901 North Moore Street, Suite 901, Arlington, VA 22209, 703–243–5900.

Taking Time—Support for People with Cancer and the People Who Care about Them, National Cancer Institute, Office of Cancer Communications, Bethesda, MD 20205, 1-800-4-Cancer.

Groups

Cancer Care, Inc., 1180 Avenue of the Americas, New York, NY 10036, 212–286–5571.

Cansurmount, 90 Park Avenue, New York, NY 10016, 212–736–3030, Contact the social work department of your local health care agency.

I Can Cope—Contact your local unit of the American Cancer Society.

Make Today Count, PO Box 222, Osage Beach, MO 65065.

National Coalition for Cancer Survivorship, National Hospice Organization. 1901 North Moore Street, Suite 901, Arlington, VA 22209, 703–243–5900.

Books

Benjamin, H.H.: From Victim to Victor. New York, Dell Publishing, 1987.

Cousins, N.: Head First—The Biology of Hope. New York, E.P. Dutton, 1989.

Garrision, J.G., and Shepard, S.: Cancer & Hope: Charting a survival course. Minneapolis, MN, CompCare Publisher, 1989.

Lazlo, J.: Understanding Cancer. New York, Harper & Row, 1987.

LeShan, L.: Cancer as a Turning Point. New York, E. P. Dutton, 1989.

Morra, M., and Potts, E.: Choices: Realistic Alternatives in Cancer Treatment. New York, Avon Books, 1987.

Morra, M., and Potts, E.: Trumph: Getting Back to Normal When You Have Cancer. New York, Avon Books, 1990.

Pepper, C.B.: We the Victors. New York, New American Library, 1984.

Seigal, B.S.: Love, Medicine & Miracles. New York, Harper & Row, 1986.

Siegal, B.S.: Peace, Love & Healing. New York, Harper & Row, 1989.

"Taking Time—Support for People with Cancer and the People Who Care About Them. National Cancer Institute, Office of Cancer Communications, Bethesda, MD 20205, 800–4–CANCER.

Grieving

Catherine D. Harvey and Sue P. Heiney

Population at Risk

- Individuals with a diagnosis of cancer and their families/significant others
- Patients/families during all stages of disease where physical, psychosocial, and life style changes result in losses

LEVEL 1: *Potential For Grieving*

EXPECTED OUTCOME

1. Patient/family identify areas of real and potential loss significant in relationship to diagnosis.
2. Patient/family is able to recall past experiences and responses to stressful situations and able to utilize appropriate responses to:
   - communicate feelings of anger, guilt, fear, sadness, and so on.
   - develop additional coping skills.
3. Patient/family demonstrate verbal and nonverbal concern for each other.
4. Patient/family identify normal roles and changes in relationship patterns.

NURSING MANAGEMENT

Assessment

1. Assess patient's/family's previous roles and handling of stressful situations and losses (particularly recent):
   - Have patient/family experienced loss (e.g., from relocation, death, divorce) of a close relative, friend, pet, or job?
   - Have dietary, sleep patterns changed?
   - Has schoolwork been affected?
   - Have social contacts been maintained or new ones started?
   - Has family been able to continue with activities of daily living?
2. Assess current coping strategies and their effectiveness.
3. Determine sources of strength for the patient/family and how support is defined.
4. Observe each family member's reaction to changing roles resulting from cancer.
5. Note patient's/family's spiritual, social, and economic status, usual life style and cultural ethnic factors that may affect grief reaction.
6. Observe pattern of interactions among family members for changes to indicate development of potential problems.
7. Observe physical health of each family

member now and as patient's disease progresses.

Nursing Interventions

1. Provide private atmosphere for discussion and learning.
2. Show concern, express availability, and develop trust by displaying empathy, maintaining a nonjudgmental attitude, and by listening.
3. Notify ancillary resource persons as agreed upon with the patient/family.
4. Reinforce evidence of positive communication among family members.

Patient Teaching

1. Normal responses to loss include denial, anger, fear, isolation, bargaining, depression, acceptance.

2. Grieving is a normal response to a real or potential loss.
3. Grieving begins at the time of patient's diagnosis and family grieving can continue after patient's death.
4. Individuals within the family unit may experience the grief responses differently (e.g., timing, duration, intensity, behaviorally).
5. Information on diagnosis, role change, physical loss should be shared among all family members because it builds the foundation of mutual understanding and trust.
6. Touching, holding, hugging, caressing, and doing special favors are ways of communicating concern and caring (not acceptable in some subcultures).
7. Note availability of supportive community resources.
8. Plan an organized activity schedule according to patient's/family's needs and desires.

LEVEL 2A: Anticipatory Grieving

EXPECTED OUTCOME

1. Family members communicate impending loss.
2. Patient/family share responses to impending loss.
3. Patient/family express feelings and reactions of normal grief.
4. Patient/family identify future life changes and take actions to cope with changes.
5. Patient/family identify important life memories and develop ways to maintain family integrity following patient's death.

NURSING MANAGEMENT

Assessment

1. See Assessment, Level 1.
2. Assess patient's/family's understanding of current health status and potential for death.

Nursing Interventions

1. Give patient/family permission to grieve.
2. Discuss reality of actual loss with patient/family.
3. Explore losses secondary to disease pro-

cess and life style changes with patient and family.

4. Initiate family meetings in a private area.
5. Promote positive communications among family members.
6. Lead discussion of problems and solutions with patient and all family members.
7. Show acceptance of any response and sincere effort to change.
8. Share importance of memories and facilitate family's identification of the best methods for preserving memories (e.g., family album, gifts, memorials, last wishes, audio or visual recordings).
9. Facilitate patient's inquiry and discussion of implication of living wills and code status.
10. Provide educational materials about loss and grief.
11. Facilitate maintenance of hope.
12. Refer to support services as needed.

Patient Teaching

1. Teach importance of maintaining health and welfare of all family members.
2. Assure family of normalcy of anticipatory grief and normal responses.
3. Teach physical and psychologic responses to stress and ways to cope.

LEVEL 2B: Actual Normal Grieving

EXPECTED OUTCOME

1. Family members work together to overcome daily obstacles:
   - adjust to role changes.
   - seek support from others.
   - openly discuss problems.
   - work toward resolution of problems.
2. Patient/family recognize inhibiting responses to further growth as a unit:
   - identify lack of communication as inhibiting response.
   - identify possible feelings of alienation that may be due to reality denial, guilt, resentment, fear of being left alone, anger, financial distress, or inconsistencies in coping as inhibiting responses.
3. Family restores its supportive structure:
   - acknowledges responses of each family member.
   - renews coping behavior.

NURSING MANAGEMENT

Assessment

1. See Assessment Levels 1 and 2A.
2. Assess family's reaction to loss.
3. Assess significance of loss to patient/family:

- To what extent has patient been able to continue with usual activities?
- Has performance at work changed?
- Have social contacts been made or changed?
- Has financial situation been altered?

- Are other physical illnesses occurring within the family?
4. Note inappropriate responses leading to increasing stress among family members (e.g., quarreling, lying, name calling).
5. Determine family setting and stability prior to illness.
6. Ascertain physical well being of all members (e.g., weight loss, insomnia, anorexia).
7. Evaluate adaptive responses of family members (e.g., talking about and resolving problems with care of patient).

Nursing Interventions

1. Give permission to patient/family to grieve.
2. Initiate family meetings in a private area.
3. Carefully probe persistent denial of grief.
4. Show acceptance of any response and sincere effort to effect a change if needed.
5. Listen but don't offer false hope.

Patient Teaching

1. Teach importance of maintaining health and welfare of all family members.
2. Teach normal response to grief process.
3. Teach inhibiting responses (e.g., lack of communication, noncompliance with instructions, nonparticipation).
4. Teach adaptive responses (e.g., participation in activities of daily living, open lines of communication, working out problems as they arise).
5. Offer reassurance of the availability of self and others as resource persons.
6. Discuss need to seek support from other sources (friends, church, and the like) with encouragement not to be alone.
7. Caution against making major life changes (e.g., selling home, job change), as stability is needed.
8. Teach patient/caregivers of the need to be mutually accepting, patient, and understanding during grief process.

LEVEL 3: *Dysfunctional, Maladaptive, Prolonged Grieving*

EXPECTED OUTCOME

1. Patient/family is able to remember with appropriate emotional responses:
   - seek new opportunities.
   - participate in the living community.
   - renegotiate family roles and relationships.
2. Patient/family are able to reinvest emotional surpluses:
   - seek new opportunities.
   - participate in the living community.

NURSING MANAGEMENT

1. See Assessment Levels 1, 2A, and 2B.
2. Note family members' responses to loss/

death of a member. Initial reaction may change over a period of time.

3. Assess patient's/family's ability to participate in activities of daily living and to perform roles.
4. Determine physical well being of patient/family.
5. Observe pathologic or maladaptive grief responses:
   - signs and symptoms of psychotic depression.
   - interruptions or changes in family roles such as increasing dependency.
   - signs of regression such as thumb sucking, bed wetting in children.
   - prolonged isolation, withdrawal.
   - signs and symptoms of suicidal intent.

Nursing Interventions

1. Offer reality-oriented guidance. Allow time to be with family members individually or as a group.
2. Provide quiet area for family to express immediate feelings regarding the death of a loved one and possibly to project plans for the future.
3. Utilize other resource persons as needed.
4. Help utilize positive coping mechanisms inherent in the unit itself—recall past coping skills.
5. Assist family to restructure time and routines.
6. Plan follow-up visits by nurse, spiritual advisor, social worker at weekly intervals initially, especially with prolonged anticipatory grieving. At least one visit after death is beneficial, with follow-up visits adjusted to family's needs.
7. Make referral for counseling or therapy.

Patient Teaching

1. Time often changes family members' responses to the death of a member.
2. Teach patient/family that each person grieves differently.

3. A variety of emotional responses may be helpful.
4. Emphasize need to evaluate each family member's health periodically.
5. Reassure patient/family members that a myriad of feelings is normal during grief response.
6. Therapeutic grief is the chance to think about the loss of a loved one while developing the ability to start life again with a fuller meaning.
7. Teach patient/caregivers of the need to be mutually accepting, patient, and understanding during grief process.

SUGGESTED READINGS

Aronson, G.J.: The Meaning of Death. New York, McGraw-Hill, 1959.

Barton, D.: Dying and Death—A Clinical Guide for Caregivers. Baltimore, Williams and Wilkins, 1977.

Cohen, K.P.: Hospice-Prescription for Terminal Care. Germantown, MD: Aspen Systems Corp., 1979.

Collison, C. and Miller, S.: Using images of the future in grief work. Image 19(1):9–11, 1987.

Garfield, C.A.: Psychosocial Care of the Dying Patient. New York, McGraw-Hill, 1978.

Hickey, S.S.: Enabling hope. Cancer Nursing 9(3):133–137, 1986.

Johnson, S.E.: After a Child Dies: Counseling Bereaved Families. New York, Springer Publishing, 1987.

Koop, R.L.: Encounter with Terminal Illness. Grand Rapids, MI, Zondervan Publishing, 1980.

Kuebler-Ross, E.: Death—The Final Stage of Growth. Englewood Cliffs, NJ, Prentice-Hall, 1975.

Oates, W.E.: Your Particular Grief (Ch. 6). Philadelphia, Westminster Press, 1981.

Paston, L.: In the Midst of Winter. New York, Vintage Books, 1982.

Schneider, J.M.: The Clinical Significant Difference Between Grief, Pathological Grief and Depression. Patient Counseling and Health Education. (vol 2). Princeton, NJ, Excerpta Medica, 1980, pp.161–169.

Taking time. (NIH Publication No. 80-2059). Bethesda, MD: National Institutes of Health, 1980.

Weisman, A.: Coping with Cancer. New York, McGraw-Hill, 1979.

Worden, J.W.: Grief Counseling and Grief Therapy: A Handbook for the Mental Health Practitioner. New York, Springer Publishing, 1982.

Worden, W.: Grief Counseling, Grief Therapy. New York, Springer Publishing, 1983.

PATIENT EDUCATION MATERIALS AND COMMUNITY RESOURCES

Bell, J.: What Will I Tell the Children? Omaha, NB, University of Nebraska, Medical Center Public Affairs Office, 402–559–4353, 1986.

Knees, B., and Pattie, A.: Up from Grief Patterns of Recovery. New York, Seabury Press, 1982.

Miles, M.S.: The Grief of Parents When a Child Dies. Oak Brook, IL, The Compassionate Friends, 1980.

Price, E.: Getting Through the Night: Finding Your Way After the Loss of a Loved One. New York, Dial Press, 1982.

Upson, N.S.: When Someone You Love is Dying. New York, Simon & Schuster, 1986.

Westberg, G.E.: Good Grief. Philadelphia, Fortress Press, 1962.

COMFORT

The nurse assesses the patient's source and degree of discomfort, method of pain and symptom management, effects of disease and treatment on life style, and outcomes of interventions to alleviate discomfort to formulate actual or potential nursing diagnoses.

Appropriate patient outcomes to consider in planning nursing interventions will specify the patient's ability to:

1. communicate alterations in comfort level.
2. identify measures to modify psychosocial, environmental, and physical factors that increase comfort and promote the continuance of valued activities and relationships.
3. describe the source of the discomfort, the treatment, and the expected outcome of the proposed interventions.
4. describe appropriate interventions for potential or predictable problems such as pain, sleep pattern disturbances, and pruritus.

Evaluation of the patient's responses to nursing care is based on whether the patient identifies and manages factors that influence comfort.

Excerpted from the ANA/ONS Standards of Oncology Nursing Practice.

Alteration in Comfort: Acute Pain

Judith Paice

22

ACUTE PAIN: *Acute pain has a defined pattern of onset, usually originates from tissue damage, may or may not be accompanied by autonomic dysfunction, and is of a short duration (less than 6 months).*

Population at Risk

- All individuals diagnosed with cancer, or who are undergoing diagnostic evaluation for the potential diagnosis of cancer, due to (1) diagnostic procedures, (2) medical or surgical therapies, or (3) the disease process

LEVEL 1:   Potential

EXPECTED OUTCOME

1. Patient demonstrates knowledge related to potential alteration in comfort:
   - verbalizes role of acute pain as a protective mechanism.
   - identifies physiologic, psychologic, social, cultural, other factors that influence the perception of pain and its treatment.
   - describes conditions and procedures that may induce acute pain.
   - verbalizes the importance of reporting changes in pain perception.
2. Patient demonstrates knowledge of measures that may prevent or minimize the perception of acute pain:
   - identifies pharmacologic and nonpharmacologic therapies that potentially minimize the intensity of acute pain perception.

NURSING MANAGEMENT

Assessment

1. Assess patient's medical history, including course of illness and modalities used in treatment of cancer.
2. Identify procedures that may potentially lead to acute pain.
3. Determine patient's previous experiences with acute or chronic pain including:
   - circumstances of onset.
   - location.
   - intensity.
   - quality.
   - onset, duration.
   - aggravating factors (e.g., activity).
   - alleviating factors (e.g., medications, relaxation, heat).
   - significance of the pain.
4. Identify concerns patient may have regarding pain therapy (e.g., fear of tolerance, addiction, or side effects associated with pain therapy).

125

5. Obtain patient's history regarding usual patterns of:
   - bowel and bladder elimination.
   - cognitive function.
   - sleep.
   - ability to eat.
   - physical activity.
   - socialization and communication.
   - sexual activity.

Nursing Interventions

1. Prepare area of skin or body that is to undergo invasive examination/procedure with cold, heat, or local/topical analgesic or anesthetic agent to reduce pain.

Patient Teaching

1. Discuss that acute pain is a protective mechanism or warning signal indicating the need to seek methods to alleviate the underlying source of the pain problem.
2. Teach that the pain experience is highly individual and variable. Components of the perception of pain include:
   - physiologic (e.g., organic etiology of the pain).
   - sensory (e.g., location, intensity, quality, duration).
   - affective (e.g., psychologic reactions to pain, including anxiety/depression).
   - congitive (e.g., meaning of the pain).
   - behavioral (e.g., affect of pain on activity, facial expressions of pain, body movements).
3. Discuss that most acute pain can be controlled to an acceptable level (as defined by the patient) using pharmacologic and nonpharmacologic measures, including:
   - pharmacologic measures:
     - non-narcotics.
     - nonsteroidal antiinflammatory drugs (NSAIDs).
     - narcotics.
     - antidepressants.
     - anticonvulsants.
     - amphetamines.
     - muscle relaxants.
   - nonpharmacologic measures:
     - thermal (heat, cold).
     - transcutaneous electrical nerve stimulation (TENS).
     - mechanical (massage).
     - cognitive-behavioral methods (e.g., distraction, guided imagery, relaxation, hypnosis, biofeedback).
4. Teach patient to report all pain to nurse or physician so that treatment may be initiated before development of severe pain.
5. Explain that pain intensity will be measured using one of several available scales, including:
   - Numerical Rating Scale (e.g., 1 to 10, "0" indicating no pain, "10" indicating the worst pain imaginable).
   - Visual Analog Scale (a 10 cm line representing pain intensity. The patient marks an "x" on a spot on the line that represents his or her pain intensity).
   - Verbal Descriptor Scales (e.g., several words ranked to indicate pain intensity, including "none," "mild," "moderate," "severe," and "unbearable."
6. Explain that addiction is almost nonexistent in the treatment of pain resulting from cancer. Tolerance occurs but is managed easily in most patients with increases in narcotic dosages.
7. Teach that knowledge of the anticipated diagnostic and treatment procedures reduces discomfort and includes:
   - basic description of the procedure and its purpose.
   - equipment used.
   - sensations likely to be experienced.
   - anticipated duration of discomfort.
   - measures that will be used to reduce discomfort.
8. Explain that knowledge of the cause of the pain, the usual oral medication schedule, and the possible side effects associated with the pain medication allows for greater understanding and improved analgesia.

9. Discuss that knowledge of anticipated technologies to reduce or relieve pain, including TENS, patient-controlled analgesia (PCA) devices, and ambulatory infusion pumps for IV, SQ, or epidural administration reduces anxiety, allows for greater understanding, ultimately provides better analgesia. Important aspects include:
- basic description of the techniques and their purpose.
- equipment used.
- sensations likely to be experienced.

LEVEL 2: *Acute Pain*

EXPECTED OUTCOME

1. Patient/caregiver demonstrate knowledge related to alteration in comfort (acute pain):
   - identify source of pain.
   - verbalize plan to report changes in pain, intensity, quality.
   - describe physiologic, sensory, affective, cognitive, behavioral components of their pain experience.
2. Patient/caregiver demonstrate knowledge of measures to minimize perception of pain:
   - participate in prescribed therapy aimed at reducing tumor.
   - identify and demonstrate specific interventions to manage pain.
   - verbalize expected outcomes of pain interventions.
3. Patient achieves control of pain to an intensity that is acceptable:
   - verbalizes to nurse or physician that pain is adequately controlled.
   - participates in desired activities.
   - returns to previous levels of physiologic and psychologic function (e.g., concentration, motivation, autonomic responses).
   - exhibits absence or correction of potential and predictable side effects of pain management program.

NURSING MANAGEMENT

Assessment

1. See Assessment, Level 1.
2. Observe patient's general appearance and behavior and record presence of
   - facial grimace.
   - guarding of a body area.
   - anxiety.
3. Determine autonomic responses, although these vital signs generally return to baseline in persons who have pain for extended periods of time:
   - elevation in blood pressure, pulse, respiratory rate.
   - diaphoresis.
   - pupillary dilation.
4. Inspect painful area for erythema, inflammation, drainage, or other deviations.
5. Auscultate the painful area for deviation from normal sounds.

6. Percuss the adjacent area and the painful area very gently to assess:
   - location, size, intensity of pain.
   - quality of sounds elicited (e.g., dullness)
7. Palpate the adjacent area, then the painful area for:
   - location, quality, intensity of pain elicited.
8. If neurologic deficit is suspected, assess sensory perception, muscle strength, reflex response, and coordination.
9. Assess effect current pain therapies have on:
   - bowel and bladder elimination.
   - cognitive function.
   - sleep.
   - ability to eat.
   - physical activity.
   - socialization and communication.
   - sexual activity.
10. Assess impact that pain and the therapy has made on patient's quality of life.
11. Continue to perform complete pain assessment, as well as response to pain therapies, on a continuous schedule.

Nursing Interventions

1. Develop a trusting, professional relationship with patient/caregiver.
2. Plan and coordinate therapeutic plan to relieve pain with patient/caregiver and other health care professionals, including:
   - findings of pain assessment.
   - choice of pharmacologic/nonpharmacologic therapies, including choice of drug, dosage, route, schedule, mechanism of delivery (e.g., PCA, ambulatory pumps).
3. Implement measures to reduce pain perception when patient is unable to do so, or assist patient/caregiver in carrying out pain management plan, including:
   - administer analgesics on time.
   - titrate medication dosage/frequency within prescribed parameters. If relief is not satisfactory to patient, seek change in drug, dosage, or frequency from prescribing health care professional. Use an accepted equianalgesic table to calculate equal doses when changing from another drug.
   - minimize negative environmental stimuli.
   - administer cutaneous stimulation (e.g., massage painful area).
   - assist patient with guided imagery, relaxation techniques, distraction.
   - facilitate use of TENS units or biofeedback if appropriate.
4. Implement measures to manage or reduce side effects of pharmacologic therapy, including:
   - avoid long-term use of agents that may lead to adverse effects (e.g., meperidine or narcotic agonists or antagonists).
   - initiate measures to promote adequate bowel and bladder function.
   - institute measures to prevent or minimize nausea and vomiting.
   - implement interventions to reduce sedation. (If receiving good pain relief, reduce the dosage of narcotic and assess if pain relief continues. If pain returns upon reducing dosage, change to different narcotic or add a low-dose amphetamine in the morning. Implement safety measures).
   - report to physician respiratory depression (<8 breaths/min and evidence of poor perfusion), disorientation, hallucinations, inability to arouse patient, neuromuscular flaccidity, agitation, nausea, emesis.
   - in the rare event of respiratory depression:
     ○ stimulate the patient to breathe by shaking.
     ○ administer Naloxone only on an emergency basis. Titrate the dosage of Naloxone by diluting the drug in 10 ml of fluid and administer until respiratory rate returns to normal. Patients who have received narcotics for an extended period of time may

develop withdrawal symptoms (e.g., agitation, pruritus, rhinorrhea).
- monitor patient frequently. The duration of Naloxone is approximately 45 minutes to 1 hour. Because the duration of action of most narcotics is longer, respiratory depression may recur when the action of Naloxone is complete.

5. Discuss therapeutic plan for reducing pain and managing side effects with all health care professionals caring for the patient.
6. Evaluate the effectiveness of therapeutic plan and communicate with appropriate health care professionals (e.g., physicians, nurses, physical and occupational therapists).
7. Document the therapeutic plan, the evaluation of its effectiveness, side effects of the therapy, and patient's/caregiver's ability to implement the plan.
8. Administer therapies aimed at reducing the size of the tumor (e.g., chemotherapy, radiotherapy, biologic response modifiers).

Patient Teaching

1. See Patient Teaching, Level 1.
2. Explain that acute pain is of short duration, with anticipated resolution when underlying cause is successfully treated.
3. Discuss probable physiologic causes of acute pain that are specific to the patient:
   - tumor infiltration of bone, nerve, hollow viscus, or retroperitoneum.
   - altered body functions not directly related to cancer (e.g., abdominal distension due to constipation, preexisting conditions such as arthritis).
   - inflammation, infection, tumor necrosis.
   - effects of cancer therapy (e.g., incisional pain, stomatitis).
4. Discuss factors influencing medication effectiveness including:
   - choice of drug.
   - route of administration.

- dosage.
- frequency of administration.
- schedule of drug administration (e.g., around the clock [ATC] vs. as needed [PRN]).
- onset and duration of action.
- mechanism of action.

5. Instruct the patient on the "analgesic ladder."
   - Mild pain (use nonopioid drugs such as aspirin, or other NSAIDs).
   - Moderate pain (add a weak opioid, such as codeine, to the NSAID. Adjuvant drugs, such as anticonvulsants or antidepressants, may be given).
   - Severe pain (use a strong narcotic, such as morphine, hydromorphone HCl, levorphanol tartrate, or methadone. May also use a NSAID and an adjuvant drug).
6. Recommend measures to manage side effects of analgesics (refer to Nursing Interventions, Level 2, Step 4).
7. Instruct patient/caregiver regarding function and troubleshooting of any devices used in pain therapy (e.g., PCA pumps, ambulatory pumps).
8. Educate patient/caregiver regarding the antitumor effect, potentially reducing pain perception, of chemotherapy, biologic therapy, radiotherapy, and surgery.
9. Recommend educational community resources to patient/caregiver regarding the management of pain.

SUGGESTED READINGS

American Pain Society: Principles of Analgesic Use in the Treatment of Acute Pain and Chronic Cancer Pain: A Concise Guide to Medical Practice. Washington, DC, American Pain Society, 1987.

Cleeland, C.S.: The impact of pain on the patient with cancer. Cancer 54(11):2635–2641, 1984.

Coyle, N., Mauskop, A., Maggard, J., and Foley, K.: Continuous subcutaneous infusions of opiates in cancer patients with pain. Oncology Nursing Forum 13(4):53–57, 1986.

Donovan, M. (Ed.): Pain control. Nursing Clinics of North America 22(3):645–741, 1987.

Dorrepaal, K.L., Aaronson, N.K., and van Dam, F.S.A.M.: Pain experience and pain management among hospitalized cancer patients: A clinical study. Cancer 63(3): 593–598, 1989.

Fields, H.L.: Pain. New York, McGraw-Hill, 1987.

Foley, K.M.: The treatment of cancer pain. New England Journal of Medicine 313(2):84–95, 1985.

Kaiko, R.F., Foley, K.M., Grabinski, P.Y., et al.: Central nervous system excitatory effects of meperidine in cancer patients. Annals of Neurology 13(2):180–185, 1983.

Kane, N.E., Lehman, M.E., Dugger, R., et al.: Use of patient-controlled analgesia in surgical oncology patients. Oncology Nursing Forum 15(1):29–32, 1988.

McCaffery, M, and Beebe, A.: Pain: Clinical Manual for Nursing Practice. St. Louis, C.V. Mosby, 1989.

McGuire, D.B. (Ed.): Cancer pain. Seminars in Oncology Nursing 1(2):81–150, 1985.

McGuire, D.B., and Yarbro, C.H.: Cancer pain management. Orlando, FL, Grune & Stratton, 1987.

Payne, R., and Foley, K.M. (Eds.): Cancer Pain. Medical Clinics of North America 712:153–352, 1987.

Spiegel, K., Kalb, R., and Pasternak, G.W.: Analgesic activity of tricyclic antidepressants. Annals of Neurology 13(4):462–465, 1983.

World Health Organization: Cancer Pain Relief. Geneva, World Health Organization, 1986.

PATIENT EDUCATION MATERIALS AND COMMUNITY RESOURCES

Dubner R., and Max M.: Relieving Pain. Office of Clinical Center Communications, National Institutes of Health, Building 10, Room 1C255, 9000 Rockville Pike, Bethesda, MD 20892. 301–496–2563, 1988.

Cancer Pain Can Be Relieved: A Guide for Patients and Families. Wisconsin Cancer Pain Initiative, 3675 Medical Sciences Center, University of Wisconsin Medical School, 1300 University Avenue, Madison, WI 53706, 1988.

Questions and Answers about Pain Control: A Guide for People with Cancer and Their Families. Developed by the National Cancer Institute. Distributed by local divisions of the American Cancer Society, Inc. 1983.

Melzack, R., Paris, P., and Rogers, A.: How to Talk to Your Doctor about Acute Pain. Du Pont Pharmaceuticals, Medical Products Department, Wilmington, DE 19898, 1987.

Rogers, A.: Coping with Pain at Home: A Guide for Cancer Patients and Their Families. Du Pont Pharmaceuticals, Biomedical Products Department, Wilmington, DE 19898, 1986.

Twycross, R., and Tack, S.: Oral Morphine: Information for Patients, Families and Friends. Roxane Laboratories, Columbus, OH 43216, 1987.

Alteration in Comfort: Chronic Pain

Saundra J. Willoughby

Population at Risk

- Individuals living with cancer who are experiencing tumor infiltration of the bone, soft tissue, neural tissue, or a hollow viscus
- Individuals who have received cancer treatment with surgery, radiation therapy, or chemotherapy
- Individuals who have experienced herpes zoster

LEVEL 1: Potential Pain

EXPECTED OUTCOME

1. Patient demonstrates knowledge related to potential alteration in comfort:
   - verbalizes that pain is a protective mechanism or warning sign.
   - identifies personal physiologic, psychosocial, spiritual factors that influence the perception of pain and its treatment.
   - verbalizes importance of reporting changes in comfort state.
   - identifies factors and situations that may induce pain.
2. Patient demonstrates knowledge of measures that minimize the development and perception of pain:
   - participates in prescribed tumor treatment.
   - verbalizes that there are a variety of methods available to control pain.
   - verbalizes/demonstrates measures to prevent pain specific to individual situation.
   - participates in at least one noninvasive method of reducing stress and pain.

NURSING MANAGEMENT

Assessment

1. Assess patient's medical history, emphasizing course of illness and treatment.
2. Identify areas of potential pain (e.g., pain implications of planned treatment modalities, potential metastatic sites).
3. Determine patient's previous experiences with pain, including:
   - circumstances of onset and duration.
   - location and radiation.
   - intensity.
   - quality.
   - aggravating factors (e.g., eating, activity, separation from significant others).
   - alleviating factors (e.g., medications, distraction, meditation and prayer).
   - associated physiologic manifestations, (e.g., palpitations, dyspnea, neurologic dysfunction).

4. Evaluate meaning of pain to patient (e.g., recurrence of disease, death, punishment by God).
5. Assess patient's fears and perceptions regarding anticipated pain and pain therapy (e.g., fear of addiction).

Nursing Intervention

1. Encourage patient to select a noninvasive method of reducing stress and pain.
2. Establish setting in which patient can practice self-selected noninvasive method.
3. Arrange for appropriate health care professional to provide patient instruction regarding noninvasive methods that are not in your area of expertise after consulting with physician (e.g., clinical nurse specialist, physical therapist, social worker, pastoral counselor, psychologist).

Patient Teaching

1. Teach that pain is a protective mechanism or warning sign indicating need to flee from the source of pain or to seek methods to heal the underlying problem.
2. Discuss experience of pain as highly individual and variable. Factors that influence the perception of pain include:
   • physiologic (e.g., sensory responses to physical injury).
   • psychosocial (e.g., loss of roles, fear of medical procedures, anxiety, depression).
   • spiritual (e.g., loss of meaning in life, punishment by God, faith that God will sustain strength).
3. Teach that pain usually can be controlled to a tolerable level (as defined by patient) using one or more invasive/noninvasive methods.
4. Explain that pain is real, although medical science may at times have difficulty immediately establishing the physiologic cause (e.g., bone pain may precede visu-

alization of tumor on x-ray by as much as 3 months).
5. Instruct patient to report all pain to nurse or physician so that treatment may be initiated.
6. Teach that the primary treatment of cancer pain is to prevent tumor growth or reduce tumor burden by treating the disease (e.g., surgery, chemotherapy, radiation therapy).
7. Provide information regarding the multiple medications to treat pain related to cancer including:
   • nonopioid analgesics.
   • opioid analgesics.
   • antidepressants.
   • muscle relaxants.
   • anticonvulsants.
   • tranquilizers.
8. Explain that pain may be related to a physiologic problem other than cancer that requires medical intervention (e.g., bowel distention with flatus, angina).
9. Discuss noninvasive methods that assist in prevention or amelioration of pain and stress including:
   • distraction (e.g., music, reading, crafts).
   • imagery (guided by self, family member, audiotapes).
   • prayer and meditation (individual or group).
   • exercises (e.g., moderate daily exercise routine, range-of-motion exercises).
   • psychosocial counseling (e.g., social worker, psychologist, psychiatrist).
   • spiritual counseling (e.g., pastoral counselor or therapist).
10. Medication to control pain ideally should be given orally.
11. Inform patient that although tolerance to narcotic analgesics (and their side effects) may develop, psychological addiction is essentially nonexistent in the treatment of cancer pain apparently due to the antagonistic effect of pain against the narcotic (as evidenced by patient reduction of drugs as tumor burden decreases).

12. Provide information regarding the anticipated diagnostic and treatment procedures to reduce discomfort including:
    - basic description of the procedure and its purpose.
    - equipment used.
    - sensations likely to be experienced.
    - anticipated duration of discomfort.
    - measures that will be used to reduce discomfort.

LEVEL 2: Mild to Moderate Chronic Pain

EXPECTED OUTCOME

1. Patient/caregiver demonstrate knowledge of altered comfort, mild to moderate chronic pain related to disease process/previous cancer therapy:
   - identify source of pain.
   - identify characteristics of chronic pain.
   - identify difference between baseline pain and breakthrough pain.
   - identify potentially debilitating impact on normal life functions.
   - verbalize plan to report changes in pain intensity or character.
   - identify personal physiologic, psychosocial, spiritual aspects of life that have been altered as a result of living with chronic pain.
2. Patient/caregiver demonstrate knowledge of measures to manage chronic pain:
   - participate in prescribed therapy.
   - identify/demonstrate specific interventions to manage pain.
   - verbalize expected outcome of pain interventions.
   - verbalize/demonstrate measures to modify personal, physiologic, psychological, social, or spiritual factors that influence perception of pain or its treatment.
   - verbalize signs and symptoms of potential side effects associated with prescribed analgesic/adjuvant medications.
3. Patient personally achieves satisfactory control of pain:
   - verbalizes to nurse or physician that pain is adequately controlled.
   - participates in desired activities, including return to baseline, physical, psychologic, social, spiritual, sexual, and cognitive functions and patterns.
   - exhibits absence and correction of potential and predictable side effects of pain management program.

NURSING MANAGEMENT

Assessment

1. See Assessment, Level 1.
2. Assess patient's current pain experience including:
   - onset.
   - quality (e.g., dull ache, burning, piercing).
   - location and radiation.
   - intensity and severity of pain as rated

by the patient on a scale of 1 to 10 with extremes of variation (e.g., ranges from 3 to 6).

- frequency of baseline pain and breakthrough pain (e.g., occurs continuously at a level 3 with level 6 intensity 5 times per day).
- aggravating factors (e.g., position change, bowel and bladder elimination, activity).
- alleviating factors (e.g., distraction, massage, application of cold or heat, physical exercise, relaxation exercises, prayer and meditation).
- perception of pain impact on normal life function (e.g., inability to concentrate, limited activity, interference with relationships with others, anorexia, loss of sleep).
- goals and desired level of pain control using a rating scale (e.g., to have uninterrupted sleep at night, pain generally not greater than level 1).

3. Assess family's response to patient's continuing experience with pain (e.g., anger, withdrawal, sympathy, anxiety.)
4. Assess family dynamics and stressors that may be contributing to or decreasing patient's pain (e.g., role changes, psychosocial or spiritual conflict.)
5. Assess patient's use of medications for pain relief including:
   - specific medication (e.g., nonopioid or opioid analgesics, adjuvant drugs) and effectiveness.
   - patterns of medication request and self-administration related to intensity of pain (e.g., 24- to 48-hour record that ideally includes time of request, rating of pain intensity, specific medication used, activity, level of consciousness, blood pressure, pulse, respirations).
6. Identify current prescribed antineoplastic palliative therapy planned or in progress (e.g., radiation therapy, chemotherapy, surgery).
7. Obtain patient's history regarding usual patterns of:
   - bowel and bladder elimination.

- cognitive function.
- communication.
- sleep.
- socialization.
- physical activity.
- sexual activity.
- religious activity.

8. Observe patient's general appearance and behavior for:
   - ability to give detailed description of pain experience.
   - emotional depression (e.g., flat affect, withdrawal, apathy).
   - signs and symptoms of transient increased pain intensity (e.g., facial grimace, guarding of an area, anxiety, crying).
9. Assess level of consciousness (e.g., orientation to person, place, time, reality).
10. Assess presence or absence of autonomic responses including:
    - change in blood pressure.
    - tachycardia.
    - increased respiratory rate.
    - diaphoresis.
    - pupillary dilatation.
11. Inspect painful area for:
    - color (e.g., erythema, blanching).
    - deviation from normal structural appearance.
12. Auscultate the painful area, if located in a cavitary region, for deviation from normal sounds.
13. Percuss the adjacent area and then painful area to assess:
    - location and intensity of pain elicited.
    - quality of sounds elicited.
    - size (e.g., measure the area of dullness).
14. Palpate the adjacent area, then painful area for:
    - location and intensity of pain elicited.
    - configuration (of mass or lesion).
    - size.
15. If neurologic deficit is suspected, assess sensory perception, muscle strength, and reflex response.
16. Until desired level of pain control is achieved, use 24-hour pain assessment

tool that may be completed by patient/caregiver and evaluate the following on a regular basis (e.g., every shift in the hospital, daily in the home setting):
- general appearance and behavior.
- level of consciousness and cognitive function.
- location, intensity, quality of pain.
- aggravating and alleviating factors.
- duration of response to pain treatment.
- vital signs.
- bowel and bladder elimination patterns.
- communication pattern.
- sleep pattern.
- socialization.
- physical activity and neuromuscular function.
- religious activity.

17. Following initiation of primary treatment of the tumor, inspect, auscultate, percuss, and palpate the painful area on a regular basis.
18. Evaluate patient's perception of pain as compared with increasing or decreased tumor size.
19. After desired level of pain control is achieved, assess patient at regular intervals for:
- side effects of analgesic and adjuvant medications.
- decreased effectiveness of pain management program.

Nursing Interventions

1. Establish a trusting relationship with the patient, communicating your recognition that the pain is real and that the goal of the health care team is to bring the pain under control.
2. During the first 24 to 48 hours of pain assessment and intervention:
- administer the prescribed analgesics/adjuvant drugs promptly upon patient request, within the prescribed parameters.
- record the drug, time of administration, patient rating of pain intensity, associated pain manifestations.
- record response to intervention (e.g., pulse, respiration, blood pressure, sleep or relaxation).
- titrate medication dosage within prescribed parameters.

3. Following initial assessment:
- calculate the total 24-hour milligram dosage of each prescribed medication used.
- consult with physician regarding assessment findings making recommendations for regular interval scheduling of baseline analgesic/adjuvant drugs.
- initiate around-the-clock regular administration of baseline analgesic/adjuvant drugs, record patient responses.
- continue administration of prn analgesics promptly upon patient request with appropriate record notation.

4. Implement noninvasive measures to alter patient's perception of pain according to patient's preference:
- minimize negative environmental stimuli.
- assist patient with guided imagery (e.g., describe a peaceful setting and place the patient in it).
- assist patient with deep breathing and muscle relaxation exercises.
- discuss use of prayer and meditation.
- suggest distraction measures (e.g., listening to a favorite tape recording, watching TV).
- administer cutaneous stimulation concurrent with administration of analgesics (e.g., massage the painful or adjacent area).

5. Implement physical measures to protect the patient from further injury (e.g., immobilization of painful extremity, back brace).
6. Administer prescribed chemotherapy.
7. Consult with physician to:
- report continuing assessment findings.
- report effectiveness of nursing measures initiated.

- identify possible causes of increased pain perception.
- make pain management recommendations requiring physician input (e.g., medication, social work counseling, physical therapy consult).

8. Implement measures to manage or reduce side effects of analgesics:
   - measures to promote bowel and bladder elimination.
   - measures to prevent nausea and vomiting.
   - measures that promote patient's return to normal patterns of cognition, sleep, communication, socialization, spiritual expression, sexuality.
   - measures to promote optimal neuromuscular function.
9. Recommend referral to home health care agency for continued nursing assessment of patient's/family's response to pain management program, and further teaching.

Patient Teaching

1. See Patient Teaching, Level 1.
2. Teach characteristics of chronic pain:
   - persisting beyond the expected healing time.
   - difficulty ascribing the pain to effects of a specific injury.
   - absence of autonomic nervous system response to pain (e.g., sweating, tachycardia, pupillary dilatation).
   - associated manifestations of changes in personality, life style, functional ability, depression (hopelessness, helplessness, loss of libido and appetite, sleep disturbances).
3. Discuss successful management of chronic pain that requires time for thorough assessment of:
   - physiologic history and current status (e.g., determination of the underlying cause of the pain).
   - personal, physical, psychosocial, spiritual factors that may be contributing to the pain.

- family's psychosocial and spiritual stressors.
- response to the various methods used to manage the pain.

4. Teach pathophysiology associated with the chronic pain syndrome(s) specific to the patient:
   - tumor infiltration of the bone, soft tissue, neural tissue, or a hollow viscus.
   - postsurgical pain syndrome.
   - postchemotherapy pain syndrome.
   - postradiation therapy pain syndrome.
   - postherpetic neuralgia.
   - altered body functions not directly related to cancer or cancer therapy (e.g., angina, arthritis).
5. Inform patient that if tumor infiltration is the suspected cause of chronic pain and potential for tumor response to traditional therapy exists, surgery, chemotherapy/radiation therapy may be recommended in conjunction with other pain relief measures.
6. Provide information regarding analgesic medications used to control mild to moderate chronic pain that include nonopioids (e.g., acetaminophen, nonsteroidal, antiinflammatory drugs) and weak opioids (e.g., codeine, Darvocet, Percodan, Vicodin). Nonopioids and mild opioids are often prescribed in combination because their mode of action differs (e.g., nonopioids act at the site of injury to block transmission of pain impulses or to decrease the inflammatory response; opioids act in the CNS to decrease the perception of pain).
7. Discuss adjuvant drugs, which may be prescribed although their mechanism of action to induce pain relief is not always well-known, including:
   - antidepressants (e.g., tricyclics especially for pain associated with nerve injury).
   - muscle relaxants (e.g., Valium, Norflex to control muscle spasms).
   - anticonvulsants (e.g., Tegretol, Dilantin especially for neuralgias, phantom

limb pain, pain described as burning or stabbing).
- tranquilizers (e.g., Ativan, Valium, Xanax to decrease anxiety).
8. Teach specific side effects of all medications prescribed for pain management and measures to manage side effects of medications (e.g., antiemetics, stool softeners, laxatives, increased roughage in diet).
   - sedation is a common side effect for the first 24 to 72 hours of successful pain management resulting from previous sleep deprivation associated with chronic pain.
9. Inform patient that before, during, and after chronic pain is successfully managed, patient will be asked to describe the pain using a pain assessment tool or format (see Assessment, Level 2, step 16) that assists the health care team to determine if the pain management program is achieving a level of pain control consistent with the patient's goal.
10. Discuss administration schedule with patient/caregiver:
    - initially pain medications will be administered as needed within the prescribed frequency and dosage.
    - as pain control is achieved, medications may be prescribed to be taken regularly, around the clock to control baseline pain (pain occurring 12 or more hours per day).

- some medications will still be prescribed to be taken as needed for breakthrough pain (e.g., transient increased severity of pain that may be precipitated by movement, bowel or bladder elimination, medical procedures, temporary altered physical function such as bowel distention with flatus).
11. Teach specific techniques for facilitating pain management using noninvasive measures and behaviors (see Nursing Interventions, Level 2, step 4):
    - Description of potential benefits of counseling through social work, psychology, clergy to decrease patient and family stressors associated with chronic pain (may require physician's order).
    - description of potential benefit of physical therapy intervention (e.g., application of TENS units, modified exercise program, back brace):
12. Inform patient/caregiver of the need to report changes in pain intensity and frequency and all side effects to the physician or nurse to maintain safe and effective pain management.
13. Discuss potential benefit of follow-up intervention by a nurse in the home setting through a home health care agency.

LEVEL 3:   Severe Chronic Pain

EXPECTED OUTCOME

1. Patient/caregiver demonstrate knowledge of altered comfort, severe chronic pain related to disease process/previous cancer therapy:
   - identify source of pain.
   - identify characteristics of chronic pain.
   - identify difference between baseline pain and breakthrough pain.
   - identify potentially debilitating impact on normal life functions.

- verbalize plan to report changes in pain intensity or character.
- identify personal physiologic, psychosocial, spiritual aspects of life that have been altered as a result of living with chronic pain.

2. Patient/caregiver demonstrate knowledge of measures to manage severe chronic pain:
   - patient participates in prescribed therapy.
   - identify/demonstrate specific interventions to manage pain.
   - verbalize expected outcome of pain interventions.
   - verbalize/demonstrate measures to maintain safe administration of strong opioids via elected route.
   - verbalize/demonstrate measures to modify personal physiologic, psychological, social, spiritual factors that influence perception of pain or its treatment.
   - verbalize signs and symptoms of potential side effects associated with prescribed analgesics/adjuvant medications.

3. Patient personally achieves satisfactory control of pain:
   - verbalizes to nurse or physician that pain is adequately controlled.
   - participates in desired physical, psychosocial, spiritual, sexual, cognitive activities within limitations of underlying disease process.
   - exhibits absence or correction of potential and predictable side effects of pain management program.

NURSING MANAGEMENT

Assessment

1. See Assessment, Levels 1 and 2.
2. Assess patient/family ability to acquire knowledge and skill necessary to maintain safe administration of analgesics through most effective route of administration.
3. Assess willingness and financial ability of patient/family to adhere to prescribed pain management program.
4. Assess community resources for patient accessibility to prescribed medication(s) (e.g., pharmacy within a reasonable distance that supplies prescribed drugs; infusion company for supplies, drugs, and equipment).
5. During first 2 hours of continuous opioid infusion, assess patient's response:
   - every 30 minutes for subcutaneous route.
   - every 15 to 30 minutes for intravenous route.
   - every 30 minutes for intrathecal or epidural (intraspinal) route.
6. Following the initial induction phase of opioid infusion:
   - assess vital signs, level of consciousness, patient's assessment of effectiveness of pain control every 4 hours until desired level is achieved.
   - assess for signs and symptoms of systemic infection (e.g., elevated temperature, tachycardia).
   - inspect insertion site for presence or absence of erythema, tenderness, swelling, local fever, drainage.

Nursing Interventions

1. See Nursing Interventions, Levels 1 and 2.
2. If subcutaneous, intravenous, or intraspinal infusion is the selected route of opioid administration:

- adhere to institutional/agency policies and procedures related to infusion administration via prescribed route (e.g., care of an indwelling intravascular or intraspinal access catheter or port, care of subcutaneous infusion device).
- arrange for the same models of equipment and supplies that will be used in the home, to be available for patient/caregiver instruction in the hospital.
- notify the home health care agency of patient's anticipated discharge and probable need for home visit on day of discharge (try to arrange patient discharge early in week to maximize potential for smooth transition from hospital to home).
- notify infusion company of anticipated discharge date to facilitate delivery of equipment and supplies to patient's home before discharge.
- recommend that physician prescribe short-acting equianalgesic opioid that can be administered orally, sublingually, or rectally in the event of infusion disruption.
- prioritize patient/caregiver instruction to ensure procedure competency relative to potential complications of infusion (e.g., starting and stopping the pump, irrigation of an intravascular catheter or port, knowledge of pump alarms and procedures to resolve or correct problems, reporting of pump disruption to nurse and infusion company).

3. If respiratory rate is less than 10 respirations per minute when patient is awake:
- assess level of consciousness for presence or absence of confusion.
- report change in patient's status to physician.
- decrease dosage of opioid as prescribed.
- monitor vital signs and level of consciousness every 15 minutes until normal level is achieved.
- be prepared to administer naloxone hydrochloride (dilute one ampule in 10 ml

of normal saline and administer slow intravenous push).

Patient Teaching

1. See Patient Teaching, Levels 1 and 2.
2. Discuss use of nonopioid drugs for severe chronic pain:
   - nonopioids/adjuvant drugs may be the most effective means of controlling severe chronic pain (e.g., NSAIDs for bone pain, anticonvulsants for pain secondary to nerve injury).
   - nonopioids/adjuvant drugs may be prescribed in combination with strong opioids to control severe chronic pain.
   - nonopioid analgesics and adjuvant drugs have known dosage and frequency limitations that must be adhered to in order to avoid toxic effects.
3. Teach use of strong opioids for severe chronic pain:
   - recent research has indicated that some strong opioids (e.g., morphine, hydromorphone), analgesics are dosage-limited only by the exhibition of undesirable or toxic side effects for the individual patient (e.g., myoclonic jerking, nausea and vomiting, confusion, seizure activity, sedation, respiratory depression). Severe chronic pain may serve as an antagonist to counteract toxic effects such as respiratory depression (e.g., less than 10 respirations per minute while awake and alert).
   - dosage and frequency of opioids are increased (e.g., every 24 to 48 hours) to reduce potential for undesired side effects and to obtain accurate assessment of full analgesic effect.
   - rapid reduction of strong opioids, whether intentional (e.g., reluctance to take the medication) or accidental (e.g., occlusion of infusion tubing) may produce symptoms of physical withdrawal (e.g., nausea and vomiting,

abdominal cramping, severe anxiety, diaphoresis, seizures).

- if signs and symptoms of physical withdrawal occur, report immediately to physician or nurse to facilitate prompt intervention.

4. Discuss route of administration that is determined by:

- ability to ingest and absorb adequate quantities of analgesics to control baseline pain.
- ability of patient/caregiver to acquire knowledge of safe administration for the elected route. Note that MS Contin is not effective as a timed-release tablet if crushed.
- availability of support programs in community to maintain safe administration (e.g., skilled nurse from a home health care agency, infusion company for supplies, drugs, equipment).

5. Teach potential routes of opioid administration that include oral, sublingual, rectal, continuous subcutaneous, and intravenous infusion with bolus, continuous, or intermittent intraspinal administration.

- intermittent subcutaneous and intramuscular administration are *not* recommended due to resultant peak and valley effects.

6. Discuss the schedule for administration of pain medication:

- difference between short-acting opioids (begin to control pain within 30 minutes, last 2 to 4 hours) long-acting opioids (peak in about 2 hours, generally last for 6 to 12 hours).
- during initial period of severe chronic pain assessment and intervention, immediate-release or short-acting strong opioids will be administered orally, subcutaneously, or intravenously within prescribed dosage and frequency.
- when control of baseline pain is achieved, prescribed analgesic will probably be converted to slow-release or long-acting strong opioid (e.g., MS

Contin, Roxanol SR, methadone) that is taken on a regular schedule around the clock to facilitate a more consistent control of the pain. Short-acting analgesics will also be prescribed for breakthrough pain.

7. Explain that if morphine is the drug selected, nausea is a common side effect for the first 72 hours and does *not* necessarily indicate an allergic reaction. Efforts will be made to control nausea with antiemetic until tolerance to this side effect develops.

8. Discuss that if swallowing is not feasible, short-acting strong opioids may be administered sublingually or rectally (e.g., after inserting tablet in gelatin capsule, morphine and hydromorphone are available in suppository form), but this requires frequent, regular administration and may result in peak and valley effects as well as sleep deprivation.

9. Provide general instruction for infusion therapy:

- name and phone number of home health care agency.
- name of infusion company with 24-hour telephone number for emergency service.
- irrigation of intravascular catheter or port upon discontinuance of infusion.
- operation of the pump including start and stop, warning signals (e.g., occluded line, air in line), and how to manage the problem.
- bolus administration including prescribed frequency, need to press button as frequently as needed to assist with assessment process.
- cleansing of the insertion site and dressing changes (may be deferred to the home health care nurse).
- changing the tubing and pouch/cassette that contains medication using aseptic technique.
- programming the pump.
- titration of medication within prescribed parameters.
- universal precautions when handling

and disposing of needles and other contaminated supplies.

10. Provide information regarding subcutaneous infusions:
    - advantage as an infusion method is that it does not require a port.
    - technique for aseptically inserting needle subcutaneously (may be deferred to home care nurse).
    - rotation of needle insertion sites.
    - observe for signs and symptoms of subcutaneous plaque formation (e.g., erythema, leakage, pain, swelling, induration) necessitating needle site change.
    - change needle insertion site every 7 days or more often as needed.
    - bolus injection requires 30 minutes to reach peak effect (e.g., administer 30 minutes prior to activity that is known to produce breakthrough pain.

11. Provide information regarding intravascular infusions:
    - signs and symptoms of systemic or local infection to report to the nurse or physician (see Assessment, Level 3, step 4).
    - signs and symptoms of needle displacement from the port to report to the nurse or physician.
    - bolus injection requires 6 to 10 minutes to reach peak effect.

12. Provide information regarding intraspinal infusions:
    - only nonpreservative injectable medications can be used because of potential irritation of the meninges; check the labels.
    - signs and symptoms of needle displacement from the port (e.g., swelling and erythema, pump alarm indicates occlusion although tubing appears unobstructed) to report to the nurse or physician.
    - signs and symptoms of local infection, meningitis, encephalitis to report to the nurse or physician.
    - bolus injection requires 30 to 60 minutes to reach peak effect.

- preparation for and insertion of needle into port, or insertion of an indwelling catheter should be performed by a skilled nurse or physician (exception may be considered if caregiver in home repeatedly demonstrates adherence to sterile technique and expresses willingness to become independent with this procedure).

13. Discuss neurologic procedures including cordotomy, rhizotomy, sympathetic nerve block as alternative treatment options that alter perception of pain by disrupting sensory neuron pathway.

14. Provide information regarding other community resources for the management of severe chronic pain including hospice, pain clinics, palliative care units.

SUGGESTED READINGS

Adams, F., Cruz, L., Dreachman, M.J., and Zamora, E.: Focal subdermal toxicity with subcutaneous opioid infusion in patients with cancer pain. Journal of Pain and Symptom Management 4(1):31–33, 1989.

Barbour, L.A., McGuire, D.B., and Kirchoff, K.T.: Nonanalgesic methods of pain control used by cancer outpatients. Oncology Nursing Forum 13(6):56–60, 1986.

Blue, C.L., and Purath, J.: Home care of the epidural analgesia patient: The nurse's role. Home Healthcare Nurse 7(4):23–30, 1989.

Brena, S.F., and Chapman, S.L.: Management of Patients with Chronic Pain. New York, Spectrum Publications, Inc., 1983.

Bruera, E., Brennies, C., and MacDonald, R.: Continuous SQ infusion of narcotics for the treatment of cancer pain: An update. Cancer Treatment Reports 71(10):953–958, 1987.

Coyle, N., Mauskop, A., Maggard, J., and Foley, K.M.: Continuous subcutaneous infusions of opiates in cancer patients with pain. Oncology Nursing Forum 13(4):53–57, 1986.

Dupen, S.L., Peterson, D.G., Bogosian, A.C., et al.: A new permanent exteriorized epidural catheter for narcotic self-administration to control cancer pain. Cancer 59(5):986–993, 1987.

Ferrell, B., and Schneider, C.: Experience and management of cancer pain at home. Cancer Nursing 11(2):84–90, 1988.

Ferrell, B., Wisdom, C., Wenzl, C., and Brown, J.: Effects of controlled-release morphine on quality of life for cancer pain. Oncology Nursing Forum 16:521–526, 1989.

141

Johanson, G.A.: Physicians' handbook of symptom relief in terminal care. Santa Rosa, 1988. (Available from Home Hospice of Sonoma County, 558 "B" Street, Santa Rose, CA 95401).

Kendrick, E.D.: Pain: A review of physiology and management options. Home Healthcare Nurse 7(6):9–17, 1989.

Lapin, J., Portenoy, R.K., Coyle, N., et al.: Guidelines for use of controlled-release morphine in cancer pain management: Correlation with clinical experience. Cancer Nursing 12(4):202–208, 1989.

Lindley, C.M., Dalton, J., and Fields, S.M.: Narcotic analgesics: Clinical pharmacology and therapeutics. Cancer Nursing 13(1):28–38, 1990.

Loescher, L.J., Welch-McCaffrey, D., Leigh, S.A., et al.: Surviving adult cancers. Part 1: Physiologic effects. Annals of Internal Medicine 111:411–432, 1989.

McCaffery, M.: Patient-controlled analgesia: More than a machine. Nursing 17(11):62–64, 1987.

McCaffery, M., and Beebe, A.: Pain: Clinical Manual for Oncology Nursing. St. Louis, C.V. Mosby, 1989.

McCaffery, M., Ferrell, B., O'Neil-Page, E., and Lester, M.: Nurses' knowledge of opioid analgesic drugs and psychological dependence. Cancer Nursing 13(1):20–27, 1990.

Melzack, R., and Wall, P.: The challenge of pain. New York, Basic Books, 1982.

Miaskowski, C.: Pain management. In Supportive Care for the Patient with Cancer. Valley College, NY, 1988. (Available from Oncology Nursing Society, 1016 Greentree Road, Pittsburgh, PA 15220-3125.)

Oates, W.E., and Oates, C.E.: People in Pain: Guidelines for Pastoral Care. Philadelphia, Westminster Press, 1985.

Paice, J.A.: Cancer pain management: When side effects occur. In Miaskowski, C.A. (Moderator): Oncology Nursing Perspectives: Management of Treatment-induced Side Effects. Symposium presented in San Francisco, 1989. (Available from Smith Kline & French Laboratories).

Paice, J.A.: Intrathecal morphine infusion for intractable cancer pain: A new use for implanted pumps. Oncology Nursing Forum 13(3):41–47, 1986.

Portenoy, R.K.: Continuous infusion of opioid drugs in the treatment of cancer pain: Guidelines for use. Journal of Pain and Symptom Management 1(4):223–228, 1986.

Portenoy, R.K., and Hagen, N.A.: Breakthrough pain: Definition and management. Oncology Special Supplement 3(6):25–30, 1989. (Available from Kominus Publishing Co., Inc., 331 Willis Avenue, PO Box 86, Williston Park, NY 11596.)

Principles of Analgesic Use in the Treatment of Acute Pain and Chronic Cancer Pain: A Concise Guide to Medical Practice. American Pain Society, 1987. (Available from American Pain Society, 1200 17th Street, NW, Suite 400, Washington DC 20036.)

Rankin, M.A. and Snider, B.: Nurses' perceptions of cancer patients' pain. Cancer Nursing 7:149–155, 1984.

Scheetz, J., and Shell, B.: Physical therapy in the symptomatic management of pain. Dimensions in Oncology Nursing 2(3):9–13, 1988.

Twycross, R.G.: Incidence of pain. Clinical Oncology 3(2):5–15, 1984.

Walsh, T.D.: Control of pain and other symptoms in advanced cancer. Oncology Special Supplement 1(2):1987. (Available from Dominus Publishing Co., Inc., 331 Willis Avenue, PO Box 86, Williston Park, NY 11596.)

Wilkie, D., Lovejoy, J., Dodd, M., and Tesler, M.: Cancer pain control behaviors: Description and correlation with pain intensity. Oncology Nursing Forum 15:723–731, 1988.

World Health Organization: Cancer Pain Relief, 1986. (Available from WHO Publications Center USA, 49 Sheridan Avenue, Albany, NY 12210.)

PATIENT EDUCATION MATERIALS AND COMMUNITY RESOURCES

Children's Cancer Pain Can be Relieved: A Guide for Parents and Families. 1989 (Available from the Wisconsin Cancer Pain Initiative.)

Melzack, R.: The tragedy of needless pain. Scientific American 262(2):27–33, 1990.

Twycross, R.G., and Lack, S.A.: Oral Morphine: Information for Patients, Families, and Friends. Beaconsfield, Bucks, England, Beaconsfield Publishers Ltd, 1987. (Available from Roxane Laboratories, Inc., Columbus, OH 43216.)

Alteration in Comfort: Pruritus

Mary Anne Bord, Noella Devolder McCray, and Suzanne Shaffer

24

Population at Risk

- Individuals with polycythemia vera, Hodgkin's disease, non-Hodgkin's lymphoma (including T-cell cutaneous), multiple myeloma, leukemia, malignant melanoma, adenocarcinoma, squamous cell carcinoma, inflammatory breast carcinoma, carcinoid syndrome, intracranial tumors involving the fourth ventricle, graft-versus-host disease, AIDS and AIDS-related Kaposi's sarcoma
- Individuals with treatment-related side effects: surgery, radiation, chemotherapy, biotherapy, and opiate therapy
- Individuals with complications including iron deficiency anemia, renal failure, biliary obstruction
- Individuals with concurrent conditions including diabetes mellitus, mastocytosis, history of allergic dermatitis, psychogenic pruritus, pregnancy, advanced age

LEVEL 1: Potential

EXPECTED OUTCOME

1. Patient identifies personal factors that predispose to pruritus.
2. Patient exhibits nonirritated, healthy skin.
3. Patient demonstrates knowledge of measures to promote and maintain skin health:
   - identifies measures to promote good skin hydration.
   - describes good fluid and nutritional intake.
   - identifies possible skin irritants.

NURSING MANAGEMENT

Assessment

1. Assess fluid and nutritional status.
2. Evaluate skin care practices.
3. Assess skin turgor, texture, color, temperature, and lesions.
4. Determine presence of pruritus risk factors (e.g., previous radiation therapy or biliary obstruction).
5. Obtain relevant laboratory data based on assessment.

Patient Teaching

1. Teach signs and symptoms of skin changes to report to health care team (e.g., dryness, jaundice, rash, lesions, itch).
2. Explain rationale and measures to maintain adequate nutrition and hydration.
3. Discuss rationale and measures to promote skin hydration:
   - emollients/protectants (e.g., Keri Lotion, Nivea Cream, Eucerin Cream.
   - mild soaps (e.g., Aveeno Bar).
   - importance of rinsing soap off well, especially after bed bath.

4. Describe rationale and measures to prevent skin irritation:
   - avoid harsh detergents.
   - avoid irritating, binding clothing.
   - wear soft cotton clothing.
   - use adhesives and dressings with caution.
   - avoid cold, wind, hot and dry conditions.
   - thoroughly wet skin before soap application.

LEVEL 2: Mild to Moderate

EXPECTED OUTCOME

1. Patient identifies/demonstrates measures to control pruritus:
   - identifies/demonstrates measures to promote hydration and nutrition.
   - eliminates skin irritants.
   - identifies/demonstrates appropriate relief measures.
   - demonstrates knowledge of medication administration.
   - maintains appropriate environmental conditions.
2. Patient reports relief of itching.
3. Patient maintains skin integrity.

NURSING MANAGEMENT

Assessment

1. See Assessment, Level 1.
2. Assess pruritus:
   - physical findings.
   - onset.
   - characteristics (e.g., continuous, burning).
   - factors that relieve or aggravate condition.
   - distribution and location.
   - treatment(s) used previously.

3. Identify possible causes and conditions.
4. Assess for allergic responses to medications.

Nursing Interventions

1. Prevent dry skin:
   - keep room humidity at 30 to 40%.
   - avoid frequent bathing.
   - avoid hot baths, showers, saunas, steam baths.

- avoid alkaline (e.g., lye-based soaps).
- use emollients and apply while skin is damp.
- protect from cold, wind, dry, and heat.

2. Prevent skin irritation:
   - avoid irritating clothing.
   - avoid irritating bed linen.
   - avoid use of harsh detergent and starch.
   - neutralize clothing and linen by rinsing in solution of 1 tsp vinegar per qt water.
   - avoid use of scented products on skin if there is known sensitivity.
   - use baking soda in place of deodorants.

3. Decrease potential for infection or trauma:
   - cut nails short.
   - clean hands and nails.
   - use mittens as needed, especially at night.

4. Decrease perspiration:
   - use cotton clothing to allow evaporation.
   - ensure adequate room ventilation and temperature.
   - change bed sheets frequently.
   - avoid exertion.

5. Prevent tissue hypoxia:
   - get adequate rest.
   - eat balanced diet with adequate iron, zinc, protein.
   - maintain adequate fluid intake.

6. Prevent vasodilation:
   - keep room temperature 60 to 70° F.
   - avoid alcohol, coffee, hot foods.
   - avoid hot baths.
   - treat fever.
   - treat hypoxemia.

7. Control anxiety:
   - provide enjoyable distraction.
   - offer positive suggestions rather than admonitions about scratching.
   - administer tranquilizers.
   - use purposeful relaxation techniques.

8. Employ relief measures:
   - use cool tap water, soaks and compresses.
   - place oil in bath water, or use Aveeno Colloidal Oatmeal baths.
   - apply emollient when skin is damp.
   - use rubbing, pressure, vibration instead of scratching.
   - control environment (e.g., humidity, temperature).

9. Administer medication and medical treatment as ordered (antihistamines, corticosteroids, antineoplastics, antibiotics, antidepressants, aspirin/cimetidine [for polycythemia vera], naloxone/cholestyramine [for cholestasis and uremia], or PUVA [psoralen plus long-wave ultraviolet]).

10. Apply topical agents properly:
    - powder (dry surface area before applications, light dusting).
    - lotion (firm stroke versus dabbing to obtain thin, even coat).
    - aerosol (prevent inhalation).
    - gel (apply as directed).
    - cream (may need to reapply if there is perspiration/drainage over area).
    - ointment (apply thin layer).

11. Employ general measures:
    - baths or soaks should precede application of topical agents.
    - if no baths or soaks have been ordered, gently wash site with mild, nondrying soap and warm water. For acutely inflamed skin, use warm water rinse only: pat skin dry or air dry. If skin is excessively dry, apply topical agents while damp.
    - use topical agents sparingly.
    - avoid use of starch-based powders in intertriginous eruptions infected with Candida.
    - avoid use of petroleum-based preparations in intertriginous areas.

12. Suspect allergic contact dermatitis when any dermatologic condition worsens after application of a topical agent.

Patient Teaching

1. See Patient Teaching, Level 1.

2. Substitute rubbing, pressure, vibration for scratching.
3. Teach hygienic measures to prevent contamination or trauma, including good handwashing and nail care.
4. Provide rationale and measures to control pruritus (see Nursing Interventions, Level 2).
5. Explain administration, scheduling, and side effects of medication.
6. Teach patient relaxation techniques.

LEVEL 3: Intractable

EXPECTED OUTCOME

1. Patient/caregiver identify/demonstrate measures to control severe pruritus:
   - identify/demonstrate measures to promote hydration and nutrition.
   - eliminate skin irritants.
   - identify/demonstrate appropriate relief measures.
   - demonstrate knowledge of medication administration.
2. Patient/caregiver identify measures to control or prevent complications of severe pruritus:
   - no trauma or infection.
   - no abnormal behavioral reactions.
3. Patient reports tolerable level of itching as evidenced by:
   - ability to perform activities of daily living.
   - ability to sleep or rest.

NURSING MANAGEMENT

Assessment

1. See Assessment, Levels 1 and 2.
2. Assess complications of pruritus:
   - impaired skin integrity.
   - infection.
3. Assess impact on patient's mental status, coping abilities, and activities of daily living.

Nursing Interventions

1. See Nursing Interventions, Level 2.
2. Administer medications as appropriate.
3. Arrange for anxiety management:
   - assure patient of continued effort to effectively treat itching.
   - make special provision for continuity of care.
   - use sedation only if necessary for anxiety management.

Patient Teaching

1. See Patient Teaching, Levels 1 and 2.
2. Teach signs and symptoms of infection.
3. Explain rationale and measures to control pruritus. (Refer to Nursing Interventions)
4. Discuss administration, scheduling, and side effects of medication.
5. Instruct to report difficulties in performing activities of daily living and inability to sleep or rest as a result of itching.

SUGGESTED READINGS

Anders, J., and Moller, P.: Topicals: A welter of options calls for refined application techniques. RN *45*(9):33–42, 1982.

Campbell, J.: Management of pruritus in the cancer patient. Oncology Nursing Forum, *8*:40–41, 1982.

Dangle, R.B.: Pruritus and cancer. Oncology Nursing Forum *13*(1):17–21, 1986.

Demis, J., Dobson, R., and McGuire, J. (Eds.): Clinical Dermatology, Vol 4. Hagerstown, MD, Harper & Row, 1988.

Flaxman, A.: Pruritus: Identifying and treating the causes. Postgraduate Medicine *69*(5):177–188, 1981.

Gilchrest B.: Pruritus: Pathogenesis therapy, and significance in systemic disease states. Archives of Internal Medicine *142*:101–105, 1982.

Gilman, A.G., Goodman, L.S., and Gilman, A. (Eds.): Pharmacological Basis of Therapeutics. New York, Macmillan, 1985.

Jillson, O.: Pruritus. Cutis *29*:335–339, 1981.

Johnson, B., and Gross, J.: Handbook of Oncology Nursing. New York, Wiley Medical, 1985.

Jones, D., Dunbar, C., Jirovec, M. (et al.): Medical-Surgical Nursing. A Conceptual Approach. New York, McGraw-Hill, 1978.

Shafer, K., Sawyer, J., McCluskey A., et al.: Medical-Surgical Nursing, (6th ed.). St. Louis, C.V. Mosby, 1975.

Weltman, R., and Sheepack, J.: Pruritus in the cancer patient, Part I, II, III. *In* Your Patient and Cancer. For Oncology Nurses. Fall: 10–24, 1984.

Winkleman, R.K.: Pharmacy control of pruritus. Medical Clinics of North America *66*(5):1119–1113, 1982.

Yasko, J., and Hogan, C.: Pruritus. *In* Yasko (Ed.) Guidelines for Cancer Care: Symptoms Management. Reston, VA, Reston, 1983.

Zeigfield, C.R.: Core Curriculum for Oncology Nursing. Philadelphia, W.B. Saunders, 1987, pp. 308–309.

25

Alteration in Comfort: Sleep Pattern Disturbance

Michaelyn A. Page

Population at Risk

- Patients at time of diagnosis
- Patients receiving active treatments such as surgery, biotherapy, radiotherapy, chemotherapy
- Patients experiencing serious insults secondary to tumor growth
- Patients experiencing end-stage symptomatology both iatrogenic and organic in nature

LEVEL 1:   Potential

EXPECTED OUTCOME

1. Patient demonstrates absence of unacceptable sleep disturbances:
   - reports intact, restful, restorative sleep.
   - verbalizes feeling rested.
   - demonstrates ability to function and pursue desired and required activities during waking hours.
2. Patient identifies factors related to potential impairment of sleep:
   - verbalizes symptoms and potential side effects of tumor growth and therapies that may affect sleep.
3. Patient identifies/demonstrates measures to prevent impaired sleep integrity:
   - reports symptoms that may affect sleep (e.g., pain, nocturia, night sweats).
   - implements measures to reduce stress.
   - avoids stimulants.
   - avoids hunger at bedtime.

NURSING MANAGEMENT

Assessment

1. Assess usual sleep behavior of patient:
   - time of retirement.
   - minutes needed to fall asleep.
   - number of times patient awakens during night.
   - intrusive thoughts.
   - total hours of sleep.
   - time of morning awakening.
   - satisfaction with sleep.
   - degree of restfulness felt by patient.
2. Observe number, time, and duration of daily naps.

3. Note use of sleep aids:
   - name of drug(s).
   - dosage of drug(s).
   - frequency of use.
   - length of time used.
4. Determine presence of symptoms that may affect sleep:
   - pain.
   - respiratory distress.
   - gastrointestinal disturbances.
   - genitourinary disturbances.
   - night sweats.
   - tension.
   - anxiety
   - depression.
   - CNS condition, mood changes.
5. Note use of drugs that may decrease sleep:
   - corticosteroids.
   - caffeine.
   - atropine.
   - amphetamines.

Patient Teaching

1. Explain that all persons experience daily (circadian) rhythmic changes in physiologic function and behavior.
2. Explain that the sleep-wake cycle is the most important circadian rhythm.
3. Describe the two distinct phases of sleep: NREM (nonrapid eye movement) and REM (rapid eye movement). NREM sleep alternates with REM approximately every 90 to 100 min. REM sleep is the sleep state in which most dreaming occurs.
4. Explain that sleep is a complex biologic function that is highly variable in length and depth. Individual variation in baseline sleep need is 4 to 11 hrs. Normal sleep onset occurs with a decrease in activity and a fall in body temperature. A person's need for sleep varies according to a number of factors:
   - by age 40, sleep is normally more shallow.
   - by age 60, sleep need may have decreased sleep time further, as older persons have shorter and lighter sleep cycles.
   - a linear positive correlation exists between age and number of awakenings.
   - during highly productive periods, sleep needs may decrease.
   - moderate exercise may reduce sleep latency and increase sleep length and depth.
   - anxiety and stress may cause normal shortening of sleep time.
   - poor sleep is usually self-limiting.
   - good sleep usually follows poor sleep.
5. Describe potential side effects of treatment that may affect sleep:
   - pain.
   - respiratory disturbances.
   - gastrointestinal disturbances.
   - genitourinary disturbances.
   - night sweats.
   - tension.
   - anxiety.
6. Teach rationale and measures to prevent impairment of sleep:
   - maintain daily routine of activity compatible with energy level by pacing to prevent fatigue.
   - begin routine of daily exercise if tolerated.
   - avoid prolonged time periods in bed if not sleeping.
   - maintain regular retirement time at night and arousal time in morning to comply with circadian rhythm.
   - maintain reduced level of sound to protect sleep integrity (e.g., quiet, soft music).
   - adjust room temperature to promote comfort (excessive heat fragments sleep; excessive cold usually does not promote sleep).
   - prevent hunger at bedtime through use of snacks (foods containing milk promote sleep integrity).
   - avoid ingesting products containing caffeine in evening.
   - administer corticosteroids no later than mid-afternoon.
   - avoid alcoholic beverages.

- utilize diversionary strategies (e.g., reading, watching TV, conversation, muscle massage, guided imagery, prayer, relaxation techniques, soft music).

- avoid administering diuretics in the evening.

LEVEL 2:   Mild to Moderate

EXPECTED OUTCOME

1. Patient demonstrates absence of unacceptable sleep disturbances:
   - reports intact, restful, restorative sleep.
   - verbalizes feeling rested.
   - demonstrates ability to function and pursue desired and required activities during waking hours.
2. Patient demonstrates knowledge of factors related to potential impairment of sleep:
   - verbalizes changes that may occur as consequences of treatment.
   - verbalizes short-term and long-term effects of sleep disturbances.
3. Patient identifies/demonstrates measures to manage impaired sleep:
   - makes judicious use of sleep-inducing drugs on short-term basis, as prescribed by physician.
   - implements regimen to control pain.
   - implements measures to control environment.
   - prevents hunger at bedtime.
   - communicates openly with family and friends.

NURSING MANAGEMENT

Assessment

1. See Assessment, Level 1.
2. Assess signs and symptoms of short-term sleep disturbances:
   - irritability.
   - loss of train of thought, inability to concentrate.
   - anxiety.
   - depression.
3. Note signs and symptoms that may affect sleep:
   - gastrointestinal:
     - anorexia.
     - dry mouth.
     - sore mouth.
     - dysphagia.
     - hiccups.
     - nausea and vomiting.
     - colicky abdominal pain.
     - flatulence.
     - constipation.
     - diarrhea.
     - loss of bowel control.
   - respiratory:
     - dyspnea.
     - cough.
     - chest pain.
   - genitourinary:
     - urgency.
     - frequency.
     - burning.
     - incontinence.
     - retention.

- CNS:
  - depression.
  - anxiety.
  - confusion.
- skin:
  - chills or fever.
  - night sweats.
  - pruritus.
  - decubitus ulcers.
4. Determine pre-existing sleep disturbances such as:
   - DIMS: disorders of initiating and maintaining sleep (insomniacs):
     - sleep latency (difficulty falling asleep).
     - multiple awakenings.
     - early morning awakening.
   - DOES: disorders of excessive somnolence:
     - narcolepsy (excessive daytime sleepiness).
     - associated with use of central nervous system depressants.
     - associated with psychiatric disorders, especially affective.
     - nocturnal myoclonus and "restless legs" syndrome.
     - sleep apnea.
   - disorders of the sleep-wake schedule:
     - rapid time zone change ("jet lag" syndrome).
     - work shift change.
     - non-24-hour sleep-wake syndrome.
     - irregular sleep-wake pattern.
   - parasomnias:
     - sleep walking.
     - sleep terror.
     - nocturnal enuresis.

Nursing Interventions

1. Administer sleep-inducing drugs, as ordered by physician.
2. Administer pain medication on an around-the-clock schedule to prevent or control pain (awaken patient if requested).
3. Use drugs to control night sweats (e.g., indomethacin).

4. Administer expectorants or suppressants for cough.
5. Control nausea and vomiting with anti-emetic.
6. Prevent constipation through increased fluids, fiber in diet, and use of laxatives and stool softeners.
7. Adjust environment to promote rest (good ventilation; quiet, low lighting).
8. Implement comfort measures to promote rest:
   - avoid awakening once asleep.
   - provide snack, especially milk-based product if tolerated.
   - oral hygiene to relieve dry mouth with small drinks of crushed ice to suck; treat monilial infections.
   - keep patient's skin clean and dry.
   - administer back rub.
   - massage bony prominences with lanolin-based skin lotion.
   - keep bedding clean, dry, free of wrinkles and crumbs.
   - dress patient in soft, loose clothing.
   - offer bedpan just before sleep.
   - reposition patient and support with pillows.
   - apply adequate bed covers to keep patient warm.
   - use condom catheter or disposable incontinent product for nocturnal incontinence.
9. Promote communication with patient:
   - encourage openness among patient, family, health care team in discussing thoughts and feelings.
   - be an active listener and encourage patient to share thoughts, fears, concerns.

Patient Teaching

1. See Patient Teaching, Level 1.
2. Advise patient that sharing of emotions related to disease process may broaden support system and lead to sleep integrity.
3. Identify strategies used in past to promote sleep and to assist patient to integrate into present situation.

4. Note that weight loss may interfere with sleep integrity, and that weight gain may lengthen sleep.
5. Teach rationale and measures to control or prevent pain:
   • pain medication can be administered around-the-clock or by continuous infusion.
   • waking patient at night for dose of medication may promote rather than interfere with sleep.

• increasing the dosage of current pain medication may improve pain control.
6. Note signs and symptoms of sleep disturbance to report to health care team:
   • irritability.
   • fatigability in daytime.
   • loss of train of thought.
   • anxiety.
   • depression.
   • aggressiveness.
   • confusion

LEVEL 3: Severe

EXPECTED OUTCOME

1. Patient experiences satisfactory rest and sleep behavior:
   • has uninterrupted periods of sleep and quiet rest.
   • has meaningful interaction, both verbal and nonverbal, with significant others.
2. Patient/caregiver identify signs and symptoms of severe sleep disturbances including those to report to the health care team.
3. Patient/caregiver identify measures to control severe sleep disturbances:
   • state drugs prescribed to promote sleep.
   • take/administer drugs as prescribed to control severe sleep disturbances.

NURSING MANAGEMENT

Assessment

1. See Assessment, Levels 1 and 2.
2. Assess signs and symptoms of severe sleep disturbance:
   • irritability.
   • mental confusion.
   • inability to carry on conversation and make decisions.
   • loss of train of thought.
   • anxiety.
   • depression.

Nursing Interventions

1. See Nursing Interventions, Level 2.
2. Administer prescribed drugs for manage-

ment of signs and symptoms of severe sleep disturbance:
• psychotropic drugs (e.g., thioridazine [Mellaril], haloperidol [Haldol], chlorpromazine [Thorazine]).
• sedatives (e.g., barbiturates).
• hypnotics (e.g., flurazepam [Dalmane], chloral hydrate [Beta-Chlor], triazolam [Halcion]).
• antianxiety agents (e.g., diazepam [Valium], chlordiazepoxide [Librium], oxazepam [Serax], lorazepam [Ativan], buspirone [BuSpar]).
• antidepressants (e.g., tricyclics such as amitriptyline [Elavil], imipramine [Tofranil], desipramine [Norpramin], trazodone [Desyrel]). May require smaller

doses than doses used in psychiatric population for trial period of 10 to 14 days as necessary.
- antihistamines (e.g., diphenhydramine [Benadryl]), when liver disease is present.

3. Assign a primary caregiver so that patient has a familiar face and voice providing care.
4. Sit quietly with patient. Engage in active listening or conversation if initiated by patient.

Patient Teaching

1. See Patient Teaching, Levels 1 and 2.
2. Discuss increased need for restful behavior as disease progresses.
3. Note signs and symptoms of severe sleep disturbances to report to health care team:
   - irritability.
   - fatigability in daytime.
   - loss of train of thought.
   - anxiety.
   - depression.
   - mental confusion.
   - inability to carry on conversation and make decisions.
   - hand tremors.
   - poor coordination.
4. Explain effects and side effects of psychotropic CNS drugs:
   - rationale for use:
     o control agitation.
     o control combativeness.
     o control hyperactivity.
     o potentiate action of other CNS drugs.
   - potential side effects:
     o extrapyramidal reactions: acute dystonia (muscle spasms: tongue, face, neck, back), akathisia (motor restlessness), pseudoparkinsonism (motor retardation and rigidity), tardive dyskinesia (protrusion of the tongue, puffing cheeks, chewing movements, involuntary movements).

- sedation.
- postural hypotension.
- lowering of seizure threshold.
- photosensitivity.
- blood dyscrasias.

5. Explain effects and side effects of sedative-hypnotics:
   - rationale for use:
     o induce sleep faster.
     o maintain longer sleep.
   - potential side effects:
     o tolerance.
     o mild withdrawal symptoms (e.g., nightmares, daytime agitation, "shaky" feeling) after short-term use.
     o severe withdrawal symptoms (e.g., grand mal seizures, delirium) with severe drug dependency.
     o potentiation of other CNS drugs.
6. Explain effects and side effects of antianxiety drugs:
   - rationale for use:
     o relieve muscle spasticity.
     o control agitation.
   - potential side effects:
     o sedation.
     o somnolence (more common and severe in older patients and patients with impaired liver function).
     o tolerance.
     o potentiation of other CNS drugs.
7. Explain effects and side effects of antidepressants:
   - rationale for use:
     o treat depression, which may manifest itself as feelings of hopelessness, helplessness, or worthlessness, or decreased ability to concentrate.
     o treat insomnia from depression (does not interfere with normal sleep pattern).
   - potential side effects:
     o anticholinergic (dry mouth [may be a major problem for patient with stomatitis], urinary retention).
     o sedation.
     o potentiation of other CNS drugs.
     o tricyclics contraindicated with chemotherapy drug procarbazine, which

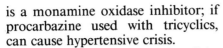

is a monamine oxidase inhibitor; if procarbazine used with tricyclics, can cause hypertensive crisis.

8. Explain effects and side effects of antihistamines:
   - rationale for use:
     - promote drowsiness.
     - useful as an alternative drug when altered liver function is present.
   - potential side effects:
     - atropine-like effects.
     - sedation.
     - potentiation of other CNS drugs.

SUGGESTED READINGS

Baines, M.M.: Control of other symptoms. *In* Sanders, C. (Ed.): The Management of Terminal Disease, Vol I. Chicago, Yearbook Medical, 1978, p. 115.

Beszterczey, A., and Lipowske, Z.J.: Insomnia in cancer patients. Canadian Medical Association Journal *116*:355, 1977.

DeLoughery, M.N.: Chronic insomnia. Nurse Practitioner *7*(2):8–11, 1982.

Karacan, I., Williams, R.L., and Moore, C.A.: Sleep disorders. *In* Kaplan, H.I., and Sadock, B.J. (Eds.): Comprehensive Textbook of Psychiatry. Baltimore, Williams & Wilkins, 1989, pp. 1105–1135.

Levy, M.H., and Gatalano, R.B.: Control of common physical symptoms other than pain in patients with terminal illness. Seminars in Oncology *12*(4):411–430, 1985.

Lokich, J.J.: Management of constitutional symptoms. *In* Lokich, J.J.: Primer of Cancer Management. Boston, Hall and Co., 1978, p. 160.

Massie, M.J.: Psychopharmacologic management of psychiatric syndromes in cancer patients. *In* Gall, R.J. (Ed.): Supportive Care of the Cancer Patient (Proceedings from symposium sponsored by Memorial-Sloan Kettering Cancer Center). New York, Biomedical Information Corp., 1983.

Sanders, C.: Principles of symptom control in terminal care. Medical Clinics of North America *66*:1169–1183, 1982.

Smith, P.L.: Approach to the patient with sleep disorders. *In* Kelley, W.N. (Ed.): Textbook of Internal Medicine. Philadelphia, J.B. Lippincott, 1989, pp. 2536–2538.

Thomas, C.D.: Insomnia: Identification and management. Seminars in Oncology Nursing *3*(4):263–266, 1987.

Alteration in Comfort: Fatigue

Barbara F. Piper

26

Population at Risk:

- Individuals (adult/pediatric) at risk for or with the diagnosis of cancer and who are experiencing its related diagnostic and therapeutic (curative, rehabilitative, palliative) procedures
- Individuals or family members serving as primary caregivers for a person with cancer

> ### LEVEL 1: Usual or Expected Tiredness: Potential for Acute/Chronic Fatigue States

EXPECTED OUTCOME

1. Patient demonstrates an awareness of being at risk for fatigue:
   - verbalizes that fatigue is a protective mechanism that serves as a warning sign of decreased energy reserves/impending illness.
   - identifies potential causes of fatigue.
   - identifies symptoms that may warn of impending acute or chronic fatigue.
2. Patient demonstrates knowledge about methods that may prevent transient tiredness states from progressing to the more intransient states of acute/chronic fatigue:
   - varies stimuli.
   - uses distraction techniques and other methods to dissipate negative effects of stressors.
   - adheres to an exercise program.
   - ingests a nutritionally balanced diet, adequate fluids.
   - schedules activities to prevent tiredness.
   - reduces unnecessary exposure to fatiguing environmental stressors.
   - reduces unnecessary energy expenditure.

NURSING MANAGEMENT

Assessment

1. Determine life style patterns:
   - usual methods of dealing with stressors, current emotional state.
   - adequacy of social support system.
   - usual patterns of mobility, exercise, activities of daily living, rest.
   - usual social, work, play-related activities.
   - adequacy of sleep/wake cycles, nutritional patterns.

155

- note any changes that may have occurred in the six months preceding diagnosis/treatment/nursing assessment.
2. Assess medication history that may predispose to fatigue such as a history of use of alcohol, caffeine, nicotine, antihypertensives, narcotics, sedatives, hypnotics.
3. Assess past experiences with tiredness or fatigue to establish baseline patterns:
   - determine if tiredness and fatigue are perceived as being similar or dissimilar states.
   - determine usual tiredness frequency, time of occurrence during the day or week, duration.
   - determine physical, emotional, mental symptoms that occur when individual is tired.
   - determine what causes individual to become tired.
   - determine what prevents or relieves the tiredness.
4. Review medical history/physical examination to determine the presence of cancer or other coexisting disease factors that place the individual at risk for fatigue (e.g., diseases involving the neurologic, pulmonary, cardiac, hematopoietic, gastrointestinal systems).
5. Identify fatigue-related risk factors associated with diagnostic workup and medical therapies:
   - anxiety and fear of the unknown.
   - type of physical preparation required for procedure (e.g., enemas until clear).
   - length of the test/procedure.
   - side effects of anesthesia, surgery, radiation therapy, chemotherapy, biotherapy.

Patient Teaching

1. Teach individual to think about personal energy stores as a bank. Deposits and withdrawals need to be made over the course of a day, the course of a week to ensure that a balance is achieved between energy conservation, restoration, expenditure.

2. Teach the patient potential causes of fatigue:
   - inadequate rest or pacing of activities.
   - inadequate nutritional intake, exercise, social support.
   - inadequate sleep.
   - any symptoms or side effects of the disease, medications, medical treatments, surgical/diagnostic procedures.
   - developmental/situational/environmental stressors (i.e., adolescence, divorce, illness, occupational, caregiver stressors).
3. Discuss symptoms that may warn of impending acute or chronic fatigue:
   - tired eyes, legs, whole body tiredness.
   - stiff shoulders.
   - lack of energy or decreased energy.
   - inability to concentrate.
   - general malaise or weakness.
   - boredom or lack of motivation.
   - sleepiness.
   - increased irritability, nervousness, anxiety, impatience.
4. Teach the individual about what others have experienced regarding fatigue symptoms (e.g., anticipated timing, duration, perceived causes, relief measures) so that this knowledge becomes part of the repertoire when dealing with fatigue.
5. Teach rationale and measures that may prevent transient tiredness states from progressing to the more intransient states of acute or chronic fatigue:
   - vary type of stimuli by changing activities to prevent boredom, lack of motivation, eye strain.
   - use distraction techniques to focus on things other than tiredness, disease or treatment side effects (e.g., reading, listening to music, visiting friends, watching television, going for walks).
   - use methods to dissipate negative effects of stressors (e.g., exercise, progressive relaxation, visual imagery, meditation, talking with others, therapeutic counseling).
   - adhere to some form of individually tailored/prescribed aerobic endurance ex-

ercise program (e.g., for healthy individuals under 40 years without physical limitations, this may include walking, jogging, swimming, cycling, or stair-climbing, three to five times per week for 30 to 45 minutes).

- ingest balanced, nutritionally complete diet emphasizing complex carbohydrates (grains, legumes, vegetables) that provide sustained source of energy supply.
- drink at least 8 to 10 glasses of water per day to maintain adequate hydration and to excrete cell destruction end products/toxins that may be associated with fatigue.
- schedule activities during the day and throughout the week to avoid becoming unusually tired. Pace self and plan adequate rest and sleep periods to allow for full energy recovery before undertaking additional activities.

- reduce unnecessary exposure to fatiguing environmental stressors (e.g., noise, allergens, lack of adequate fresh air circulation).
- reduce unnecessary energy expenditure by using assistive devices or by placing equipment and supplies within easy reach.

6. Teach individual to communicate immediately with health care professionals if tiredness becomes:
- unusually severe or disproportionate to type of activity undertaken, or unrelated to any form of activity/physical exertion.
- unrelieved by rest or sleep.
- disruptive to social activities, activities of daily living, or quality of life.
- constant or recurrent.

LEVEL 2: Acute Fatigue

EXPECTED OUTCOME

1. Patient demonstrates knowledge of acute fatigue:
   - communicates that usual tiredness has become unusually severe or disproportionate to the type of activity undertaken, or is unrelated to any form of activity/physical exertion.
   - recognizes that fatigue is unrelieved by rest or sleep.
   - states that fatigue is disruptive to social activities, activities of daily living, quality of life.
   - identifies that fatigue has been constant or recurrent for a period of less than one month.
   - acknowledges that fatigue is short term and will resolve when therapy ends.
   - identifies perceived causes of fatigue.
   - identifies physical, emotional, mental symptoms of fatigue.
2. Patient uses a variety of strategies, alone or in combination, to decrease or alleviate fatigue.
   - becomes more selective in determining type of activities undertaken, when and for how long.
   - schedules rest periods at specific times for one week.
   - delegates specific activities/responsibilities to others in order to conserve energy.

NURSING MANAGEMENT

Assessment

1. See Assessment, Level 1.
2. Obtain baseline data: age, physical performance status, stage and location of disease, disease prognosis, underlying cause(s) of fatigue.
3. Monitor patient/family response over time to medical therapies that are designed to cure or control the underlying disease process(es). Fatigue in many instances may be a cumulative, gradually worsening phenomenon in patients receiving chemotherapy, radiation therapy, and biotherapy.
4. Assess the subjective dimensions of fatigue:
   - intensity/severity dimension: determine how severe and intense fatigue is and its degree of distress and disruption in activities of daily living.
   - sensory dimension: determine location and type of physical, emotional, mental symptoms attributable to fatigue.
   - affective dimension: determine what fatigue means to the individual. Is it perceived as normal, usual, or protective; or is it perceived as being abnormal and associated with lack of treatment response or disease progression/recurrence? The perceived meaning of fatigue and its causes may influence the individual's belief about relieving fatigue when it occurs.
   - temporal dimension: determine time course of fatigue. Has it been experienced for less than one month; does it fluctuate during the day; what time of day is it most likely to occur? (Fatigue related to depression typically occurs in the morning upon waking in contrast to other causes of fatigue.)
5. Determine aggravating and alleviating factors.
6. Determine presence of other symptoms that may herald disease progression, recurrence, or side effects of treatment (e.g., headache, dizziness, weakness, dyspnea, pain, nausea, vomiting, pruritus, unintentional weight loss or weight gain, fever, infection).
7. Determine behavioral manifestations of fatigue:
   - changes in physical appearance: slumped shoulders, non-erect posture, droopy eyelids, lack of eye sparkle, frequent yawning.
   - changes in communication patterns: slowed responses to questions, short, terse responses resulting from irritability, infrequent initiating of conversation, decreased desire to socialize with others.
   - changes in activity level or pattern of activity: decreased performance status, inability to perform certain activities, walking more slowly, taking longer to accomplish activities, requiring longer or more frequent rest periods, delegating or having difficulty delegating to others.
   - changes in affect/attitude: flat or depressed affect, disinterested, irritable, impatient, apathetic, unmotivated.
8. Determine physiologic manifestations/factors related to fatigue:
   - decreased hematocrit or hemoglobin values.
   - decreased or increased blood glucose values.
   - decreased oxygen saturation levels.
   - abnormal electrolyte values.
   - abnormal thyroid or other hormonal values.
   - unintentional weight loss or weight gain (10% or more of usual body weight).
9. Assess the presence of biochemical manifestations/factors related to fatigue (e.g., changes in pH, hydrogen ion concentration, lactate or pyruvate levels).

Nursing Interventions

1. Implement exercise program individual-

ized to patient's physical and psychosocial status. Exercise prescription must take into account specific risk factors such as lytic bone lesions, thrombocytopenia, and fever that may contraindicate aerobic exercise. Passive range-of-motion exercises may be all that the patient can do safely during certain stages of disease or when experiencing side effects from treatment.

2. Monitor the timing, adequacy of dosage, and effectiveness of therapies that are designed to reduce disease and treatment-related side effects (e.g., nausea/vomiting, pain, dyspnea).
   - give certain medications at night, such as cisplatin or interferon, to reduce fatigue and other side effects that may contribute to fatigue.
   - refer to relevant standards on circulation, comfort, coping, elimination, knowledge deficit, mobility, nutrition, protective mechanisms, sexuality, ventilation for interventions specific to the underlying cause(s) of the fatigue.

3. Serve as an advocate for the patient/family by:
   - questioning need for multiple diagnostic tests.
   - obtaining orders for effective pain and other symptom relief measures.
   - minimizing phone calls or visits from family and friends.
   - initiating multidisciplinary/community service referrals to reduce fatigue directly or indirectly using such interventions as:
     ○ physical therapy referral for bed and strengthening exercises, overhead trapezes, walker, cane, stair-climbing instruction.
     ○ occupational therapy referral for assistive equipment, energy conservation activities, self-care instruction.
     ○ American Cancer Society for transportation and supplies.
     ○ social services referral for discharge planning, financial, and psychologic counseling, support groups for patients and caregivers.

○ home health agency/hospice referral for nursing, respite, attendant care.
○ religious/spiritual referral.

Patient Teaching

1. Discuss that fatigue is short-term (less than one month) and most likely will resolve when therapy has ended, or when effective treatment of the underlying cause of the fatigue has occurred (e.g., treatment of infection, anemia, pain, malnutrition).

2. Teach patient/caregivers to anticipate certain sensations that might be experienced while undergoing diagnostic testing and cancer therapies to reduce anxiety resulting in negative energy losses. Sensory preparation reduces anxiety more effectively in certain individuals than the imparting of factual information about what the test will involve. Refer to the specific knowledge deficit standard for appropriate teaching strategies.

3. Prepare the patient/caregiver to anticipate the time periods during chemotherapy treatment when acute fatigue is more likely to be experienced. Teach patient/caregiver to plan work and social activities accordingly:
   - fatigue may be greatest during the first 2 to 3 days following intravenous push (IVP) chemotherapy since anxiety about the treatment, effects of antiemetic coverage, sleep pattern disturbances may be greatest during this time.
   - schedule chemotherapy administration toward the end of the week for working patients to permit recovery during the weekend.
   - the high-risk period that occurs during the mid-cycle or nadir periods of each chemotherapy treatment cycle when bone marrow suppression is likely to be the greatest.
   - teach patient to plan or schedule to reduce risk factors for bleeding and infection during the nadir that may accentuate fatigue.

4. Teach patient to avoid exercising 24 hours before chemotherapy because false laboratory values may result (e.g., an increased white blood cell (WBC) count resulting from release of marginated WBCs).
5. Teach patient to avoid exercising 24 hours after receiving IVP chemotherapy. The increased cardiac output can stimulate more rapid excretion of drug that may not be desirable.

6. Instruct patient to maintain a diary for one week to identify fluctuations in energy levels and aggravating and alleviating factors, preplan activities and schedule rest periods for one week to determine effects on energy levels. Several short rest periods may be more beneficial than one long rest period.

LEVEL 3: Chronic Fatigue

EXPECTED OUTCOME

1. Patient/caregiver demonstrate knowledge of chronic fatigue:
   - verbalize that constant or recurrent fatigue for a month or more is unrelieved by rest or sleep, unrelated to any form of activity or exertion, and disruptive to social activities, ADLs, quality of life.
2. Patient/caregiver demonstrate knowledge of measures to manage chronic fatigue:
   - identify those activities that give greatest satisfaction or personal meaning to life.
   - delegate all nonessential activities to others.
   - pace self and conserve energy in order to accomplish activities that are most meaningful.

NURSING MANAGEMENT

Assessment

1. See Assessment, Levels 1 and 2.
2. Assess whether fatigue and other fatigue characteristics that may suggest a more chronic pattern have existed for a month or more. Little is known about differences in acute and chronic fatigue states; the time differential (less than one month vs. one month or longer) may be an artificial or arbitrary one.
3. Assess the type of interventions patient/family member(s) have tried to relieve fatigue.

Nursing Interventions

1. See Nursing Interventions, Level 2.
2. Help patient to interpret fatigue symptoms accurately. Provide reassurance, when appropriate, that chronic fatigue does not necessarily mean disease recurrence, lack of treatment response, or disease progression.
3. Encourage the combined use of several strategies to relieve fatigue, since chronic fatigue is most likely multicausal.
4. Information about effective interventions for fatigue is limited; therefore, stimulate

160

and participate in well-designed research studies that test fatigue interventions. Such studies might address:

- identifying adequate rest periods and determining how to pace activities. Pressure-rate product studies conducted with cardiac patients (multiply heart rate and systolic blood pressure together; divide the product by 100) may provide a useful research and practice model to follow in cancer patients.
- using distraction, support groups, cognitive-behavioral approaches to reduce fatigue.
- testing nutritional approaches such as smaller, more frequent feedings and types of supplements.
- tailoring exercise prescriptions to stage of disease, determining effects of exercise on fatigue (e.g., walking, bicycling, bed or strengthening exercises).
- testing different drug therapies in formal clinical trials that anecdotally are reported to be effective in treating fatigue in cancer and other populations, such as amantadine, corticosteroids, tricyclic antidepressants, monoamine oxidase inhibitors, nifedipine, vitamin B_{12}, dopamine agonists/antagonists (methylphenidate and metoclopramide hydrochlorides, and prostaglandin inhibitors (aspirin, indomethacin). As with all drug therapies, one must be alert to the side effects that may limit the effectiveness of such interventions.

Patient Teaching

1. See Patient Teaching, Levels 1 and 2.
2. Prepare patient/caregiver for the more cumulative, chronic forms of fatigue that may occur with radiation therapy, chemotherapy, surgery, and biotherapy.
3. Explain that chronic fatigue may occur simply as a function of the cumulative effects of treatment, cell destruction end products, and other factors that occur over time and may not necessarily be a function

of disease progression or lack of tumor response to treatment.

4. Teach surgical patient/caregivers that fatigue may last more than one month resulting from the combined effects of preoperative anxiety, anesthesia, changes in activity and nutritional status, the nature of the cancer diagnosis, and the effects of pain medications.
5. Teach radiation therapy patient/caregivers that fatigue symptoms may begin the second week of treatment and may progressively worsen over the course of treatment. Symptoms may persist for 2 to 3 months following therapy in some individuals.

SUGGESTED READINGS

Adolphe, A.B.: Chronic fatigue syndrome: Possible effective treatment with nifedipine (Letter to the editor). American Journal of Medicine 85:892, 1988.

Agre, J.C., Rodriquez, A.A., and Sperling, K.B.: Symptoms and clinical impressions of patients seen in a postpolio clinic. Archives of Physical Medicine and Rehabilitation 70:367–370, 1989.

Aistars, J.: Fatigue in the cancer patient: A conceptual approach to a clinical problem. Oncology Nursing Forum 14(6):25–30, 1987.

Bass, C.: Fatigue states (editorial). British Journal of Hospital Medicine 41:315, 1989.

Cimprich, B.: Attentional fatigue in the cancer patient (Abstract 321A). Oncology Nursing Forum (Supplement) 17(2):218, 1990.

Cohen, R.A., and Fisher, M.: Amantadine treatment of fatigue associated with multiple sclerosis. Archives of Neurology 46:676–680, 1989.

Gregersen, R.A.: Fatigue in the cardiac surgical patient. Progress in Cardiovascular Nursing 3:106–111, 1988.

Jamar, S.C.: Fatigue in women receiving chemotherapy for ovarian cancer. In Funk, S.G., Tournquist, E.M., Champagne, M.T., et al. (Eds.): Key Aspects of Comfort: Management of Pain, Fatigue, and Nausea. New York, Springer, 1989, pp. 224–228.

King, K.B., Nail, L.M., Kreamer, K., et al.: Patients' descriptions of the experience of receiving radiation therapy. Oncology Nursing Forum 12(4):55–61, 1985.

Lawhorne, L., and Ringdahl, D.: Cyanocobalamin injections for patients without documented deficiency. Journal of American Medical Association 261(13):1920–1923, 1989.

MacVicar, M.G., and Winningham, M.L.: Promoting functional capacity of cancer patients. Cancer Bulletin 38(5):235–239, 1986.

Piper, B.F.: Fatigue: Current bases for practice. *In* Funk, S.G., Tournquist, E.M., Champagne, M.T., et al. (Eds.): Key Aspects of Comfort: Management of Pain, Fatigue, and Nausea. New York, Springer, 1989, pp. 187–198.

Piper, B.F., Lindsey, A.M., and Dodd, M.J.: Fatigue mechanisms in cancer patients: Developing nursing theory. Oncology Nursing Forum *14*(6):17–23, 1987.

Piper, B.F., Rieger, P.T., Brophy, L., et al.: Recent advances in the management of biotherapy-related side effects: Fatigue. Oncology Nursing Forum (Supplement) *16*(6):27–34, 1989.

Rhodes, V.A., Watson, P.M., and Hanson, B.M.: Patients' descriptions of the influence of tiredness and weakness on self-care abilities. Cancer Nursing *11*(3):186–194, 1988.

Rhoten, D.: Fatigue in the post-surgical patient. *In* Norris, C.N. (Ed.): Concept Clarification in Nursing. Rockville, MD, Aspen, 1982, pp. 277–300.

Rieger, P.T.: Management of cancer-related fatigue. Dimensions of Oncology Nursing *2*(3):5–8, 1988.

PATIENT EDUCATION MATERIALS AND COMMUNITY RESOURCES

Chronic Fatigue Syndrome Society, P.O. Box 230108, Portland, OR 92723, 503–684–5261

NUTRITION

The nurse assesses the patient's current nutritional status, effects of disease and treatment, and past and present nutritional patterns to formulate actual or potential nursing diagnoses.

Appropriate patient outcomes to consider in planning nursing interventions will specify the patient's ability to:

1. identify foods that are tolerated and those that cause discomfort or are distasteful.
2. describe measures that enhance food intake and retention.
3. select appropriate dietary alternatives to provide sufficient nutrients when foods that were part of the customary diet are no longer tolerated.
4. describe methods of modifying consistency, flavor, or amounts of nutrients to ensure adequate nutrient intake.
5. describe dietary modifications compatible with patient's cultural, social, and ethnic practices.
6. describe interventions to relieve symptoms (e.g., nausea, vomiting, stomatitis) that interfere with nutritional intake.
7. list foods and fluids that provide optimal comfort during the terminal stage of illness.
8. identify mechanisms to assess patient's nutritional status.

Evaluation of the patient's responses to nursing care is based on whether the patient manages nutrition and hydration in a way that facilitates health and comfort in the presence of disease and treatment.

Excerpted from the ANA/ONS Standards of Oncology Nursing Practice.

Nutrition, Alteration in: Less Than Body Requirements Related to Disease Process and Treatment

Carol Sandor

Population at Risk

- All patients with cancer, especially those undergoing radiation therapy, chemotherapy, surgical intervention, or immunotherapy

LEVEL 1: *Potential*

EXPECTED OUTCOME

1. Patient demonstrates knowledge related to potential alteration in nutrition:
   - verbalizes relationship between disease process and treatment and nutritional status.
   - identifies signs and symptoms to report to the health care team.
2. Patient identifies/demonstrates measures to prevent nutritional deficit:
   - selects foods or nutrients to maintain nutritional status.
   - uses medication as prescribed to control symptoms that interfere with good nutrition.
3. Patient maintains adequate nutritional status:
   - maintains normal body weight for height or a body weight within 10 lbs of prediagnosis weight.
   - has normal lab values.
   - maintains routine level of activity or rest.
4. Patient describes a sense of well-being:
   - maintains maximum physical, social, psychologic functions.

NURSING MANAGEMENT

Assessment

1. Evaluate nutritional status:
   - measure height and weight.
   - compare to ideal body weight for height or prediagnosis weight.
   - assess lab values (e.g., serum albumin to be > 3.4 mg/100 ml, lymphocyte count

to be 1500 unless patient is undergoing chemotherapy, hemoglobin, hematocrit).

- Obtain anthropometric measurements (arm muscle circumference, triceps skin fold thickness).

2. Obtain history of food preferences, including allergies and lactose tolerance. Include cultural and religious food preferences.
3. Evaluate for presence of anxiety, depression, pain, anger, fatigue.
4. Assess condition of oral cavity for evidence of gum disease, missing or broken teeth, caries, poorly fitting dentures, stomatitis, areas of tenderness or pain.
5. Assess ability to care for self, including obtaining and preparing food, availability of facilities for food preparation.
6. Assess family and support systems.

Nursing Intervention

1. Encourage activity as tolerated to increase appetite and utilize nutrients.
2. Encourage frequent rest periods, particularly before and immediately after meals.
3. Arrange for assistance in obtaining and preparing food, if needed.
4. Emphasize good oral hygiene habits including regular dental check-ups.
5. Assist patient in setting realistic goals such as:
   - eating high-protein, high-caloric foods.
   - eating small meals every 2 to 3 hours with ⅓ of calories consumed at breakfast.
   - reducing unpleasant environmental stimuli (e.g., odors including those related to food preparation, harsh noise, extremes of temperature).
   - using a glucose polymer that does not add or alter taste (32 calories/tsp) to all foods and beverages.
   - if not contraindicated, a glass of wine or sherry before meals may be a stimulus to meal enjoyment.
6. Provide verbal and written information regarding nutrition.

Patient Teaching

1. Teach signs and symptoms of early nutritional deficit (e.g., anorexia, weight loss, nausea, vomiting, diarrhea).
2. Discuss relationship of adequate nutrition to disease process and treatment.
3. Explain relationship of nutritional state and immunocompetence to disease process and treatment.
4. Describe signs and symptoms associated with disease process and treatment that tend to alter nutritional intake (e.g., altered taste, sore mouth, dry mouth, pain, nausea).
5. Discuss anxiety and measures to alleviate it:
   - Anxiety, mood swings, difficulty concentrating, anorexia, insomnia may be recognized as distress responses related to the uncertainties of disease, treatment, anticipated outcome.
   - stimulate patient's motivation to facilitate active coping.
   - be aware of relationship between patient's emotional state and perception of attitudes and beliefs of family, friends, professionals.
   - encourage realistic hopefulness regarding care and treatment.
   - discuss tendency to use eating situations and problems as vehicle for expressing hostility and negative feelings, and ways to avoid this.
   - emphasize need to maintain routine activity level.
6. Discuss elements of a nutritious diet (basic food groups):
   - describe good nutrition as an integral part of healing, resisting or recovering from infections, and maintaining a sense of well-being—an important part of the treatment plan.
7. Explain general measures to maintain adequate nutritional status:
   - routine oral hygiene.
   - artificial saliva, if appropriate.
   - avoidance of extreme food temperatures.

- alteration of food texture to make it easy to eat.
- foods easily accessible and eating whenever hungry.
- controlling pain, nausea, other symptoms as directed by health care team.
- encouraging family to prepare favorite foods and participate in meal planning.

8. Discuss ways to overcome alterations in taste (e.g., "mouth blindness," metallic, or bitter taste):
   - describe measures to prevent or minimize ulcers and dryness of mouth.
   - suggest marinating meats in teriyaki or soy sauce.
   - encourage experimentation with different seasonings such as lemon, salt, vanilla, cinnamon.
   - sugar-free lemon drops, gum, mints may mask metallic or bitter taste.
   - substitute high-protein foods for beef or pork if these are not tolerated.
   - cold foods may be more appealing.
   - include meats in soups and sauces.

9. Discuss measures to control abdominal discomfort (e.g., feeling of fullness, bloating):
   - avoid fried and greasy foods.
   - limit fluid intake at, or immediately before, meals.
   - frequent small meals may be better tolerated than 3 regular meals.
   - rest after eating.
   - avoid gas-producing foods (e.g., beans, cabbage, beer, carbonated beverages).
   - encourage eating in a sitting position.

10. Discuss measures to control constipation:
    - increase amount of high-fiber foods in diet.
    - drink 8 to 10 glasses of fluids per day.
    - limit fluids containing caffeine.
    - avoid cheese products and refined grain products.
    - increase physical activity as tolerated.

11. Discuss measures to control cramps, diarrhea:
    - low-residue diet, high in calories and protein, low in fat and fiber.
    - avoid gas-forming foods and beverages.
    - frequent small meals may be better tolerated than 3 regular meals.
    - limit simple sugars.
    - potassium-rich and iron-rich foods may be helpful if weakness and fatigue are present.
    - avoid very hot or very cold foods.

12. Describe measures to control dry mouth (xerostomia):
    - increase liquid intake, sipping water or nonirritating juice several times each hour.
    - avoid starchy foods.
    - add sauces, syrups, broths to food.
    - moisten dry foods in liquid prior to eating.
    - instruct patient to suck on smooth, flat, sugarless candy or lozenges.
    - use oral lubricants, artificial saliva, lip balm, as appropriate.
    - humidify room air unless contraindicated.
    - emphasize importance of regular dental care and oral hygiene.

13. Describe measures to prevent stomatitis and mucositis:
    - soft, cold foods may be preferred.
    - avoid acidic foods.
    - frequent oral hygiene with nonabrasive fluid (e.g., baking soda and water, normal saline).

14. Discuss measures to control dumping syndrome.
    - decrease amount of carbohydrates to 150 gm daily.
    - increase protein.
    - eat frequent, small meals.
    - eliminate candies, jellies, chocolate, sugars.
    - consume liquids between meals rather than with meals.

Nutrition, Alteration in: Less Than Body Requirements Related to Disease Process and Treatment

LEVEL 2: Mild to Moderate

1. Patient demonstrates knowledge of altered nutrition related to disease process and treatment:
   - verbalizes signs and symptoms of inadequate nutritional status.
   - verbalizes measures to promote adequate nutrition.
   - identifies complications of altered nutrition and possible limitations of oncologic treatment.
2. Patient identifies/demonstrates measures to correct or control altered nutrition related to disease process and treatment:
   - performs oral hygiene measures.
   - obtains dental care.
   - controls symptoms and side effects appropriately.
   - maintains adequate nutritional intake.
3. Patient exhibits control of alterations in nutrition:
   - returns to near normal weight or ceases continued weight loss.
   - maintains serum albumin levels of 3.2 to 3.5 g/dl and lymphocyte count of 1500.
   - evidences routine or near-routine activity level.

Assessment

1. See Assessment, Level 1.
2. Evaluate weight loss* over time to determine degree of malnutrition:

Time	None	Mild	Moderate	Severe
1 wk	—	1%	<1–2%	>2%
1 mo	<2%	2%	5%	>5%
3 mo	<5%	5%	7.5%	>7.5%
6 mo	<7.5%	10%		>10%

* % weight change
$$= \frac{\text{usual wt.} - \text{actual wt.}}{\text{Usual wt.}} \times 100$$

3. Evaluate serum albumin levels to assess degree of nutritional deficit: Mild: 3.4 to 3.0 mg/100 ml; Moderate: 3.0 to 2.1 mg/100 ml; Severe: 2.1 mg/100 ml.
4. Monitor total iron binding capacity, ferritin, electrolyte balance, hydration status, calorie intake.
5. Assess intake and output for dehydration secondary to diarrhea, vomiting, fistula drainage, and the like.
6. Note pain, anxiety, depression, fatigue.
7. Assess side effects related to disease process and treatment (e.g., stomatitis, mucositis, changes in taste sensation, constipation).
8. Ascertain need for modified diet.

Nursing Interventions

1. See Nursing Interventions, Level 1.
2. Provide oral hygiene before and after meals.
3. Refer patient to clinical dietitian/nutritionist.
4. Provide high-calorie, high-protein dietary supplements that are most appropriate to patient's needs (e.g., add milk powder to whole milk, malts, eggnogs, puddings, Isocal, Polycose, Carnation Instant Breakfast, Ensure, Ensure Plus).
5. Offer small, frequent feedings when food intake decreases.
6. Eliminate or limit non-nutritious foods.
7. Assist with maintenance of activity and independence in activities of daily living.
8. Administer prescribed medications and treatments to control side effects of dis-

ease process and treatment (e.g., oral care, antiemetics 30 minutes before eating, chewing gum, fluids, artificial saliva to help relieve dry mouth).

9. Plan care so that painful or unpleasant procedures do not take place before or immediately after meals.

10. Provide psychologic support by listening to nutritional and related problems of patient/caregiver. Encourage continued effort in supporting nutritional regimen and control of symptoms and side effects as prescribed.

11. Encourage continuation of therapy to control disease.

12. Suggest follow-up dental consult for ill-fitting dentures secondary to weight loss.

13. Refer to home care and community support agencies such as Meals on Wheels, as appropriate.

Patient Teaching

1. See Patient Teaching, Level 1.
2. Teach signs and symptoms of altered nutritional status and dehydration. Emphasize those that should be reported to the health care team.
3. Recommend eating high-protein, high-calorie snacks (e.g., peanut butter and crackers, eggnog) to increase nutrient intake.
4. Emphasize need to ingest foods high in electrolytes (e.g., Gatorade, fruit juices, salty broths, soups, milk, green leafy vegetables) to control electrolyte loss associated with vomiting and diarrhea, excessive wound or fistula drainage.
5. Instruct regarding medications to control or minimize side effects.
6. Discuss need to follow prescribed treatment protocols.
7. Suggest ways to adjust meal size to appetite, enhance or minimize food odors, coordinate meals with antiemetics/pain medications and create a relaxed, pleasant environment.
8. Advise regarding availability of support groups for patient/caregiver. (Local chapters of the American Cancer Society and the Oncology Nursing Society and local mental health agencies are good resources.)

LEVEL 3: Severe

EXPECTED OUTCOME

1. Patient/caregiver demonstrate knowledge about severe alterations in nutrition related to disease process and treatment:
   - verbalize factors that cause or contribute to malnourishment.
   - identify signs and symptoms to report to health care team
2. Patient/caregiver demonstrate measures to manage severe alteration in nutritional status:
   - patient takes medications as prescribed to maintain comfort and control symptoms.
   - demonstrate proper administration of enteral or parenteral nutrition.
   - identify bowel regimen appropriate to needs.
3. Patient exhibits stable or improved nutritional status consistent with disease process:
   - achieves stable weight.
   - maintains adequate hydration.
   - exhibits stable laboratory values.

4. Patient/caregiver verbalize plans for life style that may be anticipated after cancer therapies are completed.
5. Patient/caregiver name foods and fluids that provide optimal comfort during terminal stages of illness.

NURSING MANAGEMENT

Assessment

1. See Assessment, Levels 1 and 2.
2. Assess for edema that may accompany advanced cancer:
   - daily weight may be misleading as to actual nutritional status.
   - accurate monitoring of intake and output is essential.
   - anthropometric measurements are required.
3. Obtain leukocyte count. Profound leukopenia is often accompanied by infection. Fever, chills, anorexia, and increased energy consumption accelerate deterioration of nutritional status.
4. Assess for confusion, agitation, lethargy, hallucinations, apathy, or dysphagia that can result in impaired intake and consequent dehydration.
5. Assess for signs and symptoms of fluid and electrolyte imbalance.
6. Assess bowel status.

Nursing Interventions

1. See Nursing Interventions, Levels 1 and 2.
2. Encourage rest before and immediately after meals.
3. Encourage or provide mouth care before and after meals and as needed to maintain moist, unimpaired mucous membrane integrity.
4. Feed patient to conserve energy as necessary.
5. Administer enteral/parenteral feedings as prescribed to provide or augment nutrition.

6. Promote rehabilitation based on prognosis and patient's ability to participate.
   - provide opportunity to discuss fears regarding altered feeding methods.
   - provide opportunity for patient to discuss self-concept and altered body image.
   - develop exercise program to improve utilization of nutrients, improve and maintain strength.
   - offer diversional activities.
   - as appropriate, offer opportunities to discuss life style, employment, anticipated alterations in activities of daily living as they apply to postcancer treatment.
7. Initiate social service and home care referral, as appropriate.

Patient Teaching

1. See Patient Teaching, Levels 1 and 2.
2. Teach elements of enteral nutritional support delivery system:
   - purpose and location of tube.
   - techniques for insertion and attachment of tube.
   - nutritional products to be used and advantages and drawbacks of each.
   - procedures for determining tube placement/location, patency, including need to reposition nasal tube as necessary to prevent pressure necrosis.
   - selection of appropriate formula:
     ○ blenderized formula is less expensive, individually formulated, contains dietary fiber to prevent constipation.

- commercially prepared enteral formulas are convenient and may be complete (containing all necessary nutrients) or incomplete (lacking in one or more essential nutrients).
- methods and schedule of administration:
  - check placement of tube before initiating any feeding and every 8 to 10 hours during continuous feeding.
  - elevate head of bed 30 to 45 degrees to prevent reflux or aspiration, unless tube is in jejunum.
- signs and symptoms of complications to report to health care team:
  - aspiration (dusky color, cough, noisy breathing, restlessness, agitation, wheezing, rapid pulse).
  - diarrhea, nausea, vomiting, dumping syndrome, gastric retention (bloating), increasing lethargy.

3. Teach elements of total parenteral nutrition support system:
   - necessary equipment.
   - catheter care and dressing changes according to physician's orders.
   - maintaining patency of catheter with normal saline heparin flush.
   - sterile IV solution containing glucose, amino acids, additional ingredients as ordered.
   - IV fat supplement to provide essential fatty acids, if ordered.
   - monitoring blood and urine for glucose.
   - daily temperature and weight (if appropriate).
   - signs and symptoms of complications to report to health care team:
     - temperature above 100° F.
     - redness, swelling, leaking around catheter insertion site.
     - problems related to infusion pump.
     - swollen neck veins, arm or shoulder pain, or decreased circulation on catheter side.
     - clotting of catheter.
     - edema.
4. Describe measures to promote comfort.

5. Demonstrate active/passive exercises to maintain muscle tone.
6. Suggest methods to involve patient participation in family activities at mealtime whenever possible.
7. As appropriate, instruct caregiver in methods to promote rehabilitation such as encouraging self-care activities, outings, visits with friends, assisting in care of home.

SUGGESTED READINGS

Donoghue, M. Nunnally, C., and Yasko, J.P.: Nutritional Aspects of Cancer Care. Boston, VA, Reston, 1983.

Dudjak, L.A.: Mouth care for mucositis due to radiation therapy. Cancer Nursing 10(3):131–140, 1987.

Konstantinides, N., and Shronts, E.: Tube feeding: Managing the basics. American Journal of Nursing 83:1311–1323, 1983.

Kouba, J.: Nutritional care of the individual with cancer. Nutrition in Clinical Practice 3:175–182, 1988.

Padilla, G.V.: Psychological aspects of nutrition and cancer. Surgical Clinics of North America 66(6):1121–1135, 1986.

Ropka, M.E.: Nutrition. In Johnson, B.L., and Gross, J. (Eds.): Handbook of Oncology Nursing. Bethany, CT, Fleschner, 1985, pp. 185–227.

Schnipper, I.M.: Symptom management: Anorexia, Cancer Nursing 8:33–35, Supplement I, 1985.

Shahert, J.K.: Nutrition and cancer. In Burkhauer, P.K., and Donley, D.D. (Eds.): Dynamics of Oncology Nursing. New York, McGraw-Hill, 1978, pp. 89–109.

Smith, S.A.N.: Theories and intervention of nutritional deficit in neoplastic disease. Oncology Nursing Forum 9(2):43–46, 1982.

Trester, A.K.: Nursing management of patients receiving cancer chemotherapy, Cancer Nursing 5(6):201–210, 1982.

Yasko, J.M., and Greene, P.: Coping with problems related to cancer and cancer treatment. CA: A Cancer Journal for Clinicians 37(2):106–125, 1987.

PATIENT EDUCATION MATERIALS AND COMMUNITY RESOURCES

Cancer Information Service: 1–800–4–CANCER.

Eating Habits—Recipes and Tips for Better Nutrition During Cancer Treatment. NIH Publication

Nutrition, Alteration in: Less Than Body Requirements Related to Disease Process and Treatment

No. 87–2079, Rev 1986. Available free and in quantity from: Office of Cancer Communication, National Cancer Institute, Bldg 31, Room 10A24, Bethesda, MD 20892

Enteral Products and Literature Guide, Mead Johnson, Evansville, IN 47721.

Ross Laboratories, Columbus, OH 43216

(The contents of this chapter are in no way meant to represent the views of the Department of Veterans Affairs.)

Nutrition, Alteration in: Less Than Body Requirements Related to Nausea and Vomiting

Barbara Hall, Ina J. Hardesty, and Rosemarie Hogan

Population at Risk

- Patients receiving cancer chemotherapeutic agents, narcotic analgesics, or biologic response modifier therapy
- Patients receiving radiation therapy to the gastrointestinal tract, head, or neck
- Patients with cancers involving gastrointestinal system

LEVEL 1: Potential

EXPECTED OUTCOME

1. Patient demonstrates knowledge related to potential alteration in nutrition:
   - identifies causes of nausea and vomiting.
   - identifies effects of nausea and vomiting on nutritional status.
   - acknowledges importance of maintaining good nutritional status.
   - verbalizes potential sequelae of altered nutritional status.
2. Patient identifies/demonstrates measures to maintain nutritional status:
   - describes measures to prevent or alleviate nausea and vomiting.
   - describes balanced diet that includes all major food groups.
   - identifies/demonstrates adequate caloric intake.
   - identifies/demonstrates adequate protein intake.
   - adjusts eating patterns and schedules as needed.
   - identifies signs and symptoms to report to health care team.
3. Patient maintains nutritional status:
   - maintains weight within normal range for height and build.
   - maintains balanced diet that includes all major food groups.
   - maintains pertinent laboratory values within normal range.
   - hair, nails, skin turgor remain of good texture and quality.
4. Patient experiences minimal nausea and no vomiting.

NURSING MANAGEMENT

Assessment

1. Assess baseline nutrition, including:
   - weight and height:
     - preillness weight and height.
     - weight 1 mo ago.
     - admission weight.
     - weight loss or gain.
     - comparison of current weight with ideal weight.

173

- skin test results (indicating anergy).
- age.
- anthropometric measurements (midarm muscle circumference, triceps skin fold).
- physical assessment:
  - hair—color, shine, amount.
  - face—skin color, edema, scaling.
  - eyes—color of membranes, fissuring of eyelid corners, dryness of eye membranes.
  - lips—redness, swelling, lesions, moisture.
  - tongue—color, swelling, texture, sores, moisture.
  - teeth—caries, pain, shine.
  - gums—color, bleeding, swelling.
  - glands—swelling, lymphadenopathy.
  - skin—color (icterus, pallor, abnormal pigmentation), eruptions, lesions, bruises, edema, turgor, excessive dryness or oiliness, abnormal hair distribution, texture, lack of fat under skin.
  - nails—firmness, color.
  - musculoskeletal system—muscle tone, ability to ambulate, appearance of muscles (wasted).
  - ability to chew or swallow.
2. Monitor laboratory values (e.g., CBC and differential, electrolytes, serum iron, TIBC, total protein, albumin).
3. Monitor vital signs.
4. Obtain diet history, including:
   - dietary habits:
     - times of day at which patient eats.
     - times that appetite is greatest.
     - types of food eaten.
     - amount of food eaten.
     - types and amount of fluid patient drinks.
     - daily food intake diary (detailed listing of foods and quantities consumed during previous day).
     - number of meals per day.
     - use of vitamin and nutritional supplements.

- meals eaten outside home.
- responses to food intake:
  - recent changes in food patterns.
  - food likes and dislikes.
  - response to odor of food.
  - present response to sweets, pork, beef, other proteins.
  - factors that cause patient to reject food.
- means and methods of food storage and preparation.
- sociocultural influences:
  - values related to food.
  - cultural practices related to food.
  - social and family patterns of eating.
  - religious beliefs related to food.
  - meals eaten outside home.
  - foods that patient considers to be a reward or to be nurturing.
5. Assess history of nausea and vomiting:
   - Is patient at high risk for anticipatory nausea?
   - Does patient have nausea alone, or is it followed by vomiting?
   - Has pattern of nausea and vomiting changed since illness? How?
   - What promotes nausea and vomiting (e.g., eating, pain, coughing, body position, ambulation, activity, drugs, specific foods)?
   - How frequent is nausea and vomiting and how long does it last?
     - Is discomfort relieved by vomiting?
     - What measures have been used to control nausea and vomiting in the past?
6. Monitor patient for:
   - anorexia.
   - altered taste.
   - nausea.
   - vomiting (type and amount).
   - sore mouth.
   - fatigue, level of energy.
   - pain.
   - obstruction.
7. Determine known or probable preexisting disease states:
   - diabetes.

- renal disease.
- CNS involvement.
- liver disease.
- malabsorption syndrome.
- hypercalcemia.
8. Note altered bowel habits and measures used to control them:
    - diarrhea (frequency, color, quantity, quality).
    - constipation.
9. Ascertain current and recent treatment:
    - chemotherapy (type, last treatment, schedule).
    - radiation (site, last treatment).
    - surgery (type, postop course).
10. Evaluate emotional status:
    - note mental status (alert, oriented, confused, lethargic).
    - assess level of anxiety.

Nursing Interventions

1. Administer antiemetics before, during, or after chemotherapy/radiation therapy on prescribed schedule if drugs have high emetrogenic properties.
2. Schedule antiemetics according to pattern of nausea and vomiting.
3. Provide adequate analgesia as needed; titrate amount of oral medications at mealtime to control pain but maintain alertness.
4. Consider giving chemotherapy at night or late afternoon, if appropriate.

Patient Teaching

1. Discuss potential causes of nausea and vomiting.
2. Discuss potential effects of nausea and vomiting on nutritional status.
3. Teach signs and symptoms to report to health care team:

- character, amount, frequency of vomiting.
- weight loss.
- decreased urine output.
- decreased food and fluid intake.
4. Teach methods to prevent nausea and vomiting:
    - small, frequent, nutritious meals.
    - attractive servings.
    - allowance of sufficient time for meals.
    - small dietary intake before treatment.
    - rest periods before and after meals.
    - avoidance of highly seasoned or greasy foods.
    - modification of food consistency or type as needed.
    - quiet restful environment.
    - analgesics as needed.
    - antiemetics as needed.
    - maintenance of comfortable position.
    - relaxation techniques.
    - need to seek dental care as necessary.
    - oral hygiene measures.
    - family avoidance of coaxing, bribing, threatening in relation to food intake.
5. Teach appropriate administration of antiemetics:
    - describe actions and side effects of antiemetics.
    - emphasize need to report effectiveness of antiemetics.
    - discuss type, frequency, method, importance of scheduled antiemetic administration.
6. Teach rationale for and measures to maintain a healthy nutritional status:
    - components of balanced diet and adequate food intake.
    - methods to increase caloric and protein intake:
        - add 1 to 2 T powdered milk to food during preparation (e.g., creamed soups).
        - use milkshakes, eggnog, whole milk.
        - use ice cubes made from juices, so drinks are not diluted.
        - encourage nutritional supplements between meals.

LEVEL 2:   Moderate

EXPECTED OUTCOME

1. Patient demonstrates knowledge related to altered nutritional status:
   - identifies cause of nausea and vomiting.
   - identifies effects of nausea and vomiting on nutritional status.
   - acknowledges importance of maintaining good nutritional status.
   - verbalizes potential sequelae of altered nutritional status.
2. Patient identifies/demonstrates measures to maintain or improve nutritional status:
   - describes measures to alleviate nausea and vomiting.
   - identifies balanced diet that includes all major food groups.
   - identifies/demonstrates adequate protein intake.
   - identifies/demonstrates adequate caloric intake.
   - identifies/demonstrates adequate fluid intake.
   - adjusts eating patterns and schedules as necessary.
   - identifies signs and symptoms to report to health care team.
3. Patient maintains or improves nutritional status:
   - maintains or increases weight consistent with age, height, condition.
   - maintains pertinent laboratory values within normal limits.
   - hair, nails of good texture and quality, skin turgor normal.
4. Patient experiences minimal nausea and vomiting.

NURSING MANAGEMENT

Assessment

1. See Assessment, Level 1.
2. Assess albumin level.
3. Take weekly weights, anthropometric measurements.
4. Monitor intake and output.
5. Monitor calorie count and food diary; individualize per diet instructions.
6. Assess emotional status.
7. Evaluate effectiveness of antiemetic regimen.

Nursing Interventions

1. See Nursing Interventions, Level 1.
2. Adjust antiemetic regimen as appropriate, in consultation with physician.
3. Introduce nonpharmacologic behavioral approaches.
4. Introduce and provide necessary resources to implement behavioral approaches to alleviate nausea and vomiting:
   - hypnosis.
   - behavior modification.
   - desensitization.
   - guided imagery.
   - biofeedback.
   - relaxation techniques.
   - diversion.
   - meditation.

Patient Teaching

1. See Patient Teaching, Level 1.
2. Teach signs and symptoms of dehydration.
3. Teach measures to improve or maintain hydration status.
4. Discuss signs and symptoms of altered nutrition.

5. Recommend foods with low potential to cause nausea (e.g., dry toast, crackers, ginger ale, cola, dry popcorn, grapes, cold plates, salads, boiled or baked potatoes).
6. Note importance of eating when food is tolerated.
7. Emphasize maintenance of accurate food diary.
8. Teach rationale for and methods of non-pharmacologic behavioral approaches to alleviate nausea and vomiting.

LEVEL 3:   *Severe*

EXPECTED OUTCOME

1. Patient/caregiver demonstrate knowledge related to severe alteration in nutritional status:
   • identify signs and symptoms of severe nutritional alteration.
   • identify potential sequelae/complications of altered nutritional status.
   • identify enteral and parenteral nutrition as alternative methods of feeding.
2. Patient/caregiver identify/demonstrate measures to control nausea and vomiting:
   • demonstrate proper knowledge and administration of medications.
   • maintain quiet atmosphere free from noxious stimuli.
   • patient identifies/ingests foods or drinks with antiemetic qualities.
3. Patient exhibits clinical improvement in nutritional/hydrational status:
   • maintains stable weight.
   • ingests adequate calories for body requirements.
   • maintains adequate intake and output.
   • skin turgor within normal limits.
   • serum albumin within normal limits.
4. Patient achieves control of nausea and vomiting.

NURSING MANAGEMENT

Assessment

1. See Assessment, Levels 1 and 2.
2. Monitor supportive care (e.g., total parenteral or enteral nutrition, IV hydration) as indicated or ordered.

Nursing Interventions

1. See Nursing Interventions, Levels 1 and 2.
2. Administer antiemetics:
   • via alternate routes during emesis.
   • around the clock as ordered.
   • evaluate effectiveness of drug regimen.
3. Keep clean emesis basin within reach, and clean promptly after use.
4. Provide for proper diet:
   • identify and provide favorite foods but avoid serving favorite foods during periods of severe nausea.
   • administer supplemental feedings and fluids as ordered.
   • administer enteral and parenteral nutrition as ordered.

177

5. Arrange for patient's comfort. Patient may require IV or IM analgesics and antiemetics.

Patient Teaching

1. See Patient Teaching, Levels 1 and 2.
2. Discuss alternate methods of administration of antiemetics.
3. Note signs and symptoms of dehydration to be reported to health care team.
4. Explain rationale and techniques for supplemental fluids and nutrition.
5. Discuss rationale and techniques of enteral and parenteral nutrition.
6. Stress health care team's commitment to symptom control and importance of ongoing assessment.

SUGGESTED READINGS

American Nurses' Association and Oncology Nursing Society: Standards of Oncology Nursing Practice. Kansas City, MO, 1987.

Burns, N.: Nursing and Cancer. Philadelphia, W. B. Saunders, 1982, pp. 211–216.

Chernoff, R., and Ropka, M.: The unique nutritional needs of the elderly patient with cancer. Seminars in Oncology Nursing 4(3):189–197, 1988.

Clark, R.A., Tyson, L.B., Gralla, R.J., and Kris, M.G.: Antiemetic therapy: Management of chemotherapy-induced nausea and vomiting. Seminars in Oncology Nursing 5 (2 suppl 1):53–57, 1989.

Coons, H.L., Leventhal, H., Nerenz, P.R., et al.: Anticipatory nausea and emotional distress in patients receiving cisplatin-based chemotherapy. Oncology Nursing Forum 14(3):31–35, 1987.

Cotanch, P.H., and Strum, S.: Progressive muscle relaxation as antiemetic therapy for cancer patients. Oncology Nursing Forum 14(1):33–37, 1987.

D'Agostino, N.S.: Managing nutritional problems in advanced cancer. American Journal of Nursing 89:50–56, 1989.

Donovan, M.I.: Relaxation with guided imagery: A useful technique. Cancer Nursing 3(1):27–32, 1980.

Dwyer, J.F.: Dietetic assessment of ambulatory cancer patients. In Proceedings of the American Cancer Society and National Cancer Institute: National Conference on Nutrition in Cancer. New York, American Cancer Society, 1979, pp. 2077–2086.

Geltman, R.L., and Paige, R.L.: Symptom management in hospice care. American Journal of Nursing 83(1):78–85, 1983.

Goodman, M.: Management of nausea and vomiting induced by outpatient cisplatin (Platinol) therapy. Seminars in Oncology Nursing 3(1 Suppl 1):23–25, 1987.

Grant, M.: Nausea, vomiting, and anorexia. Seminars in Oncology Nursing 3(4):277–286, 1987.

Groenwald, S.L.: Nutritional disorders. In Groenwald, S.L. (Ed.): Cancer Nursing Principles and Practice. Boston, Jones & Bartlett, 1987, pp. 141–170.

Hogan, C.M.: Nausea and vomiting. In Yasko, J.M.: Guidelines for Cancer Care: Symptom Management. Reston, VA, Reston Publishing, 1983, pp. 198–211.

Jordan, L.N.: Effects of fluid manipulation on the incidence of vomiting during outpatient cisplatin infusion. Oncology Nursing Forum 16:213–218, 1989.

Moore, J.M.: The influence of the time of administration in cisplatin-induced nausea and vomiting. Oncology Nursing Forum 9(3):26–32, 1982.

Morrow, G.R.: Chemotherapy-related nausea and vomiting: Etiology and management. CA: A Cancer Journal for Clinicians 39(2):89–104, 1989.

Mundinger, M.O.: Nursing diagnosis for cancer patients. Cancer Nursing 1(3):221–226, 1978.

Nunnally, C., Donoghue, M., and Yasko, J.M.: Nutritional needs of cancer patients. Nursing Clinics of North America 17(4):567–578, 1982.

Peters, C.A.H.: Myths of antiemetic administration. Cancer Nursing 12:102–106, 1989.

Shils, M.E.: Principles of nutrition therapy. In Proceedings of the American Cancer Society and National Cancer Institute: National Conference on Nutrition in Cancer. New York, American Cancer Society, 1979.

Souba, W.W., and Copeland, M.E.: Hyperalimentation in cancer. CA: A Cancer Journal for Clinicians 39:105–113, 1989.

Trester, A.K.: Nursing management of patients receiving cancer chemotherapy. Cancer Nursing 5(3):201–210, 1982.

Wickham, R.: Managing chemotherapy-related nausea and vomiting: The state of the art. Oncology Nursing Forum 16(4):563–574, 1989.

Welch, D.A.: Assessment of nausea and vomiting in cancer patients undergoing external beam radiotherapy. Cancer Nursing 3(5):365–371, 1980.

PATIENT EDUCATION MATERIALS AND COMMUNITY RESOURCES

Morra, M.E., Suski, N., and Johnson, B.: Eating Hints: Recipes and Tips for Better Nutrition During Cancer Treatment. Publication No. 87-2079. Bethesda, MD, National Cancer Institute, 1987.

Sallan, S.E., Lart, M., and Tyson, L.: Nausea, Vomiting, and You. Norwalk, CT, Purdue Fredericks Publication, 1989.

Nutrition, Alteration in: Less Than Body Requirements Related to Dysphagia

Rosemary Grady, Juanita Farnen, and Pat Ascheman

Population at Risk

- Patients experiencing functional alteration of swallowing related to tumor invasion, fibrosis, surgical resection, infectious processes, stomatitis/esophagitis, neuropathies, esophageal motility disorders, and gastroesophageal reflux

LEVEL 1: Potential

EXPECTED OUTCOME

1. Patient exhibits stable nutritional status:
   - maintains normal weight for height.
   - maintains adequate hydration.
   - maintains recommended daily caloric, protein, carbohydrate, fat intake (RDA requirements).
   - maintains laboratory values within normal limits.
   - maintains normal level activity.
2. Patient demonstrates knowledge of adequate food and fluid intake:
   - states components of four basic food groups.
   - states importance and amounts of required daily nutrients.
   - identifies potential effect of dysphagia on nutritional status.
3. Patient identifies early signs and symptoms of dysphagia including those to report to health care team.

NURSING MANAGEMENT

Assessment

1. Review historic data:
   - previous medical history.

- treatments patient has received or is expected to receive, especially:
  - radiation therapy to head and neck region.

- chemotherapy and side effects experienced.
- surgical interventions, including those to head and neck region.
- previous impairment of swallowing (e.g., swallowing toxin that caused stenosis).
- diet history, including food preferences, method of food intake.
- medications: antihistamines, anticholinergics, diuretics, antihypertensives, antidepressants that may inhibit salivary output, phenothiazines that may cause orofacial dyskinesias; prokinetic agents (e.g., metoclopramide) that increase peristalsis.

2. Assess cranial nerves and swallowing ability:
   - ask patient to swallow while palpating laryngeal elevation, observing lip closure, coughing or choking.
3. Inspect oral cavity and observe structures, mobility of tongue, saliva.
   - note strength of tongue pushing on cheek against examiner's hand.
4. Assess level of alertness and responsiveness.
5. Determine fear and anxiety about choking.
6. Assess gag reflex by stimulating lateral aspects of pharyngeal wall with a tongue blade.
7. Assess coughing reflex.
8. Assess respiratory status.
9. Check condition and fit of dentures, if present.
10. Assess nutritional knowledge of calorie, protein, carbohydrate, and fat intake.
11. Assess nutritional status:
    - nutritional and hydrational status q24h.
    - height and weight.
    - skin turgor.
    - anthropometric measurements.
    - laboratory values (total iron-binding capacity, albumin, creatinine height index, serum iron, total protein and albumin-globulin ratio, serum transferrin, electrolytes, glucose, lymphocyte count).

Nursing Interventions

1. Consult dietitian to provide instruction in basic nutrition.
2. Individualize diet to patient's food preferences and nutritional diet requirements.

Patient Teaching

1. Teach basic nutritional needs and importance of maintaining balanced daily diet:
   - components of balanced diet.
   - daily caloric and protein requirements.
2. Describe phases of swallowing:
   - oral (food is chewed and propelled to the posterior tongue).
   - pharyngeal (a reflex movement; tongue rises to palate, soft palate rises to posterior pharyngeal wall, larynx moves anteriorly and superiorly as pharynx constricts and forces the bolus of food toward esophagus. The nasopharynx and airway are closed).
   - esophageal (peristaltic contraction of esophagus and relaxation of gastroesophageal sphincter moves the bolus of food into stomach by gravity and peristalsis).
3. Discuss signs and symptoms of dysphagia to report:
   - choking when swallowing liquids.
   - fear of choking.
   - food sticking in pharynx or esophagus.
   - pain when swallowing.
   - weakness of oral musculature with lip closure, tongue control, rotary jaw movement.
   - tenderness and open lesions in oral cavity.
4. Discuss potential for aspiration of liquids or solids if dysphagia occurs.

EXPECTED OUTCOME

1. Patient identifies signs and symptoms of difficulty swallowing including those to report to the health care team.
2. Patient identifies measures to obtain adequate nutrition:
   - selects appropriate foods.
   - identifies nutritional supplements.
3. Patient exhibits stable nutritional status:
   - maintains standard for height and weight.
   - shows laboratory values within normal limits.
   - displays adequate food and fluid intake on 24 hr count.
4. Patient identifies measures to improve swallowing ability:
   - identifies textures of food to eat.
   - performs exercises to improve muscle strength.
5. Patient identifies potential risk for pneumonia, esophagitis, heartburn related to gastroesophageal reflux and aspiration.

NURSING MANAGEMENT

Assessment

1. See Assessment, Level 1.
2. Referral to speech and language therapist to determine if dysphagia is related to deficit in oral, pharyngeal, or esophageal musculature.
3. Assess oral musculature, range of motion of lips, tongue, and jaw:
   - check tongue for lateralization, protrusion, elevation.
   - check lips for protrusion, retraction, closure.
   - check jaw for closure, rotary jaw movement.
4. Observe patient during and after meals for choking, drooling, regurgitation of fluid in nose, retention of food in oral cavity, note foods not tolerated well.
5. Assess level of alertness and responsiveness before each feeding.
6. Assess respiratory status after each feeding for symptoms of silent aspiration.
7. Observe adequacy of dietary intake and note whether deficient intake results from dysfunction, lack of appetite, or food preferences.
8. Assess dysphagia related to deficit in oral musculature as follows:
   - begin with semisolids.
   - give patient a small bite and note time until laryngeal elevation (Normal swallowing is 1 to 10 sec).
   - observe for food retention in buccal area.
   - ask patient to phonate "ah" after each bite.
   - note if sound is clear or garbled (garbled indicates retention on vocal cords).
   - if garbled, have patient cough, then swallow again and repeat phonation to reevaluate.
   - give patient normal bite size, same texture, and repeat process. If satisfactory proceed to solids and evaluate as above.

9. Assess dysphagia related to pharyngeal dysfunction:
   • begin with liquids and proceed to solids.
   • note coughing during or immediately after swallowing.
   • note patient reporting that food sticks in throat.
10. Assess dysphagia related to esophageal dysfunction:
    • begin with thick liquids and evaluate in similar manner as pharyngeal dysfunction.
    • if satisfactory, proceed to liquid and evaluate.
    • note report by patient of food sticking in esophagus.
11. Monitor swallowing before and during each feeding.
12. Monitor food and fluid intake.

Nursing Interventions

1. Consult dietitian for calorie count and need for diet modification in food texture and consistency.
2. Place patient in position that best promotes swallowing (e.g., sitting upright).
3. Offer 6 to 8 small feedings daily.
4. Avoid crunchy, spicy, hot foods if inflammation is present.
5. Avoid milk products if mucus is copious.
6. Weigh every other day.
7. Explain procedures to patient.
8. Have suction available if patient is fearful of aspiration.
9. If deficiency is in one side of oral musculature, have patient take small bites on strong side.
10. Modify patient's head position by lowering chin, tilting or turning head to improve swallowing ability.
11. Place food on posterior tongue with long-handled spoon or syringe if patient has difficulty propelling food to posterior tongue.
12. Implement swallowing technique to prevent aspiration of food:

   • patient inhales.
   • place small amount of food on tongue.
   • patient swallows, then exhales/coughs.
   • wait 30 seconds between bites.
13. Have patient sit upright for 15 to 30 minutes after meal. If in bed, place at 45-degree angle. Check mouth for food retention.
14. Begin oral exercises to strengthen tongue, lips, and jaw for problems with oral musculature evidenced by food retention in buccal area, aspiration prior to laryngeal elevation, drooling.
15. Have patient eat at least 2 hours before retiring at night to decrease gastroesophageal reflux and potential aspiration.
16. Allow patient uninterrupted, unhurried time to eat.

Patient Teaching

1. See Patient Teaching, Level 1.
2. Teach exercises to strengthen lips:
   • place tongue depressor between lips and have patient hold in place for increasing amount of time.
   • ask patient to close lips as tightly as possible while examiner attempts to separate with slight resistance on tongue depressor.
3. Teach exercises to strengthen tongue:
   • instruct patient to lick roof of mouth (may apply peanut butter to palate).
   • instruct patient to go through range of motion for tongue muscle (i.e., lateralization, sweeping around buccal cavity, elevation, protrusion).
4. Teach exercises to strengthen jaw; ask patient to pretend to chew gum to facilitate rotary jaw movement.
5. Describe swallowing technique to prevent aspiration of food:
   • patient alert and responsive prior to feeding.
   • patient inhales.
   • place small amount of soft, solid food on tongue.
   • patient swallows.

- patient exhales/coughs.
- waits ½ min between bites.
6. Explain rationale and measures to promote food intake:
   - amount and types of nutrients needed daily.
   - texture and consistency of food to eat to lessen patient's swallowing deficits.
   - use of mild flavorings and seasonings (e.g., nutmeg, vanilla, cinnamon) to promote palatability.
   - supplemental high-protein, high-calorie foods.
   - small, frequent meals; larger breakfasts than dinners; adequate time allocated for meals.
7. Discuss techniques to improve swallowing:
   - oral musculature dysphagia:
     - semisolid foods (pudding, canned fruit, mashed potatoes, cooked fish) for chewing impairment.

- thin, pureed foods (tilt body to 45 degrees, do not hyperextend head).
     - place food at posterior of tongue with long-handled spoon.
   - pharyngeal dysphagia:
     - try alternating solid and liquid food.
     - do swallowing exercise.
     - modify head and trunk positions.
   - supraglottic dysfunction: teach patient to voluntarily close airway (e.g., take a deep breath, hold it tight, and swallow while holding breath, cough, then re-swallow).
   - esophageal dysphagia:
     - may use food supplements.
     - use liquefied food in small, frequent feedings.
8. Teach emergency procedures to use if patient aspirates (e.g., Heimlich maneuver, suctioning, CPR).

LEVEL 3: Severe

EXPECTED OUTCOME

1. Patient maintains optimal nutritional intake:
   - shows steady weight gain or maintains stable weight.
   - exhibits laboratory values within normal limits.
2. Patient/caregiver identify measures to obtain optimal nutrition:
   - select appropriate foods.
   - identify nutritional supplements.
   - identify enteral or total parenteral nutrition as alternate method of food intake.
3. Patient/caregiver demonstrate measures to adapt to changes in mastication and swallowing:
   - demonstrate procedures for alternative feeding methods.
   - demonstrate therapeutic exercises to improve mastication and swallowing.
   - perform oral hygiene as scheduled.

NURSING MANAGEMENT

Assessment

1. See Assessment, Levels 1 and 2.

2. Monitor food intake daily and evaluate caloric and protein intake.
3. Monitor fluid intake daily.

4. Monitor weight daily.
5. Assess swallowing ability daily.
6. Assess signs and symptoms of malnutrition (fatigue, changes in mental status, weight loss, abnormal serum albumin).

Nursing Interventions

1. See Nursing Interventions, Level 2.
2. Arrange dietary and speech therapy consults, if available, to help correct problem.
3. Encourage high-calorie, high-protein diet.
4. If patient is unable to propel food to posterior of tongue, feed with long-handled spoon or catheter-tip syringe and ask patient to swallow.
5. Administer enteral feedings or total parenteral nutrition as ordered.
6. Provide supplemental feedings between meals.
7. Provide oral hygiene before and after meals.

Patient Teaching

1. See Patient Teaching, Levels 1 and 2.
2. Explain rationale and measures to improve nutritional status:
   - enteral feedings via nasogastric, gastrostomy, jejunostomy tubes.
   - total parenteral nutrition (intravenous).
3. Teach signs and symptoms of malnutrition.
4. Reinforce teaching of exercises and techniques to improve mastication and swallowing ability.

SUGGESTED READINGS

American Dietetic Association: Handbook of Clinical Dietetics. New Haven, CT, Yale University, Halliday Lithograph Corp., 1981.

Barnett, N.K.: Identification of nutritional deficiencies. Oncology Nursing Forum 9:58, 1982.

Buchin, P.J.: Swallowing disorders. Otolaryngologic Clinics of North America 21:663–675, 1988.

Buckley, J.E., Addicks, C.L., and Maniglia, J.: Feeding patients with dysphagia. Nursing Forum 15:69–84, 1976.

Bullock, J.: Dysphagia. Nursing Times 71:191–194, 1975.

Diagnosing Dysphagia (interview). Emergency Medicine 21(1):51; 54–55, 1989.

Dobie, R.: Rehabilitation of swallowing disorders. American Family Physician 17:84–95, 1978.

Goodhart, R.S., and Shils, M.E.: Modern Nutrition in Health and Disease (6th ed). Philadelphia, Lea & Febiger, 1980.

Griffin, J. Jr., and Tollison, J.: Dysphagia. American Family Physician Practical Therapeutics 22:154–160, 1980.

Griffin, K.M.: Swallowing training for dysphagic patients. Archives of Physical Medicine Rehabilitation 55:467–470, 1974.

Griffin, K.M., Stubbert, J., and Breckenridge, K.: Teaching the dysphagic patient to swallow. Archives of Physical Medicine Rehabilitation 55:60–63, 1974.

Gritz, J.M.: Assessment and intervention techniques for the dysphagic patient in the home setting. Journal of Home Health Care Practice 4:51–65, 1989.

Kramer, P.: Dysphagia—Etiologic differentiation and therapy. Hospital Practice 125–149, March 30, 1988.

Logemann, J.: Evaluation and Treatment of Swallowing Disorders. San Diego, CA, College Hill Press, 1983.

Logemann, J.: Swallowing physiology and pathophysiology. Otolaryngologic Clinics of North America 21:613–623, 1988.

Logemann, J., and Bytell, D.: Swallowing disorders in three types of head and neck surgical patients. American Cancer Society 44:1095–1105, 1979.

Loustau, A., and Lee, K.A.: Dealing with the dangers of dysphagia. Nursing 15 (2):47–50, 1985.

McConnel, F.M.S., Cerenko, D., and Mendelsohn, M.S.: Dysphagia after total laryngectomy. Otolaryngologic Clinics of North America 21:721–725, 1988.

McNally, J.C.: Dysphagia. Oncology Nursing Forum 9:58–60, 1982.

Nursing Care of the Cancer Patient with Nutritional Problems. Report of the Ross Roundtable on Oncology Nursing, Columbus, OH, November 6, 1980. Sponsored by Ross Laboratories.

Silverman, E.H., and Elfant, I.L.: Dysphagia: An evaluation and treatment program for the adult. American Journal of Occupational Therapy 33:382–392, 1979.

Sonies, B.C., and Baum, B.J.: Evaluation of swallowing pathophysiology. Otolaryngologic Clinics of North America 21:637–647, 1988.

Splaingard, M.L., Hutchins, B., Sulton, L.D., and Chaudhuri, G.: Aspirations in rehabilitation patients: Videofluoroscopy vs. bedside clinical assessment. Archives of Physical Medical Rehabilitation 69:637–640, 1988.

Nutrition, Alteration in: More Than Body Requirements Related to Disease Process and Treatment

Carol Pappas Appel

Population at Risk

- Patients receiving androgens, steroids, and adjuvant therapy for breast cancer
- Patients with decreased mobility

LEVEL 1: Potential

EXPECTED OUTCOME

1. Patient verbalizes knowledge of potential risks of excessive weight gain on disease outcome (in adjuvant breast cancer treatment), body image, self-esteem, cardiovascular status, and general health.
2. Patient demonstrates knowledge of measures to prevent excess weight gain:
   - identifies components of balanced diet including basic food groups.
   - demonstrates ability to follow maintenance diet consistent with recommendations of the American Cancer Society (low fat, high carbohydrate, low salt).
   - identifies importance of regular exercise in maintaining pretreatment body weight.
   - establishes and maintains regular exercise program (consistent with physician guidelines).
3. Patient maintains pretreatment body weight.

NURSING MANAGEMENT

Assessment

1. Obtain baseline nutritional assessment prior to therapy, including:
   - age.
   - height.
   - current weight, ideal weight.
   - condition of hair, skin, mucous membranes.
   - laboratory values (CBC, serum albumin, total protein, chemistry profile, thyroid studies, cholesterol, serum estradiol, triglycerides).
   - dietary history (eating habits, food preferences and aversions, ethnic or cultural practices, food allergies, current and past dietary modifications and restrictions, use of diet pills or liquids, food preparation arrangements, 4-day calorie count, anthropometric measurements).

2. Obtain assessment of current exercise practices, physical activity routine.
3. Determine patient's/family's learning needs related to:
   - nutrition.
   - risk of obesity.
   - exercise.
4. Determine readiness to learn.
5. Identify psychosocial factors that may affect patient's nutritional status.

Nursing Interventions

1. Establish with patient a mutually agreeable plan to maintain pretreatment body weight:
   - review appropriate nutritional principles.
   - follow dietary modifications (low fat, high carbohydrate).
   - follow exercise program (within prescribed limits).

Patient Teaching

1. Describe basic food groups.
2. Review basic dietary components, proportions, and daily requirements.
3. Identify daily caloric needs to maintain weight.
4. Explain potential risks of excessive weight on disease outcome and therapy, body image, self-esteem, cardiovascular status, and general health.
5. Provide written materials on American Cancer Society recommended diet.
6. Explain importance of appropriate daily exercise.

LEVEL 2: *Weight Gain Less Than or Equal to 10 Pounds*

EXPECTED OUTCOME

1. Patient verbalizes knowledge of risks of weight gain.
2. Patient identifies factors influencing weight gain.
3. Patient verbalizes knowledge of appropriate dietary modifications to reduce weight and prevent further weight gain.
4. Patient establishes regular exercise program.
5. Patient returns to pretreatment weight.

NURSING MANAGEMENT

Assessment

1. See Assessment, Level 1.
2. Assess willingness to comply with diet and exercise plan.
3. Identify causes of weight gain:
   - decreased activity.
   - increased depression.
   - increased intake.
   - decreased metabolic rate.
   - decreased serum estradiol level.

Nursing Interventions

1. Adjust dietary plan with patient from a maintenance to a weight reduction diet.

2. Elicit patient's ability to comply with established plan.
3. Adjust exercise program from maintenance to weight reduction per medical guidelines.
4. Encourage participation in community diet programs that have medical approval.
5. Encourage participation in community exercise programs that have medical approval.
6. Offer referral to dietitian.

7. Allow patient to verbalize feelings related to body image and self-esteem.

Patient Teaching

1. See Patient Teaching, Level 1.
2. Provide and discuss meal plans, recipes, and cookbooks to assist patient in compliance with diet plan.
3. Discuss written exercise plan.

LEVEL 3: Weight Gain Greater Than 10 Pounds

EXPECTED OUTCOME

1. Patient identifies measures to facilitate weight loss:
   • dietary modifications.
   • exercise program.
   • behavioral changes.
2. Patient identifies appropriate community resources to assist weight reduction.
3. Patient will return to within 10 pounds of pretreatment weight.

NURSING MANAGEMENT

Assessment

1. See Assessment, Levels 1 and 2.
2. Assess effects of weight gain on socialization, sexuality, activity level.

Nursing Interventions

1. See Nursing Interventions, Levels 1 and 2.
2. Initiate dietary referral.
3. Offer patient support and explore methods of obtaining support from family and friends.
4. Encourage realistic goal setting (small easily achieved goals).
5. Referral to reputable weight loss clinic.
6. Referral to appropriate support groups

(Weight Watchers, Overeaters Anonymous).

Patient Teaching

1. See Patient Teaching, Levels 1 and 2.

SUGGESTED READINGS

Brownell, K.D., and Kramer, F.M.: Behavioral management of obesity. Medical Clinics of North America 73:185–201, 1989.

Chlebowski, R.T., Nixon, D.W., Blackburn, G.L., et al.: A breast cancer nutrition adjuvant study (NAS): Protocol design and initial patient adherence. Breast Cancer Research and Treatment 10:21–29, 1987.

Nutrition, Alteration in: More Than Body Requirements Related to Disease Process and Treatment

Foltz, A.T.: Weight gain among stage II breast cancer patients: A study of five factors. Oncology Nursing Forum *12*:21–26, 1985.

Goodwin, P.J., Panzarella, T., and Boyd, N.F.: Weight gain in women with localized breast cancer—A descriptive study. Breast Cancer Research and Treatment *11*:56–66, 1988.

Heasman, K.Z., Sutherland, H.J., Campbell, J.A., et al.: Weight gain during adjuvant chemotherapy for breast cancer. Breast Cancer Research and Treatment *5*:195–200, 1985.

Huntington, M.O.: Weight gain in patients receiving adjuvant chemotherapy for carcinoma of the breast. Cancer *56*:472–474, 1985.

Knobf, M.K., Mullen, J.C., Xistris, D., and Moritz, D.A.: Weight gain in women with breast cancer receiving adjuvant chemotherapy. Oncology Nursing Forum *10*:28–33, 1983.

PATIENT EDUCATION MATERIALS AND COMMUNITY RESOURCES

Connor, S.L., and Connor, W.E.: The New American Diet. New York, Simon & Schuster, 1986.

DeBakey, M.E., Gotto, A.M. Jr., Scott, L.W., and Foreyt, J.P.: The Living Heart Diet. New York, Simon & Schuster, 1984.

PROTECTIVE MECHANISMS

The nurse assesses the patient's immune function, hematopoietic function, integumentary function, and sensorimotor function (including level of consciousness and thought process) to formulate actual or potential nursing diagnoses.

Appropriate patient outcomes to consider in planning nursing interventions will specify the patient's ability to:

1. list measures to prevent skin breakdown, mucosal trauma, infection, and bleeding.
2. identify the signs and symptoms of infection, bleeding, mucosal trauma, skin breakdown, and sensorimotor dysfunction.
3. contact an appropriate health care team member when initial signs and symptoms of infection, bleeding, mucosal trauma, skin breakdown, or sensorimotor dysfunction occur.
4. describe measures to manage infection, bleeding, mucosal trauma, skin breakdown, and sensorimotor dysfunction.

Evaluation of the patient's responses to nursing care is based on whether the patient possesses the knowledge to prevent or manage problems related to alterations in protective mechanisms.

Excerpted from the ANA/ONS Standards of Oncology Nursing Practice.

Potential for Infection

Joan C. McNally and Joy Stair

Population at Risk (All Cancer Patients)

- Patients with leukopenia (from chemotherapy, radiation to sternum, pelvis, ribs, vertebrae, ends of long bones)
- Patients with immunosuppression from steroid therapy, malnutrition, long-standing or high-intensity stress, and the frail elderly
- Patients with leukemia, lymphoma, myeloma, AIDS
- Patients on antibiotic therapy (at risk for superimposed infections)
- Patients undergoing surgical or invasive procedures
- Patients with bone marrow transplants

LEVEL 1A: Potential Infection—General

EXPECTED OUTCOME

1. Patient remains infection-free as evidenced by:
   - temperature within normal limits.
   - laboratory values within normal limits.
   - absence of inflammation.
2. Patient demonstrates knowledge related to prevention of infection:
   - identifies predisposing factors.
   - verbalizes signs and symptoms to report to health care team.
   - identifies/demonstrates appropriate hygienic measures.
   - identifies/demonstrates adequate nutritional and fluid intake.
   - identifies measures to reduce stress.
   - alters environmental risk factors.

NURSING MANAGEMENT

Assessment

1. Obtain history:
   - immunosuppressive drugs including antineoplastic agents, steroids.
   - radiation therapy.
   - nutritional history including food intake record, changes in weight.

Potential for Infection

- chronic infections.
- current and recent stress.
2. Assess immune status response to skin testing (e.g., dinitrochlorobenzene, purified protein derivative, streptokinase, Candida).
3. Arrange for hematologic laboratory studies:
   - CBC.
   - WBC, differential (neutrophils, lymphocytes).
   - absolute neutrophil count.
4. Check baseline vital signs.
5. Examine cervical, axillary, inguinal lymph nodes for enlargement, tenderness.
6. Assess patient's/caregiver's ability to read glass thermometer.

Nursing Interventions

1. Wash hands frequently and consistently with vigorous friction before donning gloves.
2. Use clean gloves for patient care activities.
3. Care for neutropenic patients before caring for other patients and take other precautions to avoid transferring any infectious agents to neutropenic patients.
4. Encourage good nutritional intake.
5. Use only sterile equipment and supplies.
6. Use aseptic technique in patient care and treatments.
7. Keep patient separate from others exposed to infections including measles, chicken pox, herpes zoster, tuberculosis, influenza, or *Pneumocystis carinii.*
8. Develop a program with the patient to assist in stress reduction.
9. Administer medications that promote hematopoiesis (e.g., colony-stimulating factors, immunoglobulin).
10. Administer prophylactic antibiotics as ordered.

Patient Teaching

1. Explain the relationship between the incidence of infection and the level of circulating granulocytes and cellular immunity.
2. Teach rationale and measures for thorough handwashing techniques:
   - meticulous handwashing before patient contact significantly decreases incidence of infection.
3. Discuss rationale and measures for balanced diet with sufficient protein, calories, fluids, vitamins, and minerals. Include information on protein:
   - balanced diet is essential for improving cellular and humoral immunity.
4. Note need to avoid fresh unpeeled fruits, raw vegetables, uncooked eggs, flowers, houseplants in presence of neutropenia.
5. Describe role of WBC in prevention of infection:
   - neutrophils are first line of defense against microbial invasion.
6. Explain effects of treatments on immune system:
   - chemotherapy and radiation therapy to bones suppress bone marrow function.
7. Inform patient of relative risk of bacterial infection associated with absolute neutrophil counts:
   - 2500–2000/mm^3—no significant risk.
   - 1000/mm^3—minimal risk.
   - 500/mm^3—moderate risk.
   - <500/mm^3—severe risk.
8. Discuss necessity of avoiding crowds or people with known infection or recently vaccinated, particularly at time of increased risk.
9. Teach signs and symptoms to report immediately (e.g., fever, chills, sore throat, purulent drainage).
10. Outline measures to decrease stress (e.g., relaxation techniques, exercise, biofeedback).
11. Note need to avoid cleaning cat litter boxes and fish tanks and to avoid contact with dog or human excreta.

LEVEL 1B: Potential Infection—Skin and Mucous Membranes

EXPECTED OUTCOME

1. Patient remains infection-free as evidenced by:
   - maintenance of skin integrity.
   - return of skin integrity in patients with open wounds or punctures at various access sites.
   - absence of fungal infections of umbilicus or feet.
   - absence of purulent drainage.
   - absence of inflammatory changes.
   - absence of tenderness.
2. Patient demonstrates knowledge related to prevention of skin infection:
   - identifies predisposing factors.
   - verbalizes signs and symptoms to report.
   - performs necessary treatments and procedures.
   - identifies/demonstrates hygienic practices.
   - demonstrates proper knowledge and administration of medications.

NURSING MANAGEMENT

Assessment

1. Obtain history:
   - past infections.
   - venipuncture.
   - radiation therapy.
   - wounds.
   - injections.
2. Inspect skin and mucous membranes. Special attention should be given to:
   - skin folds (perineum, buttocks, axillae).
   - body cavities (mouth, vagina, rectum).
   - bony prominences.
   - umbilicus.
   - IV or puncture sites.
   - surgical wounds.
   - long-term implanted venous access devices.
   - enteral feeding tubes.
3. Check skin and mucous membranes for:
   - color.
   - lesions, wounds, fissures.
   - edema.
   - moisture.
   - note that in neutropenic patients, inflammatory response (redness, edema, heat, pus formation, pain) may be decreased or absent.

Nursing Interventions

1. Provide meticulous total body hygiene (including regular perineal care).
2. Provide thorough skin care to high-risk areas (use powders sparingly to prevent caking).
3. Arrange for thorough oral care after meals and prn.
4. Use electric razors or depilatories only.
5. Provide range-of-motion exercise and turning regimen for bedbound patients.
6. Use fingersticks for blood work, with possible coordination of blood studies to be accomplished with one venipuncture.
7. Implement bowel program to prevent constipation. Avoid enemas, rectal medi-

cations, rectal temperatures, digital rectal examinations.

8. Prevent abrasions and irritations (from tape, constrictive clothing, and the like).

9. Use precautions with venipuncture and invasive procedures:
   - wear clean gloves after thorough hand-washing.
   - careful skin cleansing with povidone-iodine before needle puncture, invasive procedures.
   - strict aseptic technique.
   - possible application of antiseptic or antibiotic ointment to venipuncture site.
   - sterile dressing.
   - change of IV tubing and solutions in accordance with individual institutional policy.

10. Use bacterial barrier dressings (e.g., Op-Site, Tegaderm).

Patient Teaching

1. Teach meticulous total-body hygiene.
2. Explain rationale and methods for maintaining skin integrity:
   - trauma and invasive procedures promote acquisition of potential pathogens.
3. Discuss signs and symptoms of infection and alterations to report to health care team (e.g., elevated temperature, tenderness, redness, nonhealing wound, odor, drainage).
4. Teach prescribed treatments and procedures.
5. Teach administration and side effects of medications.

LEVEL 1C: Potential Infection—Respiratory Tract

EXPECTED OUTCOME

1. Patient remains infection-free as evidenced by:
   - temperature within normal limits.
   - absence of inflammation or exudate in oropharyngeal or nasal mucosa.
   - sputum amount and color within normal limits.
   - lung sounds within normal limits for patient.
   - laboratory and radiologic findings reveal no infectious process.
2. Patient demonstrates knowledge related to prevention of respiratory tract infection:
   - identifies predisposing factors.
   - verbalizes signs and symptoms to report.
   - performs necessary treatments and procedures.
   - identifies/demonstrates hygienic practices.
   - demonstrates proper knowledge and administration of medications.
   - identifies/demonstrates adequate fluid and nutritional intake.

NURSING MANAGEMENT

Assessment

1. Obtain history:
   - respiratory infections or disease.
   - smoking.
   - exposure to environmental or occupational irritants (asbestos, coal tar, dust).
   - sputum production.
   - chemotherapy (bleomycin, carmus-

tine, cytarabine, methotrexate, mitomycin).
  - radiation therapy to chest, nasopharynx, head and neck implants.
2. Check pharynx:
  - color.
  - surface characteristics.
3. Monitor respirations:
  - rate.
  - type.
  - rhythm.
  - depth.
4. Note presence and type of cough.
5. Check for presence of sore throat.
6. Assess sputum (color, amount).
7. Observe for pleuritic pain.
8. Check lungs and thorax:
  - inspection for muscles used, retractions.
  - palpation for vocal fremitus, expansion.
  - auscultation of breath and whispered sounds for presence of rales and rhonchi.
9. Examine cervical lymph nodes for enlargement, tenderness.
10. Obtain laboratory values:
  - arterial blood gases.
  - sputum cultures.
11. Assess diagnostic studies:
  - chest x-ray.
  - pulmonary function tests.
  - tuberculosis skin test.
  - lung tomograms.

Nursing Interventions

1. Protect patient from exposure to droplet contamination. Visitors and staff should wear masks if indicated.

2. Use aseptic/sterile technique with tracheotomy care.
3. Use proper nasopharyngeal suction techniques to avoid trauma.
4. Decrease environmental contaminants (e.g., have room wet-mopped and dusted; increase humidification).
5. Eliminate sources of stagnant water (flower vases, denture cups, irrigating containers, respiratory equipment).

Patient Teaching

1. Teach control of environmental factors (increased humidity, decreased dust and other irritants when possible, avoidance of sources of stagnant water).
2. Discuss signs and symptoms to report (change in color of sputum, increased cough, increased sputum, elevated temperature).
3. Teach rationale for and techniques of respiratory hygiene (coughing, deep breathing).
4. Explain rationale for and plan to identify and avoid potential carriers of respiratory infection.
5. Demonstrate and teach aseptic tracheostomy care.
6. Demonstrate and teach patient suctioning techniques.
7. Teach administration and side effects of medications.
8. Explain rationale for and measures to promote adequate fluid and nutritional intake.
9. Teach rationale and plan for stopping smoking.

LEVEL 1D: Potential Infection—Genitourinary System

EXPECTED OUTCOME

1. Patient remains free from genitourinary infection as evidenced by:
  - absence of urinary signs of infection (e.g., pyuria, hematuria, flank pain).

- absence of symptoms of infection (e.g., dysuria, frequency, urgency, pruritus).
- temperature within normal limits.
- absence of nausea and vomiting.
- laboratory values within normal limits.
2. Patient demonstrates knowledge related to prevention of genitourinary infection:
  - identifies predisposing factors.
  - performs necessary treatment and procedures.
  - identifies/demonstrates hygienic practices (personal and sexual).
  - demonstrates proper knowledge and administration of medications.
  - identifies/demonstrates adequate and appropriate fluid intake.

NURSING MANAGEMENT

Assessment

1. Obtain history:
   - voiding patterns.
   - dysuria, frequency, urgency.
   - past instrumentation (catheterization, cystoscopy).
   - neurologic deficits.
   - cyclophosphamide therapy.
   - prostatic enlargement.
   - vaginal hygiene (douches, sprays).
   - contraceptive techniques.
   - presence of cystocele.
2. Monitor intake and output.
3. Check urine for:
   - color.
   - clarity.
   - odor.
   - presence of blood or casts.
4. Examine external genitalia for inflammation and discharge.
5. Note flank pain.
6. Monitor residual urine volumes if indicated (e.g., in patients with neurologic deficits).
7. Assess laboratory values:
   - urinalysis.
   - Venereal Disease Research Laboratory (VDRL) and gonococcal smears (do rectal cultures in females and homosexual males at risk for gonorrhea).

Nursing Interventions

1. Use appropriate technique for specimen collections.
2. Provide good skin care and hygiene for patients with condom catheters.
3. Provide thorough perineal hygiene (every day and following each bowel movement).
4. Arrange for measures to alkalinize urine if indicated (e.g., cranberry juice).
5. Avoid use of indwelling catheter.
6. If indwelling catheter is necessary:
   - cleanse with soap and water around urethra daily.
   - use sterile technique for irrigations of catheter when obstructed.
   - maintain intact closed urinary drainage system (bag and tubing may be changed qod to prevent ascent of bacteria from drainage bag to genitourinary tract).
   - avoid reflux of urine from collection bag.
   - provide personal receptacle for emptying drainage bag.
7. Monitor intake and output.
8. Encourage fluids as appropriate.

Patient Teaching

1. Teach signs and symptoms to report (e.g., elevated temperature, dysuria, frequency, urgency, change in urine color or odor).

2. Teach perineal care.
3. Teach and demonstrate catheter care.
4. Teach appropriate voiding patterns (e.g., encourage patient not to retain urine).
5. Teach administration and side effects of medications.
6. Teach Credé method for patients with neurologic deficits.
7. Explain rationale for and measures to promote adequate fluid intake.

8. Describe sexual hygiene:
   - contraceptive techniques and related infection risks such as IUD (increased endometrial infection); diaphragm (increased cystitis); progesterone (increased vaginal infections).
   - need to avoid trauma to mucous membranes during sexual foreplay and penetration.
   - need for adequate lubrication.
   - need to avoid routine douching.

LEVEL 1E: Potential Infection—Eyes

EXPECTED OUTCOME

1. Patient remains infection-free as evidenced by:
   - absence of conjunctivitis, iritis.
   - absence of inflammation, infection of eyelids or lacrimal glands.
2. Patient demonstrates knowledge related to prevention of external eye infection:
   - identifies predisposing factors.
   - verbalizes signs and symptoms to report.
   - performs necessary treatments and procedures.
   - identifies/demonstrates hygienic practices.

NURSING MANAGEMENT

Assessment

1. Obtain history:
   - visual aids worn (if contact lenses, type and procedures followed for use).
   - history of infections.
   - loss of hair with chemotherapy.
   - radiation therapy to or near eye.
2. Inspect external eye for
   - color (redness).
   - clarity.
   - drainage.
   - presence of eyelashes.

Nursing Interventions

1. Use thorough handwashing techniques.
2. Provide aseptic contact lens care.

3. Apply artificial lubricants if needed.

Patient Teaching

1. Teach aseptic contact lens care to prevent corneal abrasion and infection.
2. Teach administration procedure for medications.
3. Discuss signs and symptoms of infection or alterations (e.g., itching, redness, drainage).
4. Demonstrate good handwashing and hygienic measures.
5. Discuss measures to prevent cross-contamination from other body areas or environmental sources.

LEVEL 2: Localized Infection

EXPECTED OUTCOME

1. Patient exhibits resolution or control of infection:
   - temperature within normal limits for the patient.
   - absence or minimal signs and symptoms specific to site of infection.
   - no evidence of cross-contamination.
2. Patient/caregiver identify/demonstrate measures to resolve or control infection:
   - demonstrate proper knowledge of administration of medications.
   - perform necessary treatments and procedures.
   - identify signs and symptoms necessary to report to health care team.
   - demonstrate measures to prevent cross-contamination.
   - identify appropriate long-term follow-up plan of care.
3. Patient/caregiver demonstrate knowledge of rationale for drug therapy in localized infections:
   - classes of drugs selected for treatment.
   - procedures for drug therapy.
4. Patient/caregiver demonstrate knowledge related to systemic infection and treatment:
   - identify signs and symptoms of systemic infection.
   - identify causative factors.
   - identify rationale for prescribed treatment.
   - state procedures for drug therapy.
   - state expected effects and side effects of treatment.

NURSING MANAGEMENT

Assessment

General

1. See Assessment, Level 1.
2. Inspect all body sites with increased potential for infection daily.
3. Examine all secretions and excretions for suspicious changes. Culture if indicated.
4. Monitor vital signs q4h.
5. Assess pattern of temperature fluctuations.
6. Observe for chills.
7. Assess nutritional and hydration status.
8. Obtain blood culture results.
9. Observe for side effects of specific antibiotics.

Skin and Mucous Membranes

1. See Assessment, Level 1, and Chapters 37 and 38.
2. Assess wounds for drainage, odor, inflammation, and tenderness.
3. Assess oral cavity for lesions. Herpes simplex virus infections can be confused with nonspecific stomatitis. Culture if indicated.
4. Assess perianal areas, including history of pain on defecation.
5. Obtain cultures and sensitivities of wound drainage before initiation of antibiotics.

Respiratory Tract

1. See Assessment, Level 1.
2. Observe sputum color and amount, and dyspnea.

3. Obtain appropriate cultures and sensitivities based on patient complaint (before antibiotic therapy).

Genitourinary System

1. See Assessment, Level 1.
2. Observe urine for color, mucus shreds, odor, and blood.
3. Assess vaginal drainage (color, consistency, odor). See Chapter 38.
4. Obtain appropriate cultures and sensitivities based on patient complaint, before antibiotic therapy.

Eyes

1. See Assessment, Level 1.
2. Culture drainage before initiation of antibiotic therapy.

Nursing Actions

General

1. See Nursing Actions, Level 1.
2. Monitor WBC, noting differential, changes in neutrophil and lymphocyte counts.
3. Use appropriate technique for obtaining specimens for culture.
4. Monitor results of cultures and sensitivities.
5. Administer antibiotics, antifungals, antiparasitics, antiviral agents as ordered and maintain schedule.
6. Note response to treatment.
7. Maintain adequate nutrition and hydration.
8. Implement measures to control fever (e.g., acetaminophen, tepid baths/sponging, environmental temperature control).

Skin and Mucous Membranes

1. See Nursing Actions, Level 1, and Chapters 37 and 38.
2. Employ strict aseptic techniques for wound care.
3. Maintain dry sterile dressing. Change dressing as ordered and when dressing becomes damp.
4. Properly dispose of soiled dressings according to institution's policy.
5. When ordered, vigorously irrigate wounds until clean.
6. May use ostomy appliances over wounds with copious amounts of drainage.
7. Maintain wound or skin precautions or isolation as ordered in individual institution.

Respiratory Tract

1. See Nursing Actions, Level 1.
2. Properly dispose of all respiratory secretions.
3. Administer oxygen as ordered.
4. Encourage hourly use of incentive spirometer.
5. Encourage respiratory humidification (including nebulizing mist treatments).
6. Encourage hourly pulmonary hygiene (coughing, deep breathing).
7. Monitor arterial blood gases.
8. Monitor chest x-ray results.

Genitourinary System

1. See Nursing Actions, Level 1.
2. Force fluids to minimum of 3000 ml per day unless contraindicated; monitor output.
3. Administer bladder analgesics such as phenazopyridine (Pyridium) and flavoxate (Urispas).

Eyes

1. See Nursing Actions, Level 1.
2. Properly administer eyedrops, ointments.

Patient Teaching

General

1. See Patient Teaching, Level 1.
2. Explain rationale for drug selection and

procedures for drug therapy administration.

3. Teach names of drug(s), administration schedule, and side effects.
4. Discuss signs and symptoms to report to health care team:
    - inform patients on steroid therapy that fever may not occur with infection.
5. Teach appropriate technique for obtaining temperature and reading thermometer.
6. Teach rationale for cultures and sensitivities.
7. Discuss measures to control fever (e.g., tepid sponge bath, acetaminophen, increased fluids).

Skin and Mucous Membranes

1. See Patient Teaching, Level 1.
2. Teach wound care (aseptic technique, dressing change when wet, irrigations, cleansing procedures, dressing application).
3. Discuss proper disposal of soiled dressings.
4. Demonstrate good handwashing technique.
5. Teach rationale for and measures to avoid cross-contamination (e.g., use of separate washcloth and towel for area of infection.

Respiratory Tract

1. See Patient Teaching, Level 1.
2. Teach proper disposal of respiratory secretions.
3. Explain rationale for use of oxygen and importance of maintaining oxygen therapy.
4. Emphasize safety precautions for use of oxygen.
5. Teach rationale for and methods of effective coughing and deep breathing.
6. Demonstrate use of incentive spirometer.
7. Teach rationale for and describe methods of respiratory humidification (including nebulizing mist treatments).
8. Explain diagnostic procedures.

Genitourinary System

1. See Patient Teaching, Level 1.
2. Teach rationale for and measures to increase fluid intake to minimum of 3000 ml per day.
3. Teach measures to promote bladder comfort (e.g., analgesic/antispasmodic applications of heat over suprapubic area).

Eyes

1. See Patient Teaching, Level 1.
2. Teach proper administration of eyedrops, ointments.

LEVEL 3: Systemic Infection

EXPECTED OUTCOME

1. Patient exhibits resolution or control of systemic infection:
    - temperature normal or within normal limits for patient.
    - absence of signs and symptoms of dehydration.
    - vital signs within normal limits for patient.
    - absence of chilling.
    - negative blood cultures.

NURSING MANAGEMENT

Assessment

1. See Assessment, Levels 1 and 2.
2. Take vital signs q2h.
3. Do respiratory assessment q4h:
   - auscultate all lung fields.
   - observe for dyspnea, orthopnea.
4. Do cardiovascular assessment:
   - blood pressure q2h (note decreasing pulse pressure).
   - note tachycardia.
5. Do CNS assessment q4h:
   - behavior.
   - level of consciousness.
   - orientation.
   - presence of headache.
6. Monitor fluid balance:
   - intake and output q8h (may do hourly urine).
   - daily weight.
   - edema.
7. Assess laboratory studies:
   - electrolytes.
   - blood urea nitrogen, creatinine.
   - CBC with WBC differential.
   - serologic studies.
   - blood cultures (obtain at least twice before initiation of antibiotics).
   - results of lumbar puncture (if appropriate) for culture and sensitivity of cerebrospinal fluid.
8. Assess emotional status.

Nursing Actions

1. See Nursing Actions, Levels 1 and 2.
2. When fever occurs, culture all potential sites of infection (including implanted venous access device tips if all other sites are negative).
3. Change IV sites q48h. Use a metal butterfly only.
4. Antibiotic therapy is continued for at least 7 days as a general rule.
   - if fever persists, may be result of drug reactions, inflammation, tumor.

5. Monitor response to treatment.
6. Administer granulocytes as ordered:
   - may premedicate patient with steroids, acetaminophen, meperidine (Demerol) to prevent or minimize chills and fever of transfusion reaction.
   - check ABO, HLA, and Rh compatibility.
   - monitor temperature, pulse, respirations, blood pressure before initiation of transfusion q15min during first half hour; q30min during remainder of transfusion, and q24h following transfusion, or according to agency policy.
   - administer granulocytes as soon as available (donor granulocytes have 6 hr lifespan).
   - prime and flush tubing with normal saline.
   - infuse slowly—50–75 ml during first hour, 200–300 ml over 2–3 hours.
   - rinse infusion bag with 20 to 30 ml normal saline to remove remaining adhering granulocytes.
   - assess for signs and symptoms of granulocyte transfusion reaction:
     - fever and chills.
     - allergic reaction: urticaria, hives, wheezing, hypotension. If present, stop infusion of granulocytes and contact physician.

Patient Teaching

1. See Patient Teaching, Levels 1 and 2.
2. Discuss importance of rapid treatment (systemic drug treatment may be initiated before causative organism or site of infection has been determined).
3. Describe common infections and the causative organisms that occur in neutropenic and immunosuppressed patients. Teaching should be in accordance with level of understanding and should outline general differences between organisms, describing

specific organism(s) causing patient's infection:

- bacterial:
  - gram negative: *E. coli,* Proteus, *Klebsiella pneumoniae,* Salmonella, *Pseudomonas aeruginosa.*
  - gram positive: *Staphylococcus aureus,* beta-hemolytic streptococci, *S. pyogenes, S. viridans,* pneumococcus, enterococcus, *Mycobacterium tuberculosis.*
- viral: cytomegalovirus, herpes simplex, herpes zoster, DNA/RNA viruses.
- protozoan: *Pneumocystis carinii, Toxoplasma gondii.*

4. Explain rationale for combination (broad-spectrum) antibiotic therapy.
5. Explain that specific types of drugs are used for specific infections.
6. Teach indications for granulocyte transfusions:
   - neutrophils less than 500/mm^3.
   - fever unresponsive to antibiotic therapy in 48 hours.
   - neutropenia expected to last 5 days or longer.
   - disease process with potential remission.
7. Explain potential side effects of treatment.

SUGGESTED READINGS

Donovan, M., and Pierce, S.: Cancer Care Nursing. New York, Appleton-Century-Crofts, 1976.

Fuks, J.Z., Patel, H., Hornedo, J., et al.: Infections in patients with non-small-cell lung cancer treated with induction chemotherapy. Medical and Pediatric Oncology *14*(5):255–261, 1986.

Haeuber, D., and DiJulio, J.E.: Hematopoietic colony stimulating factors: An overview. Oncology Nursing Forum *16*(27):247–255, 1989.

Hertz, J., Matthay, R., and Smith, G.P.: Carinii pneumonia: Be alert to increased incidence. The Journal of Respiratory Diseases 5:70–76, 1983.

Klastersky, J.: Infection prevention in cancer patients. *In* Klastersky, J. (Ed.): Infections in Cancer Patients. New York, Raven Press, 1982, pp. 87–104.

Masur, H.: Those common candida—When to suspect trouble and what to do about it. Your Patient and Cancer *1*(3):27–33, 1981.

Morell, A., and Barandum, S.: Prophylactic and therapeutic use of intravenous administration in patients with secondary immunodeficiencies associated with malignancies. Pediatric Infectious Disease Journal *7*(5 Suppl.):87–91, 1988.

Patterson, P.: Granulocyte transfusion: Nursing considerations. Cancer Nursing 3:101–105, 1980.

Payan, D., and Rubin, R.: Invasive aspergillosis: When your patient's defenses are down. Your Patient and Cancer *1*(10):29–36, 1981.

Petrosini, B., Becker, H., and Christian, B.: Infection rates in central venous catheter dressings. Oncology Nursing Forum *15*(6):709–717, 1988.

Pizzo, P., and Young, R.: Management of infections of the cancer patient. *In* Devita., V.T.: Cancer Principles and Practices of Oncology, Volume 2. Philadephia, J.B. Lippincott, 1985, pp. 1963–1975.

Poland, J.M.: Diagnostic acumen: Differential diagnosis of oral HSV infection. Nursing Acumen *1*(1):3, 1989.

Reheis, C.E.: Neutropenia. Nursing Clinics of North America *20*(1):219–225, 1985.

Robichaud, K.J., and Hubbard, S.M.: Infection. *In* Groenwald, S.L., Hansen, M., Goodman, M., et al. (Eds.): Cancer Nursing. Boston, Jones & Bartlett, 1987, pp. 221–224.

Schmaier, A.: Oncologic emergencies. Medical Times *111*(2):87–88, 1983.

Schiffer, C.A., and Wade, J.C.: Supportive care: Issues in the use of blood products and treatment of infection. Seminars in Oncology *14*(4):454–467, 1987.

Wade, J.C., and Schimpff, S.C.: Approaches to therapy of bacterial infections in the granulocytopenic patient. *In* Klastersky, J. (Ed.): Infections in Cancer Patients. New York, Raven Press, 1982, pp. 105–129.

Yasko, J., and Nunnally, C.: Infection. *In* Yasko, J.: Guidelines for Cancer Care: Symptom Management. Reston, Va, Reston Publishing, 1983.

Injury, Potential for, Related to Thrombocytopenia

E. Joyce Alexander

32

Population at Risk

- Individuals in whom malignancy has originated in or has invaded bone marrow
- Individuals with nonmalignant bone marrow failure (aplastic anemia)
- Individuals infected with HIV virus
- Individuals experiencing immune destruction of platelets
- Individuals receiving antineoplastic drugs
- Individuals receiving radiation therapy to long bones or large body surfaces

LEVEL 1:   Mild Thrombocytopenia (Platelet Count 50,000–100,000)

EXPECTED OUTCOME

1. Patient demonstrates knowledge of potential for bleeding related to thrombocytopenia:
   - identifies relationship between platelets and bleeding.
   - lists measures to prevent bleeding.
   - contacts appropriate health care professional when initial signs and symptoms of bleeding occur.
   - states measures to manage bleeding.
2. Patient demonstrates absence of bleeding.

NURSING MANAGEMENT

Assessment

1. Monitor CBC, hemoglobin, and platelet counts.
2. Assess potential for increasing myelosuppression.
3. Observe for signs and symptoms of bleeding daily or at each visit:
   - oral cavity for bleeding from gums.
   - skin for petechiae, ecchymosis, hematomas.

203

- presence or history of epistaxis.
- eyes for scleral bleeding.
- stools for black color or bright red blood.
- urine for hematuria.
- emesis for bright red or coffee ground color.
- female patients for vaginal bleeding, pad count.
- vital signs for changes in blood pressure or heart rate.

Nursing Interventions

1. Use soft toothbrush, avoid flossing, avoid alcohol-based mouthwashes.
2. Implement measures to prevent constipation: offer fluids and high-fiber diet if tolerated, stool softeners if ordered.
3. Prevent damage to rectal mucosa by avoiding taking rectal temperatures, suppositories, enemas, and rectal examinations.
4. Avoid IM injections; when subcutaneous injections are necessary, apply ice immediately without pressure.
5. Avoid invasive procedures whenever possible; when venipuncture, arterial stick, bone marrow aspiration, or other invasive procedures are necessary, apply pressure directly for 5 minutes, then apply a pressure dressing.
6. Avoid drugs that interfere with platelet function, including aspirin and nonsteroidal antiinflammatory drugs.
7. Avoid bladder catheterization whenever possible; when necessary, use straight in-and-out technique with smallest catheter possible.

Patient Teaching

1. Explain relationship between platelets and bleeding.
2. Discuss measures to prevent bleeding:
   - use soft toothbrush, avoid flossing, avoid alcohol-based mouthwash.
   - avoid blowing nose forcefully.
   - prevent constipation: drink fluids, eat high-fiber diet if tolerated, take stool softener regularly if ordered, do not take enemas or rectal suppositories.
   - use electric razor for shaving; do not use razor blades.
   - avoid wearing tight and restrictive clothing.
   - for female patients, avoid tampons for menstrual flow; use sanitary napkins instead.
   - use water-based lubricant before sexual intercourse.
   - avoid contact sports and other activities predisposing to injury.
   - avoid taking aspirin or medications containing aspirin, nonsteroidal antiinflammatory drugs (Indocin, Advil, Motrin), blood thinners (Coumadin).
3. Describe signs and symptoms of bleeding:
   - bruising, petechiae, hematomas on skin.
   - bleeding of gums.
   - black color or bright red blood in stools.
   - blood in urine.
   - blood in emesis or coffee ground color emesis.
   - dizziness or light-headedness, especially when standing from a sitting, lying, stooping position.
   - change in mental status.
   - nose bleeds.
   - increased pad count, prolonged or heavy flow for menstruating females.
   - scleral bleeding.
4. Identify appropriate health care professional to notify when/if initial symptoms of bleeding occur. Give patient/family at least 2 phone numbers at which health care professionals may be reached in an emergency.
5. Discuss measures to manage bleeding:
   - ice packs to area of bruising, across bridge of nose for nose bleed, or to bleeding area along with pressure.
   - pressure to area of bleeding or, for nose bleed, to nostrils below bridge of nose.

EXPECTED OUTCOME

1. Patient demonstrates knowledge related to potential for bleeding related to moderately severe thrombocytopenia.
   - lists measures to prevent bleeding.
   - identifies signs and symptoms of bleeding; contacts appropriate health care professional when initial signs and symptoms of bleeding occur.
   - states measures to manage bleeding.
2. Patient demonstrates absence of bleeding.

NURSING MANAGEMENT

Assessment

1. See Assessment, Level 1.
2. Monitor CBC, hemoglobin, and platelet counts daily.
3. Assess for the presence of factors that further compromise platelet function, including fever, sepsis, and certain medications (tricyclic antidepressants, antihistamines, phenothiazines, and some antibiotics).
4. Observe for signs and symptoms of bleeding daily including:
   - oral cavity for bleeding from gums.
   - skin for petechiae, ecchymosis, hematomas.
   - stools for black color or bright red blood.
   - urine for hematuria.
   - emesis for bright red or coffee gound color.
   - female patients for vaginal bleeding, pad count.
   - vital signs for changes in blood pressure or heart rate.
   - evidence of epistaxis.
   - neurologic status or headaches.
   - eyes for scleral bleeding.

Nursing Interventions

1. See Nursing Interventions, Level 1.
2. Implement measures to prevent bleeding:
   - control nausea and vomiting to prevent retching.
   - consult with physician regarding pharmacologic control of menstrual cycle to prevent bleeding for female patients.
   - assist with ambulation if patient is unsteady, weak, confused.
   - anticipate possible need for platelet transfusion. Consider use of filters with platelet transfusion to remove leukocytes.
   - administer antihypertensives to decrease risk of intracranial bleed as ordered.
3. Implement measures to manage bleeding episodes:
   - apply pressure and cold to bleeding site.
   - elevate bleeding site if possible.
   - apply topical thrombin if ordered.
   - administer platelets when ordered. Premedicate, when ordered, to prevent reactions.

Patient Teaching

1. Explain relationship between a moderately low platelet count and increasing risk of bleeding.
2. Discuss measures to prevent bleeding.
3. Instruct patient and family to assess daily for signs and symptoms of bleeding.
4. Identify appropriate health care team member to notify when/if initial symptoms of bleeding occur. Give patient/family at least 2 phone numbers at which health care professionals may be reached in an emergency. Explain emergency nurse call system to hospitalized patients and their families.
5. Discuss measures to manage bleeding.

LEVEL 3:   Severe Thrombocytopenia (Platelet Count < 20,000)

EXPECTED OUTCOME

1. Patient/caregiver demonstrate knowledge related to severe thrombocytopenia:
   - list measures to prevent bleeding.
   - identify signs and symptoms of bleeding.
   - contact appropriate health care professional when initial signs and symptoms of bleeding occur.
   - state measures to manage bleeding.
2. Patient demonstrates absence of bleeding.

NURSING MANAGEMENT

Assessment

1. See Assessment, Levels 1 and 2.
2. Observe for signs and symptoms of bleeding every 8 hours including:
   - neurologic status (e.g., changes in level of consciousness, vision, papillary response or affect, restlessness, headache, seizures, widening of pulse pressure, confusion, ataxia).
3. Assess responses to platelet transfusion.

Nursing Interventions

1. See Nursing Interventions, Levels 1 and 2.
2. Implement measures to prevent bleeding:
   - pad side-rails (side-rails should be up).
   - remove hazardous objects from environment.
   - premedicate for platelet transfusions to prevent platelet reactions. Consider use of leukocyte removal filters.
   - transfuse platelet before major invasive procedures.
3. Implement measures to control bleeding episodes.

Patient Teaching

1. See Patient Teaching, Levels 1 and 2.
2. Explain relationship between a very low platelet count and increasing risk of spontaneous bleeding.
3. Discuss measures to prevent bleeding.
4. Instruct patient/caregiver to observe for signs and symptoms of bleeding several times a day.
5. Instruct patient/caregiver to notify a health

206

care professional immediately for any signs and symptoms of bleeding. Explain emergency nurse call system to hospitalized patients and their families.

6. Discuss measures to manage bleeding.

SUGGESTED READINGS

Abrams, R., and Deisseroth, A.: Use of blood and blood products. *In* De Vita, V., and Rosenberg, S. (Eds.): Cancer: Principles and Practice of Oncology. 2nd Ed. (Vol. 2). Philadelphia, J.B. Lippincott, 1985, pp. 1924–1930.

Clark, J., Landis, L. and McGee, R.: Nursing management of outcomes of disease, psychological response, treatment, and complications. *In* Ziegfeld, C. (Ed.): Core Curriculum for Oncology Nursing. Philadelphia, W.B. Saunders Company, 1987, pp. 174–276.

Myers, J., Davidson, J., Hutt, P., and Chatham, S.: Standardized teaching plans for management of chemotherapy and radiation therapy side effects. Oncology Nursing Forum *14*(5):95–99, 1987.

Oncology Nursing Society and American Nurses' Association Division on Medical-Surgical Nursing Practice: Outcome Standards for Cancer Nursing Practice. Kansas City, MO, American Nurses Association. 1987.

PATIENT EDUCATION MATERIALS AND COMMUNITY RESOURCES

Publications:

Chemotherapy & You: A guide to self-help during treatment. U.S. Department of Health and Human Services, Public Health Service: National Institutes of Health. (Phone 1-800-422-6237 to order).

Acute Myelogenous Leukemia. Leukemia Society of America. 733 Third Avenue, New York, NY 10017.

Acute Lymphocytic Leukemia. Leukemia Society of America. 733 Third Avenue, 10017.

McCredie, K., and Margolis, C.: Understanding Leukemia. New York: Charles Scribner's Sons, 1983.

Organizations

American Cancer Society
1599 Clifton Road,
Atlanta, GA
30320

or contact local chapter

Leukemia Society of America
National Headquarters,
733 Third Avenue,
New York, NY 10017
Telephone 212-573-8484

33

Injury, Potential for, Related to Anemia

Marcia Rostad

Population at Risk

Individuals who have

- Diagnosis of cancer, especially leukemia, lymphoma, multiple myeloma, carcinoma of the colon or ovary, or metastatic disease
- Received chemotherapeutic agents that cause bone marrow suppression
- Received bone marrow–suppressant drugs (e.g., anticonvulsants, antituberculins, certain antibiotics including the cephalosporins, sulfas, penicillins, chloramphenicol, and amphotericin B)
- Undergone prior radiation exposure to bone marrow
- Experienced chronic infections
- Undergone surgical procedures influencing red-cell production, function, or destruction, including partial or total gastrectomy, splenectomy, or resection of the lower ileum
- Protein deficiency

LEVEL 1: Potential

EXPECTED OUTCOME

1. Patient demonstrates adequate oxygen saturation of tissue:
   - laboratory values within normal limits.
   - absence of early symptoms of anemia.
   - vital signs within normal limits.
   - no evidence of obvious or occult bleeding.
   - ability to perform activities of daily living adequate within limits of current health status.
2. Patient demonstrates knowledge of relationship of red blood cells, hemoglobin, and availability of oxygen to fulfill need of body tissues for normal function:
   - identifies oxygen-carrying ability of hemoglobin and relationship between red blood cells and hemoglobin.
   - explains extra workload on heart in order to provide oxygen to tissues when supply of red blood cells/hemoglobin is decreased.
   - relates symptoms of anemia to decreased availability of oxygen to different tissues of the body.
3. Patient demonstrates knowledge of factors that contribute to anemia:
   - states that decreased erythrocyte production may be caused by inadequate diet/malabsorption problems.

- identifies suppression of erythrocyte formation in bone marrow as result of effects of certain drugs, toxins, disease.
- identifies loss of red blood cells/hemoglobin resulting from chronic or acute blood loss.
- identifies familial tendencies and anemia.
4. Patient identifies/demonstrates measures to prevent anemia:
   - compliance with proper diet and medication regimens.
   - avoidance of individuals with infection.
   - prompt reporting of any signs and symptoms of bleeding or infection.
   - avoidance of exposure to toxic agents.

NURSING MANAGEMENT

Assessment

1. Monitor the following laboratory data:
   - CBC:
     - hemoglobin and hematocrit.
     - total erythrocyte count.
     - erythrocyte indices (mean corpuscular volume, mean corpuscular hemoglobin, mean corpuscular hemoglobin concentration [MCV, MCH, MCHC]).
     - reticulocyte count.
     - white cell count and differential.
     - platelet count.
     - peripheral blood smear.
   - bone marrow aspirate and biopsy.
   - other tests that may be done and values to be monitored:
     - Schilling test for vitamin B_{12} absorption.
     - serum levels for vitamin B_{12} and folic acid.
     - erythrocyte destruction rate.
     - serum iron.
     - total iron binding capacity (TIBC).
   - other laboratory values pertinent to individual patient's problem.
2. Obtain historical data:
   - symptoms of anemia:
     - palpitations and chest pain upon exertion.
     - dyspnea upon exertion.
     - dizziness and syncope.
     - fatigue and weakness.
     - glossitis (sore mouth/tongue).
     - anorexia.
     - indigestion.
     - headache.
     - tinnitus.
     - insomnia.
     - hypersensitivity to cold.
   - signs of blood loss:
     - gastrointestinal: hematemesis, melena, hematochezia (bloody stools).
     - uterine: menometrorrhagia.
     - respiratory: hemoptysis, epistaxis.
     - genitourinary: hematuria, any change in color of urine (e.g., smoky, brown).
   - bleeding tendency following trauma (e.g., surgery, delivery, tooth extraction):
     - petechiae, spontaneous purpura.
     - bleeding into joints (joint pain).
   - exposure to drugs, toxins:
     - radiation.
     - specific drugs (e.g., anticonvulsants, antituberculins).
     - chemotherapeutic agents with dates of administration.
     - alcohol.
     - occupational chemicals, gases.
     - toxins.
     - antibiotic therapy (e.g., penicillin, sulfas, cephalosporins, chloramphenicol, amphotericin B).
   - previous history of anemia and response to therapy.
   - family history of anemia.
   - surgical history (e.g., partial or total gas-

trectomy, splenectomy, resection of lower ileum).
- changes in nutritional status (e.g., weight loss).
3. Conduct a physical assessment:
   - vital signs.
   - nailbeds: blanching, pallor, spoon-shaped nails.
   - skin: pallor, jaundice, purpura, petechiae.
   - mucous membranes: pallor, petechiae, jaundice.
   - tongue: redness, atrophy of papillae.
   - lymph nodes: swelling, tenderness.
   - bones: tenderness over sternum, ribs, vertebrae.
   - abdomen: masses, ascites, splenomegaly.
   - neurologic: paresthesias.
   - functional performance/ability to perform activities of daily living.
   - inspect IV and IM sites for signs of bleeding.
   - inspect all wound sites and dressings for active bleeding (e.g., surgical indwelling catheter) frequently.

Nursing Interventions

1. Consult with physician about advisability of discontinuing medications known to cause anemia.
2. Determine nadir and recovery of bone marrow after chemotherapy administration.
3. Report signs and symptoms of bleeding.
4. Implement precautions if thrombocytopenic (see Chapter 32).
5. Implement measures to protect patient from infection:
   - keep staff and visitors with signs and symptoms of infection away from patient.
   - maintain personal and environmental hygiene for patient.
   - report any signs and symptoms of infection to physician immediately.

- administer antibiotics as ordered.
6. Provide diet high in protein, vitamins, and iron (essential for normal erythrocyte production).
7. Arrange for oral hygiene before and after meals (to promote comfort while eating and reduce risk of infection in oral cavity).

Patient Teaching

1. Discuss importance of maintaining normal hemoglobin level and its relationship to overall health and cardiovascular status.
2. Discuss relationship between nutrients and increased erythrocyte production:
   - arrange for dietitian to teach patient/family about foods high in protein, vitamins, and minerals, which are necessary for erythrocyte production; reinforce this education.
   - foods high in iron include liver, eggs, green leafy vegetables, carrots, apricots, raisins, whole-wheat bread.
   - foods high in B_{12} include liver, milk, eggs, other animal products.
   - foods high in folic acid include liver, green vegetables.
3. Note signs and symptoms of early anemia (e.g., pallor, fatigue, shortness of breath, tachycardia on exertion, dizziness, irritability).
4. Outline signs and symptoms of rapid-onset anemia (e.g., weakness, heart palpitations, chest pain, heart failure, coma).
5. Emphasize importance of preventing infection and necessity of informing physician or nurse if any signs and symptoms of infection occur (chronic infection is associated with inhibition of marrow proliferation and red blood cell production):
   - avoid crowds and people with active infections.
   - take antibiotics as ordered.
   - report response to therapy.
   - employ oral, body, environmental hygiene.

EXPECTED OUTCOME

1. Patient demonstrates acceptable oxygen saturation of tissues:
   - laboratory values within acceptable limits.
   - absence of minimal symptoms of anemia.
   - vital signs within acceptable limits.
   - no evidence of obvious or occult bleeding.
   - acceptable performance of activities of daily living within current health status.
2. Patient demonstrates knowledge of relationship of red blood cells, hemoglobin, and availability of oxygen to fulfill the need of body tissues for normal function:
   - identifies oxygen-carrying ability of hemoglobin and relationship between red blood cells and hemoglobin.
   - explains extra workload on heart in order to provide oxygen to tissues when supply of red blood cells/hemoglobin is decreased.
   - relates symptoms of anemia to decreased availability of oxygen to different tissues of the body.
3. Patient demonstrates knowledge of factors that contribute to anemia:
   - states that decreased erythrocyte production may be caused by inadequate diet/malabsorption problems.
   - identifies suppression of erythrocyte formation in marrow as result of effects of certain drugs, toxins, disease.
   - identifies loss of red blood cells/hemoglobin resulting from chronic or acute blood loss.
   - identifies familial tendencies and anemia.
4. Patient recognizes measures necessary to reduce risks of injury associated with impaired function of circulatory, cardiac, and neurologic systems as the result of anemia.
5. Patient demonstrates knowledge of enhancement of erythrocyte/hemoglobin production and survival:
   - compliance with proper diet and medication regimens.
   - avoidance of individuals with infection.
   - prompt reporting of any signs and symptoms of bleeding or infection.
   - avoidance of exposure to toxic agents.

NURSING MANAGEMENT

Assessment

1. See Assessment, Level 1.
2. Check the results of current laboratory data: monitor hemoglobin, hematocrit, WBC, and differential.
3. Obtain historical data:
   - irritability, difficulty concentrating.
   - menstrual irregularities.
   - loss of libido or potency.
   - nausea and decreased appetite.
   - stomatitis or esophagitis.

211

- headache.
- palpitations (state if experienced on exertion or rest).
4. Conduct a physical assessment for signs and symptoms of mild to moderate anemia:
   - pallor.
   - wide pulse pressure.
   - tachycardia.
   - heart murmur.
   - impaired sensation (pain, temperature, touch discrimination).
   - cheilosis and angular stomatitis.
5. For patients with a history of gastrectomy, assess loss of position or vibratory sense.
6. Take vital signs q4h or more frequently if blood pressure decreases, pulse increases, respirations increase. Monitor for evidence of bleeding (see Assessments, Level 1), with particular attention to occult bleeding if anemia has progressed slowly from onset.
7. Monitor response to and side effects of iron therapy.

Nursing Interventions

1. See Nursing Interventions, Level 1.
2. Protect from infection.
3. Promote rest in order to lower body's oxygen requirement and decrease cardiopulmonary strain:
   - promote quiet, nonstressful environment.
   - provide warm clothing and blankets.
   - estimate energy expenditures of activities of daily living and allow patient to prioritize activities accordingly.
4. Maintain skin integrity:
   - inspect skin daily.
   - have patient turned q2h.
   - lubricate skin with nongreasy cream or lotion after daily bath.
   - avoid drying agents to the skin (e.g., alcohol rubs).
5. Maintain physical safety: provide assistance, when getting out of bed and ambulating, to patients who are dizzy or

lightheaded or who have paresthesia or loss of position or vibratory sense.
6. Avoid hot applications of any kind to prevent burns resulting from decreased pain sensation.
7. Provide diet high in protein, vitamins, and iron.
8. Provide frequent small meals if patient is unable to tolerate larger meals.
9. Have patient avoid hot, spicy, coarse foods in order to protect oral mucosa and avoid heartburn or nausea.
10. Assist or feed patient if too weak to assist or feed self.
11. Consult dietitian regarding use of food supplements.
12. Provide mouth care:
   - inspect oral cavity daily.
   - arrange for oral hygiene before and after meals and at bedtime to promote comfort, enhance appetite, prevent infection.
   - schedule frequent mouth rinses.
   - lubricate lips with petrolatum jelly to prevent dryness and cracking.
13. Administer supplements as ordered by physician according to deficiency:
   - iron (PO):
     o administer after meal or snack.
     o give orange juice with iron salt (ascorbic acid facilitates absorption).
     o obtain orders to decrease dosage or change to different iron salt or parenteral injection if side effects occur.
   - iron (IM): utilize z-track technique to avoid darkening and discoloration of skin surrounding injection.
   - vitamin B_{12} (hydroxocobalamin—IM: mandatory if total gastrectomy).
   - folic acid (usually given PO daily in small dose, as large doses can lead to increased neurologic deterioration).
14. Plan for discharge:
   - arrange for social service consultation to determine patient's socioeconomic needs.
   - arrange for home health nurse follow-

up at home as required by patient's health status.

Patient Teaching

1. See Patient Teaching, Level 1.
2. Explain need for adjustments in activities of daily living to conserve oxygen, prevent cardiorespiratory and neurologic complications, and minimize risk of physical injury:
   - take frequent rest periods; may need bed rest.
   - ask for assistance when getting out of bed and while ambulating if lightheaded, dizzy, experiencing paresthesia or loss of position or vibratory sense.
   - do not drive if weak or neurologically impaired.

3. Discuss measures to decrease pulmonary strain:
   - plan rest periods.
   - retire early for sleep.
   - perform mild exercise of short duration.
   - shorten work periods (note that patient may not be able to work).
4. Discuss need to protect from injury resulting from decreased availability of blood, oxygen, and nutrients to periphery (skin):
   - change position frequently—at least q2h.
   - lubricate skin gently with nongreasy cream or lotion after daily bath.
   - reinforce role that nutrition has in maintenance of skin integrity.
5. Describe effects of iron supplements: stools will appear black (tarry) if patient is taking iron.

LEVEL 3: *Severe (Hemoglobin <7.5 g/dl)*

EXPECTED OUTCOME

1. Patient demonstrates acceptable oxygen saturation of tissues:
   - laboratory values at acceptable level for patient.
   - improvement in symptoms of anemia.
   - vital signs within acceptable limits.
   - no evidence of obvious or occult bleeding.
   - ability to perform activities of daily living adequate within current health status.
2. Patient demonstrates knowledge of relationship between red blood cells, hemoglobin, and availability of oxygen to fulfill need of body tissues for normal function:
   - identifies oxygen-carrying ability of hemoglobin and relationship between red blood cells and hemoglobin.
   - explains extra workload on heart in order to provide oxygen to tissues when supply of red blood cells/hemoglobin is decreased.
   - relates symptoms of anemia to decreased availability of oxygen to different tissues of the body.
3. Patient demonstrates knowledge of factors that contribute to anemia:
   - states that decreased erythrocyte production may be caused by inadequate diet/malabsorption problems.
   - identifies suppression of erythrocyte formation in bone marrow as result of the effects of certain drugs, toxins, disease.

- identifies loss of red blood cells/hemoglobin resulting from chronic or acute blood loss.
- identifies familial tendencies and anemia.
4. Patient recognizes measures necessary to reduce risks of injury associated with impaired function of circulatory, cardiac, and neurologic systems as the result of anemia.
5. Patient demonstrates knowledge of enhancement of erythrocyte/hemoglobin production and survival:
   - compliance with proper diet and medication regimens.
   - avoidance of individuals with infection.
   - prompt reporting of any signs and symptoms of bleeding or infection.
   - avoidance of unnecessary exposure to toxic agents.

NURSING MANAGEMENT

Assessment

1. See Assessment, Levels 1 and 2.
2. Monitor results of current laboratory data.
3. Obtain historical data:
   - heart palpitations.
   - chest pain.
   - activity level.
   - blood loss (severe).
   - dyspnea upon exertion.
   - increased dizziness.
   - profound loss of peripheral sensation or vibratory or position sense.
3. Conduct a physical assessment, noting signs and symptoms of severe anemia:
   - vital signs: increased pulse, decreased BP, increased respirations.
   - auscultation of heart: tachycardia, murmurs, irregularities.
   - skin: pale, cold to touch, cyanotic.
   - auscultation of lungs: rales, wheezes.
   - mentation: lethargy, lack of responsiveness.
   - muscular integrity: possible muscle necrosis can occur in severe anemia.

Nursing Interventions

1. See Nursing Interventions, Levels 1 and 2.
2. Report bleeding.

3. Administer blood transfusions:
   - obtain consent for blood transfusion.
   - packed RBCs are usually given with chronic blood loss.
   - whole blood may be needed if blood loss is acute.
   - administer slowly to avoid fluid overload if blood loss has been chronic.
   - observe for amelioration of cardio-respiratory and neurologic symptoms (improvement in mentation).
4. Protect patient from infection:
   - remove sources of infection (see Chapter 31).
   - no visitors or caregivers who have infection.
   - body, oral, environmental hygiene essential.
5. Promote rest.
6. Administer oxygen as indicated in order to prevent tissue hypoxia and to decrease workload of heart.
7. Administer cardiotonic/diuretic medications as ordered according to cardiorespiratory status.
8. Implement measures to maintain skin integrity.
9. Maintain physical safety: side-rails/bed restraints if patient is restless or confused.
10. Provide nutritious diet.
11. Provide mouth care: Use sponge Toothette if mouth is sore or tends to bleed.

12. Administer supplements as ordered according to identified mineral or vitamin deficiency.
13. Limit residual disabilities:
    - arrange for evaluation and treatment by physical therapist.
    - provide range-of-motion exercises.
    - gradually increase ambulation and activities of daily living as anemia lessens.
    - monitor cardiorespiratory and neurologic status carefully as activities increase.
14. Plan for discharge:
    - assistance will usually be needed at home while patient recovers. Help patient/family obtain assistive devices (wheelchair, walker, and the like).
    - arrange for home health nurse follow-up at home.

Patient Teaching

1. See Patient Teaching, Levels 1 and 2.
2. Emphasize that strength usually will improve as number of erythrocytes and quantity of oxygen-carrying hemoglobin increases.
3. Explain rationale for blood transfusions:
    - discuss signs and symptoms of transfusion reaction to report immediately.
    - discuss possible risks of blood transfusion and explain that blood is carefully screened and tested for these possible risks.

SUGGESTED READINGS

Aistars, J.: Fatigue in the cancer patient: A conceptual approach to a clinical problem. Oncology Nursing Forum *14*(6):25–30, 1987.

Anderson, G.: Normal and altered erythrocyte production. *In* Bullock, B., and Rosendahl, P. (eds.): Pathophysiology: Adaptations and Alteration in Function. Boston, Little, Brown & Co., 1984, pp. 167–181.

American Association of Blood Banks: Blood transfusions outside the hospital. American Journal of Nursing *89* (4):486–489, 1989.

Britton, D.: Fatigue. *In* Yasko, J.M. (Ed.): Guidelines for Cancer Care: Symptom Management. Reston, VA, Reston Publishing, 1983, pp. 33–37.

Buchanan, G.R.: Hematologic supportive care. *In* Pizzo, P.A., and Poplack, D.G. (Eds.): Pediatric Oncology. Philadelphia, J.B. Lippincott, 1989, pp. 823–826.

Goodman, M.: Managing the side effects of chemotherapy. Seminars in Oncology Nursing *5*(2) Suppl 1:29–52, 1989.

Luckman, J., and Sorensen, K.C. (Eds.): Medical-Surgical Nursing. Philadelphia, W.B. Saunders, 1987, pp. 1036–1059.

Maxwell, M.B.: When the cancer patient becomes anemic. Cancer Nursing *7*(4):321–326, 1984.

Wolfe, D.W.: Hematologic complications of malignancy. Topics in Emergency Medicine *8*(2):13–24, 1986.

PATIENT EDUCATION MATERIALS AND COMMUNITY RESOURCES

Local chapter of the American Red Cross has information on the donations and transfusion of blood and blood products. Pamphlets include:

From One to Another–The Gifts of Blood

AIDS and the Safety of the Nation's Blood Supply

34

Injury, Potential for, Related to Disseminated Intravascular Coagulopathy (DIC)

Ruth Bope Dangel

Population at Risk

- Individuals with malignant neoplasms, acute bacterial or viral infections
- Individuals who have undergone cancer chemotherapy or blood component therapy

LEVEL 1:   *Precipitating Conditions**

EXPECTED OUTCOME

1. Patient identifies/demonstrates knowledge related to DIC:
    - identifies signs and symptoms to report to health care team.
    - identifies self-care methods to decrease risk of infection.
2. Patient demonstrates absence of signs and symptoms of DIC:
    - normal coagulation and fibrinogen values.
    - normal hematologic values.
    - absence of overt or occult bleeding.
    - absence of acrocyanosis (mottled cyanosis of hands or feet).

NURSING MANAGEMENT

Assessment

1. Recognize conditions associated with cancer/cancer treatment that may precipitate DIC:
    - malignant neoplasms: all cell types, but most commonly occurs in association with leukemia, especially acute promyelocytic; mucin-secreting adenocarcinomas (e.g., lung, pancreas, stomach, prostate); disseminated malignant neo-

plasms, particularly with metastasis to liver.
    - chemotherapy.
    - surgery.
    - hemolytic processes: transfusions of mismatched blood, acute hemolysis secondary to infection.
    - immunologic disorders.
    - acute bacterial and viral infections.
    - vascular stasis, shock.

---

*The precise etiology of DIC is unknown. DIC always occurs secondary to an underlying precipitating condition.

2. Assess for signs and symptoms of abnormal bleeding and coagulation:
   - occult: abdominal distention, guaiac-positive stool, heme-positive urine, skin and scleral color changes, orthopnea, frank air hunger, tachycardia, acrocyanosis (symmetric mottled cyanosis of hands or feet), malaise, weakness, altered sensorium, vision changes, headaches.
   - overt: petechiae, ecchymoses, purpura, hemorrhagic bullae, wound hematoma, gangrene, continuous oozing of blood from mucous membranes, needle punctures, wounds, epistaxis, hemoptysis, blood from gastrointestinal, genitourinary, or respiratory tract, fall in arterial blood pressure.
3. Assess for signs and symptoms of infection (see Chapter 31).
4. Monitor laboratory values for abnormalities that indicate bleeding/infection.
5. Monitor for signs and symptoms of transfusion reaction:
   - urticaria.
   - restlessness.
   - anxiety.
   - cough.
   - change in blood pressure.
   - chills.
   - tachycardia.
   - temperature 1.5°F above pretransfusion temperature.
   - lumbar pain.
   - pallor.
   - throat constriction.
   - flushing.

Nursing Interventions

1. Recognize early signs and symptoms of bleeding and infection.
2. Obtain cultures and sensitivities of blood and body sites when infection suspected.
3. Administer antibiotic therapy as ordered.
4. Administer blood component therapy following proper policies and procedures.

5. Assist in the treatment of the underlying conditions that may precipitate DIC.

Patient Teaching

1. Teach patient about signs and symptoms of bleeding:
   - petechiae.
   - ecchymoses.
   - blood in urine or stool.
   - blood from any orifice.
   - headache, changes in level of consciousness.
2. Outline signs and symptoms of anemia:
   - weakness.
   - fatigue.
   - pale skin color.
   - intolerance to cold.
   - irritability/nervousness.
   - lightheadedness.
   - shortness of breath.
   - palpitations.
3. Discuss signs and symptoms of infection:
   - redness.
   - swelling.
   - increased warmth.
   - soreness and tenderness.
   - fever.
   - coughing.
   - runny nose.
   - sneezing.
   - sore throat.
   - pain.
   - fatigue.
   - malaise.
   - burning upon urination.
4. Emphasize need for reporting above symptoms.
5. Teach self-care methods to decrease risk of infection when myelosuppressed (see Chapter 31):
   - daily baths and perineal care.
   - good oral hygiene.
   - avoidance of individuals with communicable diseases.
   - avoidance of nicks or cuts in skin.
   - avoidance of use of hard bristle toothbrush.

- avoidance of use of mouthwashes containing alcohol.
- lubrication of skin to prevent dryness and breaks in skin integrity.
- shaving only with electric razor.
- keeping nails short and trimmed.
- promotion of normal bowel elimination without straining or constipation.

LEVEL 2: Potential for Massive Diffuse Thrombosis/Hemorrhage

EXPECTED OUTCOME

1. Patient/caregiver identify/demonstrate knowledge related to DIC:
   - identify and report signs and symptoms of DIC.
   - verbalize basic understanding of disease process.
   - state basic understanding of treatment and rationale for same.
2. Patient achieves resolution of signs and symptoms of DIC as evidenced by:
   - cessation of bleeding.
   - absence of acrocyanosis.
   - return of hematologic values to normal range.
   - return of coagulation and fibrinogen levels to normal.

NURSING MANAGEMENT

Assessment

1. See Assessment, Level 1.
2. Systematically monitor for bleeding (occult, overt, sudden massive hemorrhage) and thrombosis by assessing body systems:
   - integumentary:
     - observe for skin color–pale or jaundiced; cutaneous bleeding–petechiae, ecchymoses, purpura, oozing or hemorrhage from body orifices, incisional wounds, catheters, venipuncture sites; gingival bleeding; peripheral thrombosis; sclera–jaundice or hemorrhage; skin temperature–hands and feet mottled and cold (acrocyanosis).
     - measure ecchymoses for changes in size.
   - cardiopulmonary:
     - observe for hemoptysis, tachypnea, orthopnea, frank air hunger, complaints of palpitations or angina, orthostatic hypotension.
     - auscultate for tachycardia, murmurs.
   - gastrointestinal and genitourinary:
     - observe for complaints of abdominal tenderness, numbness or pain in legs, oliguria, occult blood in stools and urine.
     - measure abdominal girth.
   - neurologic:
     - observe for irritability or confusion; complaints of headache, vertigo; changes in level of consciousness.
   - general:
     - observe for complaints of fatigue, weakness, malaise, myalgia, bone and joint pain.
   - monitor laboratory values.
   - measure vital signs, intake, output.
3. Assess for signs and symptoms of sudden massive hemorrhage:
   - general: low blood pressure, tachycardia, oliguria.

218

- gastrointestinal: free-flowing blood from mouth or bowels, increased abdominal girth or pain.
- genitourinary: hematuria, oliguria.
- cardiopulmonary: free-flowing blood from respiratory tract, dyspnea, tachycardia.
- neurologic: decreased level of consciousness, quadriplegia, conjugate deviation of eyes, eyes that do not move laterally, pinpoint pupils.

4. Assess for signs and symptoms of thrombotic vascular occlusion and organ ischemia:
   - general: localized, referred pain.
   - neurologic: syncope, hemiplegia, cerebrovascular accident-like symptoms, paresthesias.
   - cardiopulmonary: dyspnea, tachycardia.
   - renal or mesenteric vascular occlusion: progressive oliguria, bowel necrosis.
5. Monitor results of laboratory tests commonly used in DIC:

Test	Result in DIC
Platelet count	Usually decreased
Fibrinogen level	Usually decreased
Prothrombin time (PT)	Prolonged
Fibrin split products (FSP)	Elevated
Thrombin time	Usually prolonged
Partial thromboplastin time (PTT)	Usually prolonged
Protamine sulfate test	Strongly positive
Clotting factor assays	Reduced levels
Antithrombin III	Decreased

Nursing Interventions

1. Identify precipitating factors and provide nursing care for treatment of underlying causes of DIC.
2. Prevent further bleeding and trauma through careful nursing intervention:
   - check vital signs carefully as needed:
     - avoid taking rectal temperature.
     - check blood pressure by cuff only as necessary.
     - rotate blood pressure cuff to a different extremity when possible.
     - avoid overinflation of cuff.
   - maintain skin and mucosal integrity:
     - avoid needle punctures.
     - obtain blood specimens from central or arterial lines when possible.
     - prevent skin breakdown and trauma to body orifices.
     - suction with care.
     - clean skin carefully.
     - do not use adhesive tapes.
     - use paper or silk tape on nasogastric tube, IV dressing, catheters.
     - remove tape gently.
     - change dressings regularly.
     - pad side-rails, any sharp objects in environment.
   - maintain oral hygiene:
     - do not use toothbrush.
     - use soft swabs/frequent rinses with normal saline.
     - keep lips lubricated.
     - avoid use of mouthwashes containing alcohol.
   - administer medication PO or IV.
     - avoid rectal medications.
     - avoid IM or SQ injections.
     - if necessary to administer medication parenterally, use smallest gauge needle possible, maintain pressure on site for several minutes. Observe site for oozing or hematoma formation.
   - help patient prevent Valsalva maneuver: prevent excessive coughing, gagging, vomiting, straining at stool, isometric exercises.
3. Accurately measure blood loss:
   - maintain blood loss records.
4. Correctly administer blood components and medications:
   - blood products should be administered according to agency policies and procedures:
     - before beginning administration of blood components, double check patient and product identification with second person.
     - monitor vital signs before, during, after administration.

- administer blood products through saline-primed tubing with filter using 19-gauge needle or larger.
- avoid medications that contain aspirin or other products that affect platelet function.

5. Support other needs of patient and family as they arise:
   - support physical needs of patient:
     - provide adequate rest periods.
     - provide supplemental oxygen if needed for increased tissue perfusion.
     - implement treatment to correct acid-base imbalances.
   - support psychosocial needs of patient/family:
     - explain basic reasons symptoms are occurring.
     - explain reasons for interventions.
     - encourage patient/family to express concerns, ask questions.
     - stay close to patient to alleviate anxiety.
     - reassure patient/family.

6. Monitor and document resolution of DIC as determined by:
   - normalization of coagulation factors (fibrinogen and platelet count usually first laboratory values to improve).
   - improvement in clinical symptoms (bleeding slows, then stops; perfusion to skin, organs improves).

7. Implement additional supportive measu. as ordered if DIC is not resolved:
   - give blood components to maintain blood pressure and volume and to replace clotting factors:
     - platelets for severe thrombocytopenia.
     - cryoprecipitate for low fibrinogen levels.
     - fresh frozen plasma for replacement of clotting factors (commercial preparations of concentrated clotting factors II, VII, IX, X available but usually not given because of risk of thrombus formation).
   - packed red blood cells to increase red blood cell volume and clotting factors.
   - administer heparin as ordered (heparin use is controversial).
   - administer epsilon aminocaproic acid (EACA) (EACA use is controversial).

Patient Teaching

1. Explain DIC signs and symptoms (see Level 2).
2. Explain treatment measures and rationale.
3. Suggest methods to reduce undue anxiety and stress.
4. Instruct patient to report any signs and symptoms of abnormal bleeding.
5. Teach patient to save excreta for measurement and examination for blood.

LEVEL 3:   Acute-Massive Sudden Hemorrhage/Diffuse Thrombotic Vascular Occlusion

EXPECTED OUTCOME

1. Patient maintains adequate perfusion through critical period:
   - absent or diminished bleeding.
   - adequate urinary output.
   - normal laboratory values.
2. Patient/caregiver identify/demonstrate knowledge related to acute DIC:
   - identify signs and symptoms of acute DIC.
   - state critical period of care.

- state basic understanding of treatment and rationale for same.
3. Patient/caregiver prepare for convalescence and homegoing:
   - verbalize concerns, questions.
   - assist in developing home care plans.
   - understand home care instructions.
   - state signs and symptoms to report.
4. Patient/caregiver prepare for death when inevitable:
   - verbalize concerns and feelings.
   - maintain dignity and comfort.

NURSING MANAGEMENT

Assessment

See Assessment, Levels 1 and 2.

Nursing Interventions

1. See Nursing Interventions, Levels 1 and 2.
2. Provide continued nursing care following resolution of acute phase of DIC:
   - promote comfort.
   - assess for further signs and symptoms of bleeding and thrombosis.
   - mobilize patient if indicated.
   - prevent further trauma or bleeding.
   - administer medications and blood components as needed.
   - monitor laboratory values until normal.
   - continue to monitor blood loss.
   - provide emotional support to patient/family.
   - encourage patient and family to express concerns and questions.
   - provide appropriate reassurance.
3. Allow family members to assist and care in order to decrease fear and anxiety.
4. Assist patient and family in planning for convalescence and homegoing, when appropriate.

Patient Teaching

1. See Patient Teaching, Levels 1 and 2.
2. Perform prompt and thorough physical care.

3. Reassure patient/family when possible and appropriate.
4. Inform patient/family of progress and plans.
5. Discuss convalescence and homegoing needs and responsibilities.
6. Discuss patient/caregiver concerns and feelings when death is inevitable.
7. Promote comfort and dignity of patient/caregiver.

SUGGESTED READINGS

Caprini, J.A., and Sener, S.F.: Altered coagulability in cancer patients. Cancer 33:162–172, 1982.

Dangel, R.B.: Disseminated intravascular coagulation in individuals with cancer. The Hospice Journal 1(4):77–86, 1985–1986.

Findley, J.P.: Nursing management of common oncologic emergencies. In Ziegfeld, C.R.: Core Curriculum for Oncology Nursing. Philadelphia, W.B. Saunders, 1987, pp. 321–331.

Happ, M.: Life threatening hemorrhage in children with cancer. Journal of the Association of Pediatric Oncology Nurses 4(3,4):36–40, 1987.

Kirchner, C.W., and Reheis, C.E.: Two serious complications of neoplasia: Sepsis and disseminated intravascular coagulation. Nursing Clinics of North America 17: 595–604, 1982.

American Nurses Association and Oncology Nursing Society: Standards of Oncology Nursing Practice, 1987.

Perry, A.G.: Shock complications: Recognition and management. Critical Care Nursing Quarterly 11(1):1–8, 1988.

Rooney, A., and Haviley, C.: Nursing management of disseminated intravascular coagulation. Oncology Nursing Forum 12(1):15–22, 1985.

Siegrist, C.W., and Jones, J.A.: Disseminated intravascular

coagulopathy and nursing implications. Seminars in Oncology Nursing *1*(4):237–243, 1985.

Volgelpohl, R.A.: Disseminated intravascular coagulation. Critical Care Nurse *1*:131–142, 1981.

Weinstein, S.M.: Disseminated intravascular coagulation. National Intravenous Therapy Association *5*:169–172, 1982.

Yasko, J.M., and Schafer, S.L.: Disseminated intravascular coagulation. *In* Yasko, J.M.: Guidelines for Cancer Care Symptom Management. Reston, VA, Reston Publishing, 1983, pp. 324–329.

PATIENT EDUCATION MATERIALS AND COMMUNITY RESOURCES

DIC Nursing Assessment Tool (Rooney, A., and Haviley, C.: Nursing management of disseminated intravascular coagulation. Oncology Nursing Forum *12*(1):20 (Figure 5), 1985. Could be utilized as a teaching tool with patient and family to increase their understanding of the relationship between signs and symptoms, laboratory data and treatment.

Injury, Potential for, Related to Graft Versus Host Disease (GVHD)

35

Beverly Vincent Davis

Population at Risk

- Individuals undergoing allogeneic bone marrow transplantation for malignant or non-malignant conditions
- Highest risk: individuals whose donors are mismatched for 2 to 3 antigens; individuals over age 30
- Moderate risk: individuals with HLA-identical donor (35 to 50 per cent incidence of acute GVHD: 45 per cent incidence of chronic GVHD)
- Individuals who experience acute GVHD are at increased risk of developing chronic form

LEVEL 1: Potential for GVHD—Acute

EXPECTED OUTCOME

1. Patient remains free of acute GVHD:
   - intact skin.
   - normal liver function.
   - 1 to 2 stools per day.
2. Patient identifies knowledge related to prevention of GVHD:
   - identifies predisposing factors.
   - identifies early signs and symptoms to report to health care team.
   - identifies medical regimen to prevent GVHD.

NURSING MANAGEMENT

Assessment

1. Assess patient's knowledge of GVHD: cause, symptoms, and implications related to quality of life and treatment outcome.
2. Assess for baseline, before donor marrow infusion, and the status of the three systems affected: skin (integrity), liver (alkaline phosphatase, bilirubin, serum glutamic oxaloacetic transaminase), gastrointestinal (function).
3. Continue daily assessment particularly at time when GVHD is most likely to occur (median onset, day 25 post-transplant.)

Nursing Interventions

1. Administer prescribed preventive agents (e.g., methotrexate, cyclosporine).

2. Monitor renal function and magnesium levels daily (cyclosporine can induce seizures in the presence of hypomagnesium).
3. Irradiate all blood products before transfusion to avoid infusing immunocompetent T lymphocytes.
4. Bathe skin daily with warm saline or warm Hibiclens diluted 1:8 with sterile water. Pat skin dry.
5. Immediately after bathing, apply lotion (e.g., Keri) or cream (e.g., Eucerin).
6. Apply cornstarch lightly to skin folds.

Patient Teaching

1. Discuss risk factors for GVHD.
2. Teach patient to report early signs and symptoms to health care team:
   - erythematous rash on palms, soles, ears, trunk.
   - anorexia.
   - abdominal cramping, diarrhea, nausea, vomiting.
3. Teach importance and technique of skin hygiene including frequent handwashing.

LEVEL 2: Mild to Moderate GVHD (Stages I and II)— Acute

EXPECTED OUTCOME

1. Patient identifies knowledge related to early GVHD:
   - identifies signs and symptoms of early GVHD to report to health care team.
   - identifies measures to control symptoms of GVHD.
   - identifies medical regimen to prevent GVHD.
2. Patient exhibits resolution of early GVHD as evidenced by:
   - healing of skin.
   - return of liver function tests to normal.
   - resolution of diarrhea and abdominal cramping.
   - normal serum electrolytes and adequate hydration.
3. Patient achieves control of pain and discomfort related to:
   - skin lesions.
   - diarrhea.
   - increased abdominal girth or liver pain.

NURSING MANAGEMENT

Assessment

1. See Assessment, Level 1.
2. Assess skin q8h for erythematous rash on palms, soles, ears, trunk, back, axillae.
3. Assess for signs of liver involvement:
   - right upper quadrant pain.
   - hepatomegaly.
   - elevated liver function tests (especially alkaline phosphatase, bilirubin, serum glutamic oxaloacetic transaminase).
4. Assess for diarrhea and abdominal cramping.
5. Assess need for platelet transfusion before biopsy of tissue for diagnosis of GVHD in thrombocytopenic patient.

Nursing Interventions

1. See Nursing Interventions, Level 1.
2. Communicate early symptoms to physi-

cian to facilitate prompt medical management.

3. Bathe skin bid with warm saline or with Hibiclens diluted 1:8 with sterile water. Pat dry with soft cloth.
4. Lubricate dry skin bid with an emollient lotion or cream (e.g., Keri, Aquaphor, Eucerin).
5. Use nonirritating bed sheet (e.g., Soft-Kare burn sheet). The use of special beds may be indicated if integumentary discomfort is high.
6. Maintain strict record of intake and output.
7. Monitor fluid and electrolyte status, daily weights.
8. If diarrhea develops, keep patient NPO, institute total parenteral nutrition as prescribed and administer prescribed antidiarrheal agents (e.g., Lomotil, Imodium, opium tincture).
9. Monitor quantity of diarrhea.
10. Test all stools for blood.
11. Provide gentle perirectal cleansing, followed by protective ointment, after each occurrence of diarrhea.

12. Administer prescribed systemic treatment (e.g., cyclosporine, antithymocyte globulin, monoclonal antibodies, corticosteroids). Observe for adverse effects.
13. Administer systemic analgesics on regular basis (e.g., continuous infusion of morphine).
14. Provide psychosocial support to patient.

Patient Teaching

1. See Patient Teaching, Level 1.
2. Explain reasons for interventions.
3. Teach rationale and measures to maintain skin integrity including cleansing, lubricating, preventing trauma (e.g., avoid scratching skin, use of nonirritating bed sheets), using protective ointments.
4. Teach rationale and measures to maintain normal bowel elimination, including use of antidiarrheal agents.
5. Teach rationale and measures to maintain fluid and electrolyte balance including use of antiemetics.

LEVEL 3: Severe GVHD (Stages III—IV)—Acute

EXPECTED OUTCOME

1. Patient exhibits resolution of life-threatening multiorgan dysfunction, as evidenced by:
   - healing skin.
   - normal liver function tests.
   - <500 ml stool per day.
   - absence of diarrhea, emesis.
   - normal serum electrolytes.
   - adequate intravascular hydration.
2. Patient/caregiver demonstrate knowledge related to severe GVHD:
   - identify signs and symptoms to report to health care team.
   - identify measures to manage GVHD.
   - identify measures to manage symptoms of GVHD.
3. Patient identifies measures to prevent or manage the complications of GVHD.

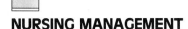

NURSING MANAGEMENT

Assessment

1. See Assessment, Levels 1 and 2.
2. Assess skin for superinfection of lesions.
3. Monitor for integumentary bleeding from desquamated skin lesions.
4. Assess intravascular fluid volume.
5. Evaluate stool and emesis for amount of blood loss from sloughing gastrointestinal tract.
6. Monitor for signs of sepsis q2–4h:
   - elevated temperatures, cardiovascular changes, change in mental status.
7. Monitor for respiratory distress.
8. Assess functional performance (activities of daily living).

Nursing Interventions

1. See Nursing Interventions, Levels 1 and 2.
2. Cover open skin areas per institutional protocol (e.g., sterile Vaseline gauze, Silvadene ointment, or antibiotic ointment–coated hydrogel dressings [e.g., Vigilon]).

3. Apply cotton mittens or gloves when sleeping to prevent scratching.
4. Maintain strict recording of intake and output, weights.
5. Provide for total parenteral nutrition and fluid replacement as prescribed.
6. Test stools and emesis for blood.
7. Transfuse platelets/RBCs as ordered.
8. Assist with oxygen therapy or mechanical ventilation as needed.
9. Provide supportive equipment and assistance with activities of daily living.
10. Provide psychosocial support to patient/family.

Patient Teaching

1. See Patient Teaching, Levels 1 and 2.
2. Frequently reinforce teaching, especially critical interventions.
3. Teach rationale and measures to maintain nutrition and fluid balance including total parenteral nutrition, fluid replacement, IV antiemetics.
4. Teach rationale and measures to prevent infection (see Chapter 31).

LEVEL 1:   Potential for GVHD—Chronic

EXPECTED OUTCOME

1. Patient remains free of chronic GVHD as evidenced by maintenance of normal:
   - skin integrity.
   - joint function.
   - swallowing.
   - visual acuity.
2. Patient demonstrates knowledge related to prevention of chronic GVHD:
   - identifies potential sites of manifestation.
   - identifies signs and symptoms to report to health care team.
   - identifies measures to prevent chronic GVHD.

NURSING MANAGEMENT

Assessment

1. Assess knowledge of chronic GVHD and potential sites of manifestation: esophagus, skin, eyes, lungs, joints, vagina, liver, gastrointestinal tract, immune system, mouth.
2. Assess patient's ability to identify and report signs and symptoms to facilitate prompt treatment.

Nursing Interventions

1. Institute plan of oral hygiene:
   * brush after eating with soft brush.
   * floss daily if platelet count >50,000.
   * routine dental visits with fluoride treatment.
   * apply lubricant to lips.
2. Institute plan for insufficient tearing:
   * routine testing for tear production (Schirmer's test).
   * facilitate ophthalmologic consultation for insufficient tearing.
   * institute use of artificial tears prophylactically.
3. Facilitate a physical therapy consultation to assess and document range of motion parameters for each joint. Monitor for changes.

Patient Teaching

1. Instruct patient in rationale and measures to prevent infections:
   * wear mask for 6 months post-transplant (practice may vary among institutions).
   * avoid contact with persons with communicable diseases.
   * avoid live virus vaccinations or contact with persons having recently received live virus vaccinations.
2. Instruct patient in rationale and measures to promote skin integrity:
   * wear sunscreen and avoid direct sunlight for 1 year post-transplant.
   * wear long-sleeve shirts and hats when outdoors in sunlight.
   * bathe with mild soap and avoid deodorant soap.
3. Teach patient to report early signs of chronic GVHD to health care team:
   * any change in skin color or texture.
   * oral burning or pain, loss of taste.
   * anorexia.
   * difficulty swallowing or painful swallowing.
   * difficulty breathing.
   * burning, grittiness, pain in eye.
   * photophobia.
   * inflammation or dryness of vagina, dyspareunia.
4. Teach patient importance of regular visits to the dentist, ophthalmologist, and gynecologist (female patients).

LEVEL 2:   Mild to Moderate GVHD—Chronic

EXPECTED OUTCOME

1. Patient demonstrates knowledge of measures to control chronic GVHD:
   * identifies signs and symptoms of chronic GVHD to report to health care team.
   * recognizes importance of early medical intervention in reducing severity and avoiding long-term dysfunctions associated with chronic GVHD.

2. Patient remains free of chronic GVHD-related infection, as evidenced by absence of:
   - fever.
   - sinus pain and drainage.
   - cough.
   - dyspnea.
   - viral skin lesions.

NURSING MANAGEMENT

Assessment

1. See Assessment, Level 1.
2. Assess for signs and symptoms during susceptible timeframe (100 to 365 days post-transplant):
   - itching and burning, especially on palms or soles.
   - rash.
   - altered pigmentation or erythema, especially on face.
   - desquamation.
   - elevated liver function tests.
   - xerostomia.
   - oral mucositis: erythema, ulcerations, lichen-like lesions, especially on buccal mucosa and tongue.
   - dysphagia, retrosternal pain.
   - weight loss.
   - reduced range of motion, contracture.
   - vaginal stricture or atrophy.
   - dyspnea.
3. Assess patient/family ability to provide care in the home.

Nursing Interventions

1. See Nursing Interventions, Level 1.
2. Assist patient to plan for activities of daily living as tolerated, allowing rest intervals.
3. Promptly report any changes in color or texture of skin.
4. Avoid harsh soaps or products that dry skin.
5. Apply lanolin-based cream to skin bid (e.g., Eucerin cream).
6. Facilitate physical therapy consultation for measures to avoid joint contracture.
7. Report joint pain, swelling, or decreased range of motion immediately.
8. Continue oral hygiene regimen and dental follow-up; add artificial saliva.
9. Monitor weight.
10. Facilitate nutritional consultation if esophageal or oral involvement interferes with eating; assist with tube feeding or total parenteral nutrition as indicated.
11. Provide support and comfort measures for patients requiring esophageal dilatation.
12. Facilitate consultation for home nursing care if needed or if required by home situation.
13. Arrange home nutritional support, enteral or parenteral, as indicated.

Patient Teaching

1. Teach patient signs and symptoms to report to health care team:
   - persistent nausea, vomiting.
   - diarrhea.
   - pain or difficulty swallowing.
   - joint pain, swelling, decreased range of motion.
   - respiratory changes.
   - fever.
   - sinus pain or drainage.
   - excessive eye dryness.
2. Teach use of water-soluble lubricants and vaginal dilator as indicated, for vaginal stenosis or atrophy.

3. Instruct patient regarding importance of prophylactic antibiotics.
4. Instruct patient/family in the performance of treatment and procedures, especially enteral or parenteral nutrition in the home.

5. When patient status indicates, discuss return to employment and activities of daily living.

LEVEL 3: Severe GVHD—Chronic

EXPECTED OUTCOME

1. Patient/caregiver demonstrate knowledge related to severe chronic GVHD:
   - identify signs and symptoms of severe GVHD.
   - recognize importance of early medical interventions in successfully managing and minimizing GVHD-related dysfunctions.
   - Identify measures to manage symptoms of severe GVHD.
2. Patient has resolution of discomfort and pain related to chronic GVHD.
3. Patient avoids or minimizes permanent disability as evidenced by maintenance of:
   - joint function.
   - skin elasticity.
   - visual acuity.
   - swallowing.

NURSING MANAGEMENT

Assessment

1. See Assessment, Levels 1 and 2.
2. Assess for signs of infection including those most common: bacterial pneumonia, sinusitis, bacteremia.
3. Assess for worsening or failure of improvement in organs and tissues susceptible to permanent disability: joints, skin, eyes, esophagus.

Nursing Interventions

1. See Nursing Interventions, Levels 1 and 2.
2. Administer prescribed antimicrobial agents. Implement appropriate nursing interventions for specific side effects of infection (see Chapter 31).

3. For patients developing herpes zoster–varicella infection, administer:
   - calamine lotion to involved skin areas.
   - cool compresses.
   - prescribed antipruritic.
   - prescribed analgesic.
4. Facilitate nutritional consultation to provide for increased nutritional requirements during infection.
5. Arrange for rehabilitative consultation regarding any organ system with persistent involvement.
6. Initiate discussion when appropriate, of survivorship issues: psychosocial, financial, employment-related, physical. Refer for appropriate consultation and counseling. Provide opportunity for patient/family to express concerns.

Patient Teaching

1. See Patient Teaching, Levels 1 and 2.
2. Explain that chronic GVHD is associated with delayed return of immune function and therefore increased risk of infections.
3. Teach signs and symptoms of infections for which patients are at high risk: bacterial pneumonia, sinusitis, and bacteremia.
4. Discuss increased risk and symptoms of herpes zoster–varicella infections (fluid-filled lesions with or without fever, chills, fatigue, pain, tingling, nausea, vomiting). Teach importance of prompt treatment with intravenous antiviral agent.
5. Tell patient to avoid exposure to individuals exposed to chickenpox.
6. Teach patient to monitor for and report effects of long-term therapy for chronic GVHD including increased risk of cataracts associated with steroids.

SUGGESTED READINGS

Anderson, J.L.: Insurability of cancer patients: A rehabilitation barrier. Oncology Nursing Forum 11(2):42–45, 1984.

Corcoran-Bushsel, P.: Ambulatory care of the bone marrow transplant patient. Puget Sound Oncology Nursing Society Quarterly, 12(1):4–7, 1989.

Corcoran-Bushsel, P.: Long-term complications of allogeneic bone marrow transplantation: Nursing implications. Oncology Nursing Forum 13(6):61–70, 1986.

de la Montaigne, M., de Mao, J., Nuscher, R., et al.: Standards of care for the patient with "graft-versus-host disease" post-bone marrow transplantation: Nursing implications. Cancer Nursing 4:191–198, 1981.

Ford, R., and Ballard, B.: Acute complications after bone marrow transplantation. Seminars in Oncology Nursing 4(1):15–24, 1988.

Freedman, S.E.: An overview of bone marrow transplantation. Seminars in Oncology Nursing 4(1):3–8, 1988.

Klemm, P.: Cyclosporin A: Use in preventing graft-versus-host disease. Oncology Nursing Forum 12(5):25–32, 1985.

McConn, R.: Skin changes following bone marrow transplantation. Cancer Nursing 10(2):82–84, 1987.

Nims, J.W., and Strom, S.: Late complications of bone marrow transplant recipients: Nursing care issues. Seminars in Oncology Nursing 4(1):47–54, 1988.

Schubert, M.M., Sullivan, K.M., Morton, T.H., et al.: Oral manifestations of chronic graft-versus-host disease. Archives of Internal Medicine 144:1591–1595, 1984.

PATIENT EDUCATION MATERIALS AND COMMUNITY RESOURCES

American Cancer Society Publication: Cancer: Your Job, Insurance, and the Law.

National Institutes of Health: Understanding the Immune System. Publication #88-529, 1988.

Cancer Information Services, Telephone 1–800–4–cancer.

Candlelighters Foundation, 2025 I Street, NW, Suite 1011, Washington, DC 20006, 202–659–5136.

Leukemia Society of America, 733 Third Avenue, New York, NY 10017, 212–573–8484.

National Cancer Information Clearinghouse, Room 10A18, Building 31 NCI/NIH, Bethesda, MD, 20205, 301–496–4070.

Skin Integrity, Impairment of, Related to Malignant Skin Lesions

Patti Owen

36

Population at Risk

- Patients with primary tumors of the breast, lung, colon or rectum, ovary, or oral cavity (squamous cell)
- Patients with malignant melanoma, Kaposi's sarcoma, lymphoma, or leukemia (common sites of cutaneous metastases include anterior chest, abdomen, head [scalp], and neck)

LEVEL 1: Potential

EXPECTED OUTCOME

1. Patient demonstrates knowledge related to potential impaired skin integrity:
   - verbalizes signs and symptoms to report to health care team.
   - identifies factors that influence maintenance of and disruption in skin integrity.
2. Patient identifies/demonstrates measures to maintain skin integrity:
   - verbalizes/demonstrates measures to limit environmental insults to high-risk areas.

NURSING MANAGEMENT

Assessment

1. Inspect skin (particularly high-risk areas) for color (note local erythema), vascularity, edema, injuries, scars, lesions, nodules.
2. Palpate high-risk areas (run palms over chest and abdomen, neck and scalp, noting masses). Metastatic skin lesions are generally hard and nonmobile.

Patient Teaching

1. Teach systematic observation and assessment of skin.
2. Explain signs and symptoms to report to health care team.
3. Discuss hygienic measures (e.g., gentle soaps, no vigorous scrubbing).
4. Explain that pressure to area of subcutaneous mass should be avoided.

LEVEL 2: *Mild to Moderate*

EXPECTED OUTCOME

1. Patient demonstrates knowledge related to impaired skin integrity:
   - verbalizes signs and symptoms of altered skin integrity.
   - identifies factors that influence impairment and maintenance of skin integrity.
   - identifies potential sequelae/complications.
2. Patient identifies/demonstrates measures to promote skin integrity:
   - performs necessary treatments and procedures.
   - demonstrates proper knowledge and administration of medications.
   - verbalizes/demonstrates appropriate hygienic measures.
   - identifies signs and symptoms to report to health care team.

NURSING MANAGEMENT

Assessment

1. See Assessment, Level 1.
2. Inspect skin lesions and note:
   - general characteristics.
   - location and distribution.
   - configuration.
   - size (measure).
   - morphologic structure (e.g., nodule, scale, crust, erosion, fissure).
   - drainage (color, amount, character).
   - odor.
3. Palpate surrounding tissue and body areas at high risk for nodules or masses.
4. Monitor for signs and symptoms of infection (temperature, pulse, respirations, change in color or odor of drainage).
5. Note associated factors that affect healing (e.g., low WBC, administration of steroids, diabetes mellitus).
6. Evaluate for associated symptoms (e.g., pain, tenderness).
7. Assess diet.
8. Note patient's physical and psychosocial responses to the lesion(s).
9. Assess patient's/family's ability to care for problems in the home.

Nursing Interventions

General

1. Implement measures to protect patient from infection (see Chapter 31).
2. Implement measures to protect patient from trauma and bleeding:
   - avoid physical irritants (pressure, friction, shearing).
   - avoid chemical irritants (body secretions, medications).
3. Implement measures to control pain associated with wound management:
   - premedicate with analgesics for dressing changes as appropriate.
   - institute noninvasive pain control measures (e.g., imagery, relaxation, hypnosis).
   - use nonadherent dressings (e.g., Telfa, Adaptic).
   - avoid frequent application of tape with use of Montgomery straps, Kerlix Wrap, Surgiflex. Stomahesive may be applied to areas lateral to wound so tape may be fastened to Stomahesive, avoiding reapplication of tape to area.

- provide sitz baths or whirlpool as appropriate.
4. Implement measures appropriate for the patient receiving radiation therapy (see Chapter 37).
5. Refer to home care agency for possible home nursing visits.

Nonulcerating Lesions

1. Limit environmental insults to affected area:
   - be gentle with skin care—avoid rubbing.
   - wash affected area with tepid water and pat dry.
   - avoid pressure to area.
   - provide nonirritating clothes.
2. Use dry dressings to protect against exposure to irritants and mechanical trauma (e.g., scratching).
3. If topical medications are being applied, occlusive dressings increase penetration of medication.

Ulcerating Lesions

1. Cleansing:
   - cleanse area with washcloth or gauze sponges, using gentle motion.
   - prevent cross-contamination if infection present (may use clean or sterile procedures).
   - use detergents containing hexachlorophene (e.g., Dial, Safeguard).
   - rinse well.
   - may irrigate with half-strength hydrogen peroxide and normal saline for effervescent cleansing.
   - rinse well with normal saline. Do not use hydrogen peroxide on healing tissue.
   - if ulceration is prone to bleeding, may elect not to debride, but irrigate only.
2. Debridement:
   - may use cotton swabs, sponges, gently applying pressure to debride ulcerating area.

- may use wet to dry dressings (wet dressings that are allowed to dry in place before they are removed) to allow gentle debridement; gently peel dressing away.
- may use continuous soaks (wet dressings) to facilitate gradual debridement of large amounts of necrotic tissue (e.g., normal saline, water, Burow's solution, hydrogen peroxide, $KMnO_4$, Dakin's solution).
- if proteolytic enzymes (e.g., Elase, Travase) are ordered, apply evenly over lesion; avoid contact with surrounding skin.
3. Prevent/manage local infection:
   - irrigate with antibacterial agents as ordered (e.g., acetic acid solution, povidone-iodine [Betadine]) in addition to previously mentioned agents.
   - use sterile procedure.
   - administer systemic antibiotics as ordered.
   - apply topical antibacterial agents as ordered (e.g., Bacitracin, Betadine).
   - obtain cultures and sensitivities of wound as ordered or if fever is present.
4. Apply dry, sterile, nonadherent dressing (e.g., Telfa, Adaptic). Change dressing and clean lesions q8h or prn.
5. Maintain hemostasis:
   - for capillary oozing, silver nitrate sticks or styptic pencils are useful.
   - for larger surface area bleeding, irrigate area and use epinephrine 1:1000 or ferrous sulfate solution (Monsel solution) if necessary.
   - consider radiation therapy consult for evaluation.
6. Control drainage:
   - change dressing as frequently as necessary.
   - use absorbent dressings for small to moderate amounts of drainage (e.g., ABD surgical pad, perineal pad).
   - apply drainage bag or ostomy pouch for large amounts of drainage (see Chapter 48).

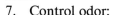

7. Control odor:
   - cleanse wound and change dressing as frequently as necessary.
   - obtain cultures and sensitivities of wound.
   - apply gauze saturated with Cepacol for 15 min. Rinse with normal saline solution.
   - may use continuous soaks of half-strength Dakin's solution (moisten prn, change q4–6h).
   - cleanse with half-strength acetic acid solution.
   - may sprinkle crushed Flagyl tablets (1 or 2) on open lesion after cleansing; physician's order is required.
   - may apply antiodor agents (e.g., baking soda, Banish, Hex-on) to outside of dressing only, as they are irritating if applied directly to skin.
   - may apply balsam of Peru to outer dressing in grid-like fashion.
8. Other nursing actions are as follows:
   - monitor nutrition and hydration.
   - encourage increased protein intake (pa-tient may be losing protein through wound drainage).

Patient Teaching

1. See Patient Teaching, Level 1.
2. Teach signs and symptoms of skin lesions.
3. Note signs and symptoms of infection and importance of monitoring temperature.
4. Explain need to avoid exposure to infection.
5. Discuss treatments and procedures:
   - clean or sterile technique.
   - handwashing technique.
   - disposal of used or soiled materials.
   - environmental hygiene.
   - good body hygiene.
   - measures to avoid cross-contamination.
   - application and side effects of medications.
   - maintenance of nutrition and hydration.
   - measures to control bleeding.
6. Instruct patient in the performance of treatments and procedures at home.

LEVEL 3:   Severe—Massive, Fungating Lesions; Large Surface Area Involvement

EXPECTED OUTCOME

1. Patient/caregiver demonstrate knowledge related to severe impairment of skin integrity:
   - verbalize potential sequelae/complications.
   - identify signs and symptoms necessary to report to health care team.
2. Patient/caregiver identify/demonstrate measures to manage severe impairment of skin integrity:
   - perform necessary treatments and procedures.
   - demonstrate proper knowledge and administration of medications.
   - verbalize/demonstrate adequate nutritional and fluid intake.

NURSING MANAGEMENT

Assessment

1. See Assessment, Levels 1 and 2.
2. Note depth of lesion(s), tissue involved.
3. Note if any vital vasculature (e.g., carotid artery) is at risk for involvement.

Nursing Interventions

1. See Nursing Interventions, Level 2.
2. Cleanse and debride:
   - may need to use jet spray (oral irrigator) or whirlpool for thorough cleaning.
   - if proteolytic enzymes are utilized, evaluate proximity of vital vasculature. Do not apply ointment near vasculature. Care must be taken to place medication on target tissue.
3. Prevent or manage local or systemic infection (see Level 2).
4. Apply dressing (see Level 2):
   - depending on amount of drainage, pack wound with sterile sponges, Iodoform gauze or petroleum-impregnated gauze.
   - to secure sterile dressing to large area, may use Montgomery straps, Kerlix Wrap, Surgiflex, or Stomahesive.
5. Protect surrounding skin from drainage:
   - change dressing frequently.
   - apply pouch or drainage bag for high output (see Chapter 48).
   - apply protective ointment or cream on surrounding skin (see Chapter 48).
6. Control bleeding:
   - use anticoagulant dressing as required; may use oxidized cellulose Surgical Absorbable Hemostat or pack wound with Gelfoam.
7. Control odor:
   - may pack wound with sponges to which balsam of Peru has been applied in grid-like fashion.
   - set tray (about 9″ × 13″) of activated charcoal (thin layer) in patient's room.
8. Other nursing actions:
   - monitor fluids and electrolytes.
   - if acidic solutions are utilized in wound management, monitor for acidosis.
9. Refer to home care agency for regular home nursing visits

Patient Teaching

See Patient Teaching, Levels 1 and 2.

SUGGESTED READINGS

Boarini, J.H., Bryant, R.A., and Irrgang, S.J.: Fistula management. Seminars in Oncology Nursing 2(4):287–292, 1986.

Brownstein, M., and Helwig, E.: Patterns of cutaneous metastasis. Archives of Dermatology 105:862–868, 1972.

Cuzzell, J.: Wound care forum: Artful solutions to chronic problems. American Journal of Dermatology 85:162, 1985.

Elewski, B.E., and Gilgox, R.S.: Eruptive lesions and malignancy. International Journal of Dermatology 24(10):617–629, 1985.

Foltz, A.: Nursing care of ulcerating metastatic lesions. Oncology Nursing Forum 7:8–13, 1980.

Hotter, A.N.: Physiologic aspects and clinical implications of wound healing. Heart and Lung 11(6):522–530, 1982.

Klaus, S., and Kierland, R.: When primary cancer spreads to the skin. Geriatrics 31:39–43, 1976.

Malasanos, L., Barkauskas, V., Noss, M., et al.: Health Assessment. St. Louis, C.V. Mosby, 1977, pp. 367–378.

Matus, N.: Topical therapy: Choosing and using the proper vehicle. Nursing 7(11):7–10, 1977.

Parrish, J.: Dermatology and Skin Care. New York, McGraw-Hill, 1975.

Roberts, S.: Skin assessment for color and temperature. American Journal of Nursing 75:610–613, 1975.

Rosen, T.: Cutaneous metastasis. Medical Clinics of North America 64(5):885–900, 1980.

Wood, D.: The draining malignant ulceration. Journal of the American Medical Association 244(8):820–822, 1980.

37

Skin Integrity, Impairment of, Related to Radiation Therapy

Joan C. McNally and Roberta A. Strohl

Population at Risk

- Patients with cancer treated with external beam radiation, especially relatively superficial cancers such as skin cancer, breast cancer, and head and neck cancer, and in whom the irradiated area includes skin folds

LEVEL 1: Potential

EXPECTED OUTCOME

1. Patient demonstrates knowledge related to potential impairment of skin integrity:
   - identifies changes that may occur to skin receiving radiation therapy.
   - identifies early signs and symptoms of skin changes.
   - identifies activities or behaviors that may potentiate skin breakdown.
2. Patient demonstrates knowledge of rationale related to potential radiation-induced skin changes:
   - identifies that larger fields and doses over a short time increase likelihood of skin reactions.
   - identifies that skin folds, bony prominences, areas subjected to pressure (axillae, perineum, under breast) are at higher risk for skin reactions.
   - identifies that, like most rapidly dividing cells, the basal layer of the epidermis is sensitive to radiation.
3. Patient identifies/demonstrates measures to prevent impaired skin integrity:
   - performs skin care in nonirritating manner within appropriate time schedules.
   - verbalizes/demonstrates adequate fluid and nutritional intake.
   - identifies signs and symptoms necessary to report to health care team.
   - identifies/demonstrates proper knowledge and application of medications/topical ointments.
4. Patient maintains skin integrity.

NURSING MANAGEMENT

Assessment

1. Inspect skin for color, moisture, scaling, temperature.

2. Assess skin for tenderness or itching.
3. Obtain history of radiation therapy (e.g., dosage, length of therapy, area irradiated, type of radiation equipment used).

236

4. Obtain history of Adriamycin therapy to assess for potential "recall" phenomenon (recurrence of skin reaction).
5. Inspect high-risk areas:
   - skin folds (e.g., buttocks, perineum, groin).
   - radiation port and exit sites.
6. Determine fluid and nutritional status.
7. Evaluate skin care practices.

Patient Teaching

1. Teach signs and symptoms of skin changes, indicating those to report to health care team (e.g., erythema, scaling, tenderness, blistering, edema).
2. Explain rationale and measures to maintain adequate nutritional and fluid status.
3. Discuss rationale and measures to prevent skin irritation and breakdown:
   - avoid constricting clothing over irradiated skin (e.g., belts, garters, restraints, brassieres, ties).
   - avoid irritating substances on irradiated skin (e.g., tape, soap, perfume, deodorants, ether, iodine, thimerosal, talcum, rough clothing).
   - wear clean soft, cotton clothing over skin at radiation port and exit sites.
   - wash clothing with mild detergents.
   - avoid heat or cold applications to area (e.g., heating pads, hot-water bottles, ice caps)
   - avoid oil-based creams, ointments, and lotions as these may contain heavy metals.
   - avoid shaving hair on skin in area receiving radiation.
   - avoid exposure to sun.
   - keep area dry and exposed to air when possible.
   - avoid swimming in salt water or chlorinated swimming pools.
4. Outline measures to control tenderness and dryness of skin:
   - use water-based, soothing topical ointments (e.g., hydrous lanolin, Aquaphor) as ordered.
   - dust on cornstarch.
   - use gentle soaps; avoid vigorous scrubbing.
   - follow skin care instructions as given by radiation therapy department.
   - use an electric razor if shaving is necessary.
   - use a sun screen agent if there is a potential for sun exposure.

LEVEL 2:   *Dry or Moist Desquamation*

EXPECTED OUTCOME

1. Patient identifies/demonstrates knowledge related to impairment of skin integrity:
   - identifies skin changes that occur in irradiated skin.
   - verbalizes signs and symptoms of impaired skin integrity, including those that should be reported to health care team.
   - identifies potential complication of impaired skin integrity.
2. Patient identifies/demonstrates measures to control or correct impaired skin integrity:
   - performs necessary treatments or procedures.
   - identifies/demonstrates measures that promote circulation and healing and prevent further skin breakdown.
   - verbalizes/demonstrates adequate nutritional and fluid intake.

237

3. Patient demonstrates control and healing of impaired skin integrity, as evidenced by:
   - absence of infection.
   - reduction or stabilization of area of impaired skin integrity.
   - decrease in drainage.
4. Patient identifies that certain chemotherapeutic agents such as DTIC and Adriamycin may enhance skin reactions if given concomitantly and that certain agents such as Adriamycin are associated with "recall" phenomenon when given after completion of radiation.

NURSING MANAGEMENT

Assessment

1. Inspect irradiated skin port and exit sites daily, especially high-risk areas (e.g., buttocks, axillae, perineum, groin, breast folds) for color, scaling, bleeding, drainage, increased temperature.
2. Assess skin for tenderness, itching.
3. Measure area of lesion.
4. Inspect drainage from lesion daily for color, odor, amount, consistency.
5. Obtain history of radiation therapy (area irradiated, dosage of radiation therapy, duration of therapy, type of equipment).
6. Obtain history of chemotherapy with Adriamycin.
7. Determine nutritional and fluid status.
8. Evaluate patient's routine skin care practices.
9. Inspect thoroughly the skin of patients receiving superficial or bolus treatment.

Nursing Interventions

1. Employ hygienic measures to protect patient from infections (e.g., good handwashing, disposal of used materials).
2. Cleanse area with saline and water.
3. Pat skin dry or blow dry with hairdryer at cool setting.
4. Expose area to air as much as possible.
5. Perform measures to prevent irritation (see also Patient Teaching, Level 1).

6. For dry desquamation:
   - apply dressings as ordered.
   - wrap dressing with gauze to eliminate tape.
   - never tape over treated area.
   - cornstarch may be applied to decrease itching and friction.
7. For moist desquamation:
   - use wet dressings of saline, water, Domeboro solution (aluminum sulfate and calcium acetate), or half-strength hydrogen peroxide solution soaks.
   - administer analgesics as ordered.
   - use topical Aquaphor or aqueous lanolin as ordered by radiation oncologist.
   - apply nonadherent dressing over area if covered by clothing.
   - rinse area with half-strength hydrogen peroxide 1 to 2 times a day as ordered.
   - avoid indiscriminate use of other ointments or solutions, which may be contraindicated.

Patient Teaching

1. Teach signs and symptoms of skin changes, indicating those that should be reported to health care team (e.g., pain, bleeding).
2. Discuss rationale and usual course of dry desquamation caused by radiation therapy:
   - identify that the epidermis divides at a rapid rate to replace the easily shed cornified layer of squamous cells.

- identify that intermediate doses of radiation will kill some but not all basal cells.
- identify that dry desquamation occurs when surviving cells replace damaged cells before the skin begins to peel 3 to 4 weeks into treatment. Thus the dermis is not exposed.
- identify that dry desquamation also occurs as a result of destruction of sebaceous (oil-secreting) glands in the treatment area.
- identify that radiation affects enzyme that produces melanin and that cells may become dark and almost black before they peel.
- identify that change in color is passed to new cells that retain it until they are shed (skin may continue to peel after treatment ends and will heal in approximately 2 weeks).
3. Discuss rationale and usual course of wet desquamation:
- identify that large dosages of radiation (such as those used in treating skin cancer) kill the entire basal layer.
- identify that for 3 to 4 weeks there are no new cells to replace the cells that existed at start of treatment and are being shed. This causes the dermis to be exposed and serum to ooze from the surface.
4. Explain treatments and prescribed procedures.
5. Describe hygienic measures to prevent contamination (e.g., good handwashing, waste disposal, perineal and perirectal cleansing).
6. Inform patient of signs and symptoms of infection (e.g., temperature elevation, purulent drainage).
7. Teach rationale and measures to maintain hydration and nutritional status.
8. Instruct patient to avoid activities and clothing that may increase irritation (e.g., shaving hair on skin, deodorants, perfumes, tight clothing, exposure to sunlight, strenuous activity).

LEVEL 3: Severe—Permanent Skin Changes

EXPECTED OUTCOME

1. Patient demonstrates knowledge related to permanent skin changes:
- identifies that new skin will always be thinner than normal skin.
- states that new skin will recover poorly from trauma.
2. Patient demonstrates knowledge of measures to manage permanent skin changes:
- identifies measures to protect skin from injury.
- states methods to prevent infection.
- describes balanced diet.
3. Patient demonstrates healing and control of impaired skin integrity:
- absence of infection.
- decrease in drainage.
- reduction or stabilization of impaired skin integrity.

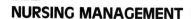

NURSING MANAGEMENT

Assessment

1. See Assessment, Levels 1 and 2.
2. Monitor for skin recovery and development of fibrosis.

Nursing Interventions

1. See Nursing Interventions, Level 2.
2. Protect skin from injury as it heals.
3. Administer analgesics as indicated.
4. Never refer to the skin reaction as a "radiation burn" as this may be suggestive of error.

Patient Teaching

1. See Patient Teaching, Levels 1 and 2.
2. Discuss rationale for permanent skin changes:
   - if reaction has been intense, dermal circulation may not recover and progressive fibrosis may develop.
   - identify that telangiectasia, slow healing, and necrosis are clinical manifestations of permanent vascular insufficiency.
   - even without an intense reaction there are permanent skin changes:
     - the new skin that develops has an epidermis that is thin and pink and will never achieve normal thickness.
     - the thinner epithelium recovers poorly from any trauma.

   - megavoltage radiation, while sparing the skin surface, can cause dermal and subcutaneous tissue reactions leading to normal-feeling skin with underlying fibrosis (common in lower abdominal wall, upper cervical and paramandibular areas, and in obese patients).
   - impairment of lymphatic drainage in the treatment field may occur to cause fibrosis of lymph glands, and lymphedema may occur.
3. Explain measures to prevent infection.
4. Discuss comfort measures.
5. Describe rationale for and measures to maintain hydration and nutritional status.
6. Explain measures to protect the skin from injury (e.g., avoidance of sun, chemicals, trauma).

SUGGESTED READINGS

Chahbazian, C.: The Skin. *In* Moss, W.T., and Cox, J. (Eds.): Radiation Oncology: Rationale, Technique, Results (6th Ed). St. Louis, C.V. Mosby, 1989, pp. 83–111.

Hassey, K., and Rose, C.: Altered skin integrity in patients receiving radiation therapy. Oncology Nursing Forum *9*(4):44–50, 1982.

Hilderley, L.: Skin care in radiation therapy: A review of the literature. Oncology Nursing Forum *10*(1):51–56, 1983.

Strohl, R.: The nursing role in radiation oncology: Symptom management of acute and chronic reactions. Oncology Nursing Forum *15*(4):429–434, 1988.

Yasko, J.: Care of the Client Receiving External Radiation Therapy. Reston, VA, Reston Publishing, 1982.

Mucous Membrane Integrity, Impairment of, Related to Stomatitis

Michelle Goodman and Carol Stoner

Population at Risk

- Individuals receiving chemotherapy that has mucous membrane toxicity (e.g., methotrexate, 5-fluorouracil, doxorubicin, bleomycin, dactinomycin, daunorubicin, vinblastine, and concurrent leucovorin and 5-fluorouracil
- Bone marrow transplant patients
- Individuals who have had radiation or who are having radiation to the head and neck area concurrent with stomatotoxic chemotherapy
- Pediatric and elderly individuals
- Individuals who are immunosuppressed
- Individuals who are nutritionally depleted
- Individuals with prolonged intubation
- Individuals with dental caries, gingival disease, xerostomia, and who have a history of persistent use of alcohol and tobacco including chewing tobacco
- Individuals with reduced metabolism/excretion of stomatotoxic drugs (impaired renal/hepatic function) or those experiencing third spacing of fluids (ascitic fluids, pleural effusions) that also prolong plasma drug levels

LEVEL 1: Potential

EXPECTED OUTCOME

1. Patient exhibits oral cavity, gums, lips free of irritation or ulceration, as evidenced by:
   - pink, moist mucosa and tongue.
   - moist, soft lips with undisrupted integrity.
   - pink and firm gingiva.
   - clean teeth with no debris.
   - watery saliva.
   - no complaints of oral burning or pain.
2. Patient demonstrates knowledge related to oral hygiene regimen:
   - performs necessary treatments and procedures.
   - identifies signs and symptoms to report to health care team.

NURSING MANAGEMENT

Assessment

1. Assess history of alcohol use, tobacco use, or other risk factors.
2. Obtain history of radiation therapy and current treatment with chemotherapy.
3. Check for oral burning, pain—change in tolerance to temperature extremes of food, change in tolerance to acidic or highly seasoned food.
4. Ascertain usual regimen for oral hygiene.
5. Evaluate oral cavity with tongue blade and light, noting color, moisture, and presence of lesions on:
   - palate.
   - gingivae.
   - dorsum of tongue.
   - inner surface of lips.
   - undersurface of tongue.
   - floor of mouth.
   - buccal mucosa.
   - oral pharynx.
6. Note color, amount, and consistency of saliva.
7. Evaluate teeth, noting if teeth are clean and free of debris.
8. Evaluate need for dental consult.

Nursing Intervention

1. Encourage prophylactic oral hygiene regimen after meals and at bedtime:
   - choice of mouthwash depends on patient preference. Avoid mouthwashes with high alcohol content.
   - patient should floss q24h with unwaxed dental floss.
   - patient should brush with soft toothbrush and nonabrasive fluoride toothpaste after meals and at bedtime.
   - remove dentures or bridge, cleanse, and replace after oral hygiene regimen.
2. Consult dentist and oral hygienist for assessment and intervention if indicated:
   - fluoride treatments are encouraged in patients receiving concurrent radiation and stomatotoxic drugs and with xerostomia.
   - xerostomia-associated caries require daily fluoride application and diet modification.
   - sucrose-sweetened foods and candies are to be avoided.
   - a neutral pH 1 per cent sodium fluoride gel is effective when applied at least once daily after brushing. The patient loads the gel into guards and places them on the upper and lower teeth for 5 minutes. The patient should not rinse, eat or drink for at least one-half hour after fluoride application.
   - removal of carious teeth may be indicated with high-risk patients before beginning therapy.
   - frequent (every 3 to 6 months) teeth cleaning and plaque removal are encouraged.
3. If patient has oral carcinoma or thick tenacious mucus, oral hygiene should include an oxidizing agent:
   - hydrogen peroxide one-fourth strength with normal saline—swish, gargle, expectorate.
   - sodium bicarbonate solution (e.g., 1 tsp in 8 oz water)—swish, gargle, expectorate (hydrogen peroxide and sodium bicarbonate may have an unpleasant taste for some patients but are good agents for mechanical debridement. Flavor with mouthwash or oil of wintergreen).
   - rinse oral cavity with warm water or saline.
   - remove mucus with a swab if necessary.
4. Patient at risk for aspiration should lean over sink or basin and use a gavage bag or oral irrigator to irrigate oral cavity. Have suction available.
5. May use lip lubricant (e.g., medicated lip ointment, water-soluble lubricating jelly, lanolin).
6. Assess need for prophylactic use of oral antifungal or antibacterial agents and request physician order if indicated.

- prophylactic nystatin oral suspension mouth rinses help prevent colonization of *Candida*. The patient swishes with 300,000 U of oral suspension for at least 2 minutes qid. If pharyngitis or any sign of gastrointestinal candidiasis is present, or if systemic antibiotics are used, the nystatin should be swallowed. The addition of dyclonine hydrochloride (5 ml 0.5 per cent solution) to 15 ml of the nystatin suspension decreases sting associated with nystatin.
7. Patients who receive leucovorin and 5-fluorouracil may experience less mucositis if ice chips are used to constrict blood vessels of oral cavity before, during, and after leucovorin and 5-fluorouracil administration (not recommended for patients with head and neck cancer).
8. Prophylactic chlorhexidine mouth rinse (Peridex)–swish, gargle (15 ml), expectorate—q8h; may be useful to minimize mucositis in high-risk (bone marrow transplant) patients; do not swallow. The therapeutic effects of chlorhexidine are related to its sustained antimicrobial properties.
9. If leucovorin is being given to minimize toxicity of methotrexate, provide written and oral instruction for administration and schedule patient for serum methotrexate level, if appropriate, to ensure compliance.

Patient Teaching

1. Teach rationale for preventive oral hygiene regimen.
2. Encourage daily oral examination.
3. Explain proper oral hygiene regimen.
4. Discuss signs and symptoms to report to health care team:
   - oral burning or pain.
   - red areas in oral cavity.
   - open lesions in oral cavity or on lips.
5. Teach patient rationale and schedule of administration of leucovorin when given to minimize toxicity of methotrexate:
   - send patient home with written schedule of when to take leucovorin.
   - send patient with all leucovorin needed.
   - inform/instruct family member to remind patient to take leucovorin as directed.
   - instruct patient to set alarm clock to ensure taking leucovorin on schedule.
6. Describe appropriate food and fluid intake.
7. Recommend dental evaluation.
8. Discourage use of tobacco of any kind including chewing tobacco.

LEVEL 2: Mild to Moderate—Grade I (Generalized Erythema of Oral Mucosa) and Grade II (Isolated Small Ulcerations/White Patches)

EXPECTED OUTCOME

1. Patient exhibits healing of oral mucosa within 5 to 7 days:
   - pink moist mucosa.
   - absence of inflammation or ulcerations.
   - moist, soft lips with integrity intact.
   - no complaints of oral burning or pain.
2. Patient remains free from progression and complications as evidenced by:
   - absence of confluent ulcerations.
   - absence of superimposed infection.
   - maintenance of adequate oral intake.

3. Patient experiences relief of oral pain, as evidenced by:
   - verbalization of comfort.
   - adequate oral intake.
4. Patient demonstrates knowledge related to oral hygiene regimen:
   - performs necessary treatments and procedures.
   - identifies signs and symptoms to report to health care team.
   - demonstrates proper knowledge and administration of medications.

NURSING MANAGEMENT

Assessment

1. See Assessment, Level 1.
2. Describe:
   - size and location of lesions.
   - degree of inflammation.
   - type of lesions.
   - presence of ulcerations, size and location.
3. Evaluate food and fluid intake.

Nursing Interventions

1. See Nursing intervention, Level 1.
2. Implement oral hygiene regimen q2h while awake and q6h during night:
   - if crusts are not present, use normal saline mouth wash.
   - if crusts and debris are present, use oxidizing agent q4h:
     - hydrogen peroxide one-fourth strength (swish and rinse with saline).
     - sodium bicarbonate solution (1 tsp in 8 oz water)—swish and rinse with saline.
     - warm saline mouth wash q2h to be alternated with either method previously described.
   - brush with soft-bristled brush, use non-abrasive fluoride toothpaste.
   - floss if bleeding does not occur.
   - rinse with saline.
   - remove dentures or bridge during procedure. Do not replace except for meals. Clean dentures or bridge after each use before storing.

3. Advise patient to use lip lubricant as needed (e.g., medical lip ointment, water-soluble lubricating jelly, lanolin).
4. Assess need for prophylactic use of oral antifungal or antibacterial agents and request physician order if indicated after culture of oral mucosa.
5. Use mild analgesic q3–4h. Suggested alternatives for oral pain include:
   - lidocaine HCl 2 per cent or 5 per cent orally (swish q2h and before meals). Swallow if throat is sore and erythematous. NOTE: If patient swallows lidocaine HCl, local anesthesia occurs, thus decreasing and obscuring gag reflex, increasing risk of aspiration).
   - Cetacaine spray and dyclonine HCl (0.5 per cent or 1 per cent) are useful but may dull gag reflex.
   - application of Orabase emollient or Gly-oxide for local pain control.
   - Zilactin—hydroxypropyl cellulose-based topical medication forms occlusive film over mucosal ulcerations.
   - "stomatitis cocktail" (mixture of equal parts lidocaine HCl, diphenhydramine HCl [12.5 mg/ml], Maalox. Using 1 oz of mixture, swish and swallow q2-4h, prn. NOTE: May cause decreased or absent gag reflex).
   - if xerostomia is not present, 50 per cent Kaopectate (kaolin 90 gm, pectin 2 gm/oz), 50 per cent Benadryl (diphenhydramine HCl) elixir (12.5 mg/5 ml) is an effective oral rinse. Swish and expectorate (q2-4h).
   - if xerostomia is present, use 50 per cent, Milk of Magnesia, Maalox, or Riopan,

and 50 per cent Benadryl (diphenhydramine HCl) elixir (12.4 mg/5 ml). Swish and expectorate (q2–4h).

- oral lubricants or "artificial saliva" (Xero-Lube, Oralube, Salivart, Moi-Ster) may be useful for patients experiencing xerostomia.
- nonsteroidal prostaglandin inhibitors such as ibuprofen (Motrin, Advil, Nuprin) and zamepirac (Zomax) with reversible decrease platelet aggregation for several hours, may be tried sparingly before advancing to narcotic analgesics that may cause nausea and vomiting.
- avoid platelet toxic analgesics with aspirin.

6. Provide appropriate nutritional and fluid intake:
   - avoid citrus fruit juices and spicy foods.

- avoid extremes in food temperatures.
- avoid crusty or rough foods.
- encourage bland foods, finger foods high in protein.

7. Arrange consultation with dietitian.

Patient Teaching

1. See Patient Teaching, Level 1.
2. Outline measures to control pain.
3. Explain administration and side effects of medication.
4. Emphasize need to eliminate tobacco use.
5. Explain proper oral hygiene as previously noted.
6. Describe appropriate nutritional and fluid components as previously noted.

LEVEL 3: Severe—Grade III (Confluent Ulcerations with White Patches Covering More Than 25 Per Cent of Oral Mucosa) and Grade IV (Hemorrhagic Ulcerations)

EXPECTED OUTCOME

1. Patient exhibits healing of severe stomatitis within 10 to 14 days, as evidenced by:
   - resolution of ulcerations.
   - decreased inflammation.
   - absence of infection.
2. Patient/caregiver demonstrate knowledge related to oral hygiene regimen:
   - perform necessary treatment and procedures.
   - demonstrate proper administration of medications.
   - maintain adequate hydration.

NURSING MANAGEMENT

Assessment

1. See Assessment, Levels 1 and 2.
2. Evaluate for infection:
   - *gingivae*-examine oral cavity for any evidence of acute necrotizing ulcerative gingivitis (ANUG). ANUG usually presents as an acute liquefaction necrosis of the interdental papillary gingiva. Spontaneous bleeding may occur.
   - *pericoronitis*-infection originating around a tooth or operculum. Area is

usually tender on palpation, inflamed and erythematous.

- odontogenic infection may present as tooth pain/fever of unknown origin.
- mucosal infections may be bacterial, fungal, or viral in origin.
- bacterial infections may present as fever and ulcerations with deep yellow core that is an ideal nidus for infection. Pseudomonas lesions are necrotizing and enclosed by a reddened halo.
- fungal infections such as *Candida albicans,* Mucormycosis, Aspergillus are common opportunistic infections.
- candidiasis (moniliasis) typically presents as white, raised, cheese-like plaques on the tongue or oral mucosa. The base appears raw, red, granular when scraped. This early vegetative phase can progress to deep tissue invasion with spiking fevers and septicemia.
- mucormycosis usually starts with vague sinonasal or dental symptoms but can progress rapidly along blood vessels to infarct large areas of bone and soft tissue.
- viral infections account for approximately 15 per cent of all mucosal infection of the oral cavity:
  ○ herpes simplex gingivitis and mucosal vesicles begin as painful itching in areas around the lips and circumoral region. Fever, anorexia, malaise may be present.
  ○ varicella presents as unilateral vesicular lesion along nerves (trigeminal).
3. Evaluate ability to chew and swallow.
4. Evaluate patient's hydration status.

Nursing Interventions

1. See Nursing Intervention, Level 2.
2. Culture suspicious ulcerations.
3. Institute aggressive and timely systemic antimicrobial therapy as ordered.
4. For oral candidiasis, administer topical medications as ordered:

- nystatin oral suspension, rinse and swallow, 300,000 U 3 to 4 times daily:
- clotrimazole troche 10 mg. Dissolve 1 tablet 5 times daily (use if no xerostomia present);
- Mycolog ointment applied to ulcerated area 2 to 3 times daily.
5. Alternate warm saline mouthwash with antifungal or antibacterial oral suspension q2h during day, and q4h at night.
6. If thick mucus and debris are present, use oxidizing agent q4h (one-fourth strength hydrogen peroxide or sodium bicarbonate solution) followed by saline rinse. (Have suction available.)
7. Gently brush teeth q4h; avoid trauma to gums. If bleeding occurs or if brushing is too painful, use moist cotton tipped applicators, Toothette, or soaked gauze for cleaning.
8. Apply lip lubricant q2h.
9. Remove dentures or bridge; do not replace.
10. For herpes infections apply acyclovir (Zovirax ointment) to lesions as ordered to prevent secondary infection and moist dressings over extraoral lesions to promote healing.
11. For odontogenic infections administer broad-spectrum antibiotics as ordered to control opportunistic and normal flora; prepare patient for tooth extraction if necessary.
12. Employ local pain control measures.
13. Parenteral analgesics may be needed, especially before meals.
14. Provide liquid or pureed diet.
15. With thick, tenacious mucus, consider diluting supplemental feedings and milk products.
16. Prevent dehydration with IV fluids or enteral feedings.
17. Apply wet saline soaks to dry, cracked, and bleeding lips.
18. Topical thrombin solution may be applied with pressure for 30 minutes to bleeding gingival surface.

Patient Teaching

1. See Patient Teaching, Levels 1 and 2.

SUGGESTED READINGS

Borsani, G., and Carl, W.: Oral care for cancer patients. American Journal of Nursing 83:533–536, 1983.

Carl, W.: Oral complications of cancer patients undergoing chemotherapy and radiation therapy. In Higby, D.J. (Ed): Supportive Care in Cancer Therapy. Boston, Martinus Nijhoff, 1983, pp. 147–167.

Carl, W.: Oral manifestations of systemic chemotherapy and their management. Seminars of Surgical Oncology 2:187–199, 1986.

Daeffler, R.: Oral hygiene measures for patients with cancer (part I, II, III). Cancer Nursing 3:347–356, 1980.

Dreizen, S., Bodey, G.P., and Rodriguez, V.: Oral complications of cancer chemotherapy. Postgraduate Medicine 58:57–82, 1975.

Dreizen, S.: Stomatotoxic manifestations of cancer chemotherapy. Journal of Prosthetic Dentistry 40:650–655, 1978.

Dudjak, L.A.: Mouth care for mucositis due to radiation therapy. Cancer Nursing 10(3):131–140, 1987.

Gainey, D., and Dose, A.M.: The use of ice chips to minimize stomatitis in patients receiving 5-fluorouracil plus leucovorin. Oncology Nursing Forum Congress Supplement 16:173, 1989.

Peterson, D.E., Sonis, S.T. (Eds.): Oral complications of cancer chemotherapy. Boston, Martinus Nijhoff, 1983.

Rosenberg, S.W.: Care of the mouth. In Wittes, R.E. (Ed.); Manual of Oncologic Therapeutics. Philadelphia, J.B. Lippincott, 1989, pp. 569–576.

Sonis, S.T.: Oral complications of cancer therapy. In DeVita, V.T., Hellman, S., and Rosenberg, S.A. (Eds.): Cancer Principles and Practice in Oncology, Third Ed., Vol 2. Philadelphia, J.B. Lippincott, 1989, pp. 2144–2152.

Ziga, S.E.: Stomatitis. In Yasko, J.M. (Ed.): Guidelines for Cancer Care: Symptoms Management. Reston, VA, Reston Publishing, 1983, pp. 212–223.

PATIENT EDUCATION MATERIALS AND COMMUNITY RESOURCES

Chemotherapy and You. National Cancer Institute, Office of Cancer Communications, Bethesda, MD 20014, 800-638-6694.

Radiation and You. National Cancer Institute, Office of Cancer Communications, Bethesda, MD 20014, 800-638-6694.

Bruning, N.: Coping with Chemotherapy. New York, Ballantine Books, 1985.

Morra, M., and Potts, E.: Choices: Realistic Alternatives in Cancer Treatment. New York, Avon Books, 1987.

39

Mucous Membrane Integrity, Impairment of, Related to Vaginal Changes

Jane C. Clark

Population at Risk

- Individuals with gynecologic malignancies, diabetes, sexually transmitted diseases
- Individuals being treated with gynecologic surgery, chemotherapy, pelvic radiation, antimicrobial therapy, immunosuppressive therapy, or who have been exposed to diethylstilbestrol (DES)

LEVEL 1: Potential

EXPECTED OUTCOME

1. Patient/significant other demonstrate knowledge of potential impairment of mucous membrane integrity related to vaginal changes:
   - describe personal risk factors for impaired vaginal membrane integrity.
   - list strategies to prevent or minimize risks of impaired vaginal membrane integrity.
   - identify signs and symptoms of impaired vaginal membrane integrity.
2. Patient demonstrates absence of impairment of vaginal mucous membrane.

NURSING MANAGEMENT

Assessment

1. Determine knowledge of patient/significant other with respect to personal risk factors for impaired vaginal membrane integrity.
2. Question patient regarding signs and symptoms of impaired vaginal membrane integrity (e.g., pain, soreness, bleeding, discharge, pruritus, odor, dyspareunia).
3. Inspect vaginal membrane for signs of impaired integrity (e.g., erythema, swelling, ulcerations, plaque, decrease in vaginal size, muscle tone/lubrication, vaginal fibrosis/stenosis).

Patient Teaching

1. Explain specific factors that place the patient at high risk for impaired vaginal membrane integrity (e.g., surgical procedures involving the vagina, pelvic radiation therapy, chemotherapy, immunosup-

pressive or antimicrobial therapy, changes in vaginal pH, exposure to sexually transmitted diseases).
2. Teach patient about preventive health practices to decrease the risks of impaired vaginal membrane integrity:
   * perineal care after each defecation or urination.

* condoms for sexual intercourse.
* cotton-lined underpants.
* avoidance of tight-fitting slacks, jeans, or pantyhose.
3. Discuss signs and symptoms of impaired vaginal membrane integrity that should be reported to health care team (see Assessments).

LEVEL 2: Mild to Moderate

EXPECTED OUTCOME

1. Patient demonstrates knowledge of impairment of mucous membrane integrity related to vaginal changes:
   * describes personal risk factors for impaired vaginal membrane integrity.
   * identifies signs and symptoms of impaired vaginal membrane.
   * lists potential complications of impaired vaginal integrity.
2. Patient identifies/demonstrates health practices to prevent further impairment and promote integrity of vaginal membranes:
   * demonstrates appropriate perineal hygiene measures.
   * performs recommended procedures and treatments.
   * complies with recommended medication regimen.
   * identifies precautions and limitations related to sexual activities, if appropriate.

NURSING MANAGEMENT

Assessment

1. See Assessment, Level 1.
2. Assess effect of impaired vaginal membrane integrity on:
   * self-care activities.
   * comfort level.
   * expression of sexuality.
3. Monitor laboratory results (wet mounts, cultures).

Nursing Interventions

1. Implement strategies to promote comfort and minimize swelling, pruritus, and pain:
   * cool compresses to perineal area.

* sitz baths.
* douches (1T vinegar in 1 qt water).
* wearing cotton panties.
* avoidance of pantyhose, tight slacks, jeans.
2. Apply topical medications as ordered, based on etiology, to promote vaginal membrane integrity:
   * nonspecific vaginitis: sulfonamide creams, douches (1T vinegar in 1 qt water, instill gently).
   * atrophic vaginitis: estrogen creams and suppositories
   * Candida vaginitis: nystatin cream or suppositories, gentian violet.
3. Administer systemic medications as or-

dered to promote vaginal membrane integrity:
- Trichomonas vaginitis: metronidazole (Flagyl) for patient and partner.
- water-soluble lubricant.
- estrogen creams or suppositories per physician order.
- systemic desensitization.

Patient Teaching

1. See Patient Teaching, Level 1.
2. Explain rationale for medication administration techniques, side effects.

3. Describe rationale for length of treatment and treatment of partner if indicated.
4. Discuss strategies to minimize dyspareunia associated with decreased vaginal lubrication:
- use of water-soluble lubricant.
- use of estrogen creams or suppositories per physician order.
- female-on-top position for intercourse.
- systemic desensitization.
5. Describe rationale and measures to manage decreased vaginal size and tone:
- rear entry position or elevation of female hips for intercourse.
- vaginal dilators.
- Kegel exercises.

LEVEL 3: Severe or Chronic

EXPECTED OUTCOME

1. Patient demonstrates knowledge of severe impairment of mucous membrane integrity related to vaginal changes:
- describes personal risk factors for impaired vaginal membrane integrity.
- identifies signs and symptoms of impaired vaginal membrane integrity.
- describes potential complications of impaired vaginal membrane integrity.
- discusses effect of chronic or severely impaired vaginal membrane integrity on personal hygiene, comfort, activities.
2. Patient demonstrates positive coping strategies to promote rehabilitation and adaptation to chronic impaired vaginal membrane integrity.
- engages in self-care activities as possible.
- identifies alternate methods of both giving and receiving sexual pleasure with partner.
- acknowledges need for counseling if appropriate.
3. Patient/caregiver demonstrate health practices to prevent further impairment and promote integrity of vaginal membranes:
- comply with recommended procedures to decrease risk of involvement of anus/urethra.
- comply with recommendations to prevent secondary infection and reinfection.

NURSING MANAGEMENT

Assessment

1. See Assessment, Levels 1 and 2.
2. Assess effect of chronic impaired vaginal membrane integrity on personal hygiene, comfort, activities of daily living, and expression of sexuality.
3. Assess compliance of patient and partner with medical plan of care.
4. Assess need for vaginal dilator (e.g., fibrotic or scarred vaginal tissue).
5. Ascertain need for psychological or sexual counseling.

Nursing Interventions

1. See Nursing Actions, Levels 1 and 2.
2. Encourage expression of frustration, fears, anxieties regarding severity and chronic nature of problem.
3. Encourage compliance with medical plan of care.
4. Encourage patient and partner to communicate feelings regarding effect of chronic nature of impairment on sexual activity.
5. Assist patient in identifying methods for minimizing symptomatology (perineal pads for discharge, sitz baths) to allow for normal activities of daily living.
6. Administer analgesics as needed.

Patient Teaching

1. See Patient Teaching, Levels 1 and 2.
2. Teach practices that decrease risks of secondary infection or reinfection, and minimize trauma:
   - avoidance of scratching.
   - compliance with medical treatment including dosage and duration of medications by patient and partner.
   - use of condoms for sexual intercourse.
   - use of water-soluble lubricants.
   - perineal care after each bowel and bladder movement.
   - general health measures such as diet, rest.
3. Explain rationale and use of vaginal dilator, if appropriate.
4. Describe alternative methods of giving and receiving sexual pleasure.
5. Inform patient of resources available for psychological or sexual counseling.

SUGGESTED READINGS

Anderson, B.L.: Sexual functioning complications in women with gynecologic cancer. Cancer 60:2123–2138, 1987.

Breslin, E: Genital herpes simplex. Sexually Transmitted Diseases 23(4):907–915, 1986.

Grant, M.M., and Davidson, S.B.: Vaginitis. In Frank-Stromborg, M.: Instruments for Clinical Nursing Research. Norwalk, CT, Appleton & Lange, 1988, pp. 401–414.

Handsfield, H.H., Judson, F., and Stone, K.M.: What's new in genital herpes? Patient Care 47–54, December 15, 1987.

Jenkins, B.: Sexual healing after pelvic irradiation. American Journal of Nursing 86(8):920–922, 1986.

Jusenius, K.: Sexuality and gynecologic cancer. Cancer Nursing 4(6):479–484, 1981.

Rubin, D.: Gynecologic cancer: Cervical, vulvar, and vaginal malignancies. RN 56–63, May 1987.

Shell, J.A., and Carter, J.: The gynecological implant patient. Seminars in Oncology Nursing 3(1):54–66, 1987.

Yasko, J.M.: Care of the client receiving external radiation therapy. Reston, VA, Reston Publishing, 1982, pp. 199–201.

PATIENT EDUCATION MATERIALS AND COMMUNITY RESOURCES

American Cancer Society: Sexuality and Cancer: For the Woman Who Has Cancer and Her Partner. New York, 1988.

Richards, S., and Hiratzka, S.: Vaginal dilatation post-pelvic irradiation: A patient education tool. Oncology Nursing Forum 13(4):89–91, 1986.

Herpes Resource Center. P.O. Box 13827, Research Triangle Park, NC 27709.

Herpetics Engaged in Living Productively (HELP). Organization for support of persons with Herpes.

40

Sensory/Perceptual Alterations Related to Peripheral Neuropathy

Mary Ogrinc

Population at Risk

- Cancer patients receiving chemotherapeutic agents that alter peripheral nervous system response to sensation (Vinca alkaloids: vincristine and vinblastine, cisplatin, procarbazine)
- Patients with paraneoplastic syndrome, especially in small-cell lung cancer

LEVEL 1: Potential

EXPECTED OUTCOME

1. Patient demonstrates knowledge related to potential sensory/perceptual alteration:
   - identifies causative factors.
   - identifies signs and symptoms of peripheral neuropathy.
   - may not be reversible if caused by cisplatin.

NURSING MANAGEMENT

Assessment

1. Determine chemotherapy protocol, including use of Vinca alkaloids (especially vincristine and cisplatin):
   - dosage.
   - frequency.
   - expected duration of treatment.
2. Obtain baseline information regarding peripheral nervous system:
   - sensory responses.
   - motor activity (especially gait).
   - hearing tests.
   - vision tests.
   - deep tendon reflexes.
   - bowel function.
   - bladder function.
   - sexual function (especially male's ability to have erection).

Patient Teaching

1. Name drugs that can cause peripheral neuropathies.
2. Discuss signs and symptoms of peripheral neuropathies:
   - paresthesia (numbness, tingling in hands and feet).
   - hoarseness (jaw or throat pain; may indicate trigeminal facial nerve pain; occurs 3 to 4 days after large dosage).
   - taste changes.
   - motor weakness:

- gait changes (e.g., foot drop).
- wrist drop.
- loss of fine motor control (e.g., buttoning, tying shoes).
- abdominal (colic-type) pain with or without constipation.
- difficulty urinating.
- inability of males to have erection.
3. Discuss fact that symptoms are usually dose-related:
  - loss of reflexes and minor paresthesia are not indications for discontinuance of drug therapy.
  - some impairment anticipated in most patients.
  - therapy is discontinued only when severe toxicity ensues (jaw pain, constipation, motor weakness).
  - drug dosage may be reduced to permit repeated administration of agent.

LEVEL 2: *Mild to Moderate*

EXPECTED OUTCOME

1. Patient demonstrates knowledge related to sensory/perceptual alteration:
   - identifies causative factors.
   - identifies signs and symptoms of peripheral neuropathy.
   - identifies potential sequelae/complications.
2. Patient/caregiver demonstrate measures to manage sensory/perceptual alteration:
   - demonstrate proper administration of medications.
   - identify signs and symptoms to report to health care team.
   - verbalize/demonstrate appropriate safety measures.
   - identify measures to maintain bowel and bladder function.
   - perform necessary treatments and procedures.
3. Patient achieves sensory/perceptual function within normal limits or with minimal deficit:
   - verbalizes absent or minimal symptoms of peripheral neuropathy.
   - neurologic examination is within normal limits or shows minimal deficit.
   - shows independence in activities of daily living.

NURSING MANAGEMENT

Assessment

1. See Assessment, Level 1.
2. Inspect skin for cuts, burns, abrasions, bruises.
3. Evaluate neurologic status:
   - assess sensory function:
     - inquire if pain is present (continuous or intermittent, usually tingling, cramping, or burning).
     - check pain response (e.g., pin prick).
     - check touch response (e.g., place object in patient's hand, eyes closed; have patient identify object).
     - check sense of vibration (e.g., tuning fork on interphalangeal discs of fingers and toes).
     - assess sensation of other body parts by having patient close eyes while light touch is applied.
     - check position sense.

253

- assess motor function:
  - check Romberg's sign.
  - observe strength, stability, type of gait; check if patient can walk on heels.
  - observe fine motor control (e.g., buttoning and unbuttoning clothes).
  - note voice changes.
- check deep-tendon reflexes; note decrease in response.
4. Note subjective reports of falling.
5. Assess need for assistive devices (e.g., cane, walker, bedside commode, raised toilet seat).

Nursing Interventions

1. If patient presents with signs and symptoms of peripheral neuropathy, withhold chemotherapeutic agent and notify physician.
2. Assist patient as necessary in carrying out activities of daily living.
3. Obtain physical therapy and occupational therapy referrals to assist patient to maintain functioning.

Patient Teaching

1. See Patient Teaching, Level 1.
2. Instruct patient regarding actions to promote safety:

- avoid exposing fingers and toes to extremes in temperature (e.g., use tepid bath water, no heating pads).
- protect feet by wearing foot covering at all times.
- protect hands and feet during inclement weather.
- utilize potholders in kitchen.
- visualize an area before placing hand or foot in area.
- encourage patient to be as active and independent as possible with deficits.
- inspect skin daily for cuts, abrasions, bruises (particularly toes, between toes, fingers, arms, legs).
- use prescribed assistive devices.
- avoid foods that are too hot or too cold.
3. Teach measures to maintain bowel function:
- regularly scheduled use of stool softeners/cathartics (see Chapter 48).
- high-fiber diet.
4. Explain measures to maintain bladder function: fluid intake of 2000 to 3000 ml/day.
5. Discuss potential sequelae/complications (especially alteration in bowel function if constipation is not managed).
6. Tell patient that recovery may be complete or partial, and is slow (months).
7. Provide sexual counseling for diminished ability of males to achieve erection (see Chapter 53).

LEVEL 3: Severe

EXPECTED OUTCOME

1. Patient/caregiver demonstrate knowledge related to severe sensory/perceptual alteration:
   - identify signs and symptoms of severe peripheral neuropathy.
   - identify potential sequelae/complications.
2. Patient/caregiver demonstrate measures to manage, facilitate adaptation to and promote rehabilitation of severe sensory/perceptual alteration:
   - demonstrate proper administration of medications.

- perform necessary treatments and procedures.
- identify signs and symptoms to report to health care team.
- verbalize/demonstrate appropriate home and life style adaptations.
- identify appropriate long-term follow-up care.

3. Patient achieves stable sensory/perceptual function, as evidenced by:
   - improvement and stability in symptoms of peripheral neuropathy.
   - improved neurologic examination.
   - absence of complications related to peripheral neuropathy.

NURSING MANAGEMENT

Assessment

1. See Assessment, Levels 1 and 2.
2. Determine patient's level of functioning, including amount of assistance required.
3. Evaluate bowel function and observe for signs and symptoms of intestinal obstruction.
4. Evaluate any change in self-image.

3. Discuss need to maintain optimal mobility and to comply with rehabilitative program.
4. Instruct regarding safety precautions at home:
   - remove throw rugs.
   - wear sturdy slippers/shoes.
   - remove obstacles from pathways.

Nursing Interventions

1. See Nursing Interventions, Level 2.
2. Implement safety measures:
   - avoidance of extreme heat and cold to toes and fingers.
   - assistance with ambulation as appropriate.
3. Refer to physical therapy and occupational therapy for evaluation and treatment in rehabilitative techniques.
4. Use footboards or other measures to prevent or control foot drop.
5. Maintain good body alignment of the patient.
6. Provide active or passive range of motion exercises as appropriate (including digits).
7. Make home care nursing referral to assist patient with home adaption and safety.

Patient Teaching

1. See Patient Teaching, Levels 1 and 2.
2. Explain use of assistive devices.

SUGGESTED READINGS

Bates, B.: A Guide to Physical Examination (2nd ed). Philadelphia, J.B. Lippincott, 1970.

Deasi, A., Van der Berg, H., Bridges, J., et al.: Can severe vincristine neurotoxicity be prevented? Cancer Chemotherapy and Pharmacology 8:211–214, 1982.

Dorr, R., and Fritz, R.: Cancer Chemotherapy Handbook. New York, Elsevier, 1980.

Goodman, M.: Managing the side effects of chemotherapy. Seminars in Oncology Nursing 5(2 Suppl.1):29–52, 1989.

Groenwald, S.L.: Cancer Nursing: Principles and Practices. Boston, Jones & Bartlett, 1987.

Holden, S., and Felde, G.: Nursing care of patients experiencing cisplatin-related peripheral neuropathy. Oncology Nursing Forum 14(1):12–18, 1987.

Johnson, B., and Gross, J.: Handbook of Oncology Nursing. New York, Wiley Medical Publications, 1985.

Reville, B., and Almadrones, L.: Continuous chemotherapy in the ambulating setting: The nurses's role in patient selection and education. Oncology Nursing Forum 16(4):529–535, 1989.

Rosenthal, S., and Kaufman, S.: Vincristine neurotoxicity. Annals of Internal Medicine 80:733–737, 1974.

Vander, A., Sherman, J., and Luciano, D.: Human Physiology. New York, McGraw-Hill, 1980.

PATIENT EDUCATION MATERIALS AND COMMUNITY RESOURCES

Bass, B.: Utilization of chemotherapy card. Oncology Nursing Forum *12*(6):83, 1986.

U.S. Department of Health and Human Resources literature

Chemotherapy and You

Eating Hints—Recipes and Tips for Better Nutrition During Cancer Treatment

MOBILITY

The nurse assesses the patient's level of mobility and potential for sequelae to formulate actual or potential nursing diagnoses.

Appropriate patient outcomes to consider in planning nursing interventions will specify the patient's ability to:

1. explain the cause of fatigue or immobility, the treatment, and the outcome of the treatment.
2. describe an appropriate management plan to integrate alteration in mobility into patient's life style.
3. describe optimal levels of activities of daily living in keeping with patient's disease state and treatment.
4. identify health services and community resources available for managing changes in mobility.
5. use measures to aid or improve mobility.
6. demonstrate measures to prevent the complications of decreased mobility.

Evaluation of the patient's responses to nursing care is based on whether the patient maintains the optimum mobility level consistent with disease and therapy.

Excerpted from the ANA/ONS Standards of Cancer Nursing Practice

Mobility, Impaired Physical, Related to Disease Process and Treatment

Sr. Karin DuFault, Sharon Cannell Firsich, Anne Gardner, Margaret B. Jones, Jean R. Moseley, Sandra Stone and Mary Jo Pearl

Population at Risk

- Individuals with primary bone tumors (multiple myeloma, osteogenic sarcoma, chondrosarcoma, Ewing's sarcoma, giant cell sarcoma)
- Individuals with metastases to bones
- Individuals with primary CNS malignancies
- Individuals with known cerebral metastasis
- Individuals with primary tumors that frequently metastasize to CNS:
  - primary tumors of lung (especially small cell), breast, prostate, colon
  - melanoma
  - leukemia and lymphomas
  - plasma cell neoplasms
- Individuals having surgical, radiation, or chemotherapeutic treatment with disruptive CNS effects:
  - radiation: head and neck, brain
  - surgery: intracranial surgery (biopsy, decompression, tumor removal, lobectomy)
  - chemotherapy: chemotherapy with L-asparaginase, vincristine, procarbazine, cisplatin, cytosine arabinoside, methotrexate, intrathecal drugs, glucocorticoids (myopathy, osteoporosis)
  - CNS infections secondary to neutropenia, meningitis, brain abscess, shunt infections, encephalitis
  - Individuals with profound fatigue and muscle weakness from high-dose interferon or interleukin-2

LEVEL 1: Potential

EXPECTED OUTCOME

1. Patient verbalizes/demonstrates knowledge related to potential alteration in physical mobility.
   - identifies signs and symptoms of impaired mobility.
   - identifies factors that influence mobility.
   - identifies potential sequelae/complications of impaired mobility.
2. Patient identifies/demonstrates measures to prevent impairment in mobility:
   - demonstrates knowledge of proper administration of medication.
   - performs necessary treatments and procedures.

259

- identifies signs and symptoms necessary to report to health care team.
- identifies/utilizes appropriate community resources.
- verbalizes/demonstrates necessary life style adaptations.
- manipulates environmental factors to minimize joint stress and provide for home safety.
- identifies activities to be avoided.
- demonstrates proper body mechanics.
3. Patient maintains physical mobility as evidenced by:
   - normal range of motion for all joints.
   - independent ambulation.

NURSING MANAGEMENT

Assessment

1. Obtain history of risk factors for impaired mobility including use of steroids, estrogens, high-dose radiation; and history of osteoporosis or arthritis.
2. Obtain history of symptoms of physical mobility problems.
3. Check laboratory values (e.g., CBC, hemoglobin, serum calcium) and x-ray scan reports.
4. Assess for bone pain and pain on movement.
5. Examine motor system:
   - muscle strength (ankles, legs, feet, flexors and extensors of hip).
   - walk on heels, then toes.
   - posture: lying, sitting, standing, walking—degree of erectness.
   - gait.
   - ability to lift feet.
   - length of stride.
   - width of base.
   - eye gaze and visual fields.
   - evenness of walking pace.
   - abnormal movements of legs (involuntary or uncoordinated).
   - tremors.
   - chorea (irregular, involuntary movement, increased tone).
   - athetosis (slow, writhing movement).
   - coordination of legs: knee to ankle while lying (e.g., run heel of one foot down shin of other leg); tandem walk; walk straight line heel to toe.

- equilibrium and balance (e.g., stand upright with feet together, first with eyes open, then with eyes closed).
- ease of mobility: movements of joints, comfort of joints with movement and rest, joint deformity or swelling, degree of range of motion of each joint.
6. Examine sensory status:
   - proprioception.
   - kinesthetic sense (touch).
   - vibration.
   - pain.
   - temperature.
7. Assess function of cranial nerve XI (spinal accessory):
   - ability to flex head against resistance and turn head from side to side (sternocleidomastoid function).
   - ability to elevate shoulders (trapezius muscle function).
8. Examine mobility patterns:
   - interest in mobility.
   - preferred activities.
   - medications affecting mobility.
   - walking distance without discomfort:
     ○ usual amount each day.
     ○ number of stairs without discomfort.
     ○ assistive devices needed.
   - ability to change position.
   - participation in activities of daily living.
   - ability to leave environment and travel elsewhere.
   - perceived mobility and activeness.

9. Assess environmental facilitators to mobility:
   - handrails.
   - height, design of chairs, furnishings.
   - lighting.
   - space.
   - elevated seats, commodes, bathing aids, "no skid" treads.
   - clear, wide passageway.
   - location of supportive devices.
10. Assess environmental barriers to activity (e.g., coping styles; support systems; patient's outlook regarding present health, therapy, and prognosis; patient's ability to ask for help with activities of daily living; social activities; reactions of significant others; financial situation).

Patient Teaching

1. Note importance of mobility and ways to increase mobility, include information on minimizing calcium loss.
2. Outline measures to improve posture.
3. Teach active range-of-motion exercises.

4. Describe proper positioning in normal anatomic position.
5. Discuss proper body mechanics for lifting and activities of daily living.
6. Discuss potential obstacles to mobility:
   - loose rugs and free edges of carpets, highly polished floors.
   - spills on floor.
   - extension cords in highly traveled areas.
   - improperly fitting clothes or shoes.
   - inadequate physical setting (e.g., shower too small to hold shower chair).
7. Teach patient/family signs and symptoms of impaired mobility, pain, and fatigue to report to health care team.
8. Discuss administration, effects, and side effects of current medication.
9. Discuss importance of balanced diet including foods high in protein and calcium.
10. Teach administration of pain medication before exercises and movement as needed.

LEVEL 2: Moderate

EXPECTED OUTCOME

1. Patient demonstrates/verbalizes knowledge related to impaired physical mobility:
   - verbalizes signs and symptoms of impaired mobility.
   - identifies factors that influence mobility.
   - identifies potential complications.
   - identifies relationship between psychological status and physical mobility.
   - identifies safety precautions.
   - identifies activities to avoid.
   - verbalizes signs and symptoms to report to health care team.
2. Patient identifies/demonstrates measures to promote mobility:
   - performs activities of daily living with approved adaptive devices.
   - makes environmental adaptations to provide safety.
   - identifies ways to conserve energy/prevent fatigue.
   - demonstrates ability to cope with limitations.
   - avoids activities that could increase immobility.

- performs necessary exercises and treatments.
- demonstrates proper knowledge and administration of pain medication.
3. Patient achieves optimal physical mobility:
    - manages activities of daily living with assistance.
    - transfers made independently or with assistance.

NURSING MANAGEMENT

Assessment

1. See Assessment, Level 1.
2. Assess and classify changes in patient's level of mobility:
    - mobile with use of equipment or device.
    - mobile with help of another person.
    - mobile with help from equipment and another person.
    - dependent and does not participate in mobility.
3. Monitor results of diagnostic testing (e.g., computed tomography scan, electroencephalogram, angiography, air studies, brain scan, spinal tap). Assess respiratory, and cardiac status.
4. Assess pain (e.g., intensity, duration, precipitating factors, relief measures, location). Check immobilized area for edema and circulation deficit, effect of movement.
5. Assess performance status using Karnofsky scale. Determine muscle strength in extremities; observe gait and difficulty ambulating.
6. Note psychological and behavioral response to immobility.

Nursing Interventions

1. Implement activities that facilitate mobility:
    - open, adequately illuminated spaces.
    - side-rails.
    - solid supports for grasping where needed.
    - nonslip rubber mats or adhesive strips in bathtub.
    - bath or shower chair.
    - furniture designed for ease in sitting and standing.
    - low-heeled, well-fitted shoes in good repair.
2. Maintain environmentally beneficial atmosphere (e.g., bed placement close to supportive devices, clear passageways).
3. Encourage patient to maintain optimal physical activity (e.g., encouragement of activities of daily living, self-care, use of supportive devices, exercise to maintain muscle strength, and balance of rest and activity). Assist patient to cough and breathe deeply.
4. Develop diet plan with patient to ensure adequate food and fluid intake to maintain muscle strength and provide energy for physical activities.
5. Promote comfort (e.g., premedicate before painful activities, use assistive or supportive devices, position for comfort, use air or water mattress, sheepskins as indicated).
6. Promote self-esteem (e.g., usual hygiene, shaving, use of own clothes, feeding self, makeup).
7. Assist with anticipatory or actual grieving related to losses or altered body image.
8. Encourage patient to maintain muscle strength and joint mobility (e.g., active and passive range-of-motion exercise against resistance, upright position, standing use of supportive or assistive devices).
9. Refer to physical therapy and occupational therapy for evaluation and treatment of deficit in mobility.
10. Refer to appropriate support group, social service, pastoral care.

11. Work with employer to keep patient working fulltime or part-time if possible.
12. Refer to vocational rehabilitation services, as appropriate.

Patient Teaching

1. See Patient Teaching, Level 1.
2. Discuss change in safety needs (e.g., recognition of unsafe environment and corrective actions to take).
3. Outline measures to maintain optimal mobility. Discuss use of assistive or supportive devices, teach transfer techniques, instruct regarding active and passive range-of-motion exercises.
4. Teach signs and symptoms to report to health care team (e.g., increasing difficulties with activities of daily living, headaches, nausea and vomiting, blurred vision, weakness, numbness and tingling, forgetfulness, onset of or increase in pain, respiratory changes, changes in limb mobility).
5. Explore relaxation techniques.
6. Describe medications (e.g., name, purpose, dosage, side effects, administration). Explain use of pain medication.
7. Educate regarding safe and adequate food and fluid intake.
8. Explain methods to promote open communication.
9. Help family members to recognize psychologic changes that may occur with decreased physical mobility (e.g., depression related to losses, anger, denial); coping strategies for behavior changes; family role in promoting optimal mobility.
10. Explain effectiveness of treatment of bone metastasis with radiation, chemotherapy, and hormonal therapy.

LEVEL 3: Severe Motor Weakness (Increased Dependence in Activities of Daily Living, Decreased Level of Consciousness, Behavioral Changes)

EXPECTED OUTCOME

1. Patient/caregiver verbalize/demonstrate knowledge related to severe impairment in mobility:
   - identify signs and symptoms of impaired mobility.
   - identify factors that influence mobility.
   - identify potential sequelae/complications of impaired mobility.
   - identify signs and symptoms to report to health care team.
   - identify rationale and schedule for pain medication administration.
2. Patient/caregiver demonstrate measures to manage impairment in mobility:
   - demonstrate proper knowledge and administration of medications.
   - perform necessary treatment and procedures.
   - report signs and symptoms of complications to health care team.
   - identify/utilize appropriate community resources.
   - verbalize/demonstrate necessary life style adaptations.
   - manipulate environment to provide for home safety.
   - seek assistance for activities that are beyond patient's capabilities or that aggravate condition.

- use proper positioning and transfer techniques.
- verbalize/demonstrate adequate food and fluid intake.

3. Patient/caregiver demonstrate behaviors to minimize or manage complications of impairment in mobility:
   - demonstrate measures to prevent or manage skin breakdown.
   - demonstrate measures to prevent or manage respiratory dysfunction.
   - demonstrate manipulation of environment to provide adequate sensory stimulation.
   - demonstrate measures to maintain bowel and bladder function.
   - demonstrate measures to promote adequate circulation to tissues.
   - verbalize control of pain.
   - exhibit adequate hydration and electrolyte balance.

4. Patient achieves or maintains optimal mobility consistent with advanced disease process, as evidenced by:
   - transfers made with assistance.

5. Patient/caregiver demonstrate optimal coping abilities:
   - identify methods to manage stress.
   - verbalize/demonstrate minimal frustration.
   - maintenance of health in family members.
   - maintenance of community support systems.

NURSING MANAGEMENT

Assessment

1. See Assessment, Levels 1 and 2.
2. Determine strengths and stressors of support system.
3. Evaluate immobilized area for pain or edema/circulation deficit.
4. Evaluate need for assistive devices (e.g., cane, walker, wheelchair, bath or shower chair, Hoyer lift, van with hand controls).
5. Assess complications of immobility (e.g., signs and symptoms of thrombophlebitis, pneumonia or atelectasis, constipation or gastrointestinal obstruction, urinary tract infection, skin breakdown, muscle and joint fibrosis, contracture).
6. Assess for signs and symptoms of hypercalcemia; check serum calcium level, change in mental status, increased lethargy.

Nursing Interventions

1. See Nursing Actions, Level 2.
2. Take appropriate nursing measures to prevent complications of immobility.
3. Assist patient to set own priorities about activities.
4. Use assistive transfer techniques.
5. Obtain referral to appropriate health professionals, especially occupational therapist, physical therapist, social worker, and therapeutic recreationist.
6. Eliminate environmental hazards.
7. Consult with speech pathologist for severe communication problems.
8. Supervise medication regimen as necessary.
9. Help family recognize and deal with disruption of roles.

10. Review personal and environmental safety measures with patient/caregiver:
    - immobilize affected extremity or site with sling, splint, belt, as ordered.
11. Prepare family for need to supervise patient's activities closely.
12. Assist family/patient with continuing grief.
13. Help family learn ways of coping with behavioral changes.
14. Give patient/family clearly written instructions.

Patient Teaching

1. See Patient Teaching, Levels 1 and 2.
2. Teach patient/caregiver preventive measures for complications of immobility.
3. Discuss energy conservation and self-pacing techniques.
4. Inform patient/caregiver about available community resources.
5. Explain transfer techniques and assistive devices as needed.
6. Describe methods of dealing with specific problems such as incontinence (e.g., positioning, turning methods, administration of pain medication).
7. Teach caregiver to observe and report changes in coordination and gait.
8. State how to eliminate environmental hazards.
9. Present patient with one concept at a time, verifying cognition by asking for demonstration.
10. Instruct patient/caregiver to report severe or progressively worsening headaches to physician.
11. Teach patient/caregiver signs and symptoms to report to health care team: changes in mentation, severe or progressively worsening headache or other pain, signs and symptoms of hypercalcemia.
12. Teach patient/caregiver to recognize symptoms of impending seizure (e.g., aura).
13. Explain how to manage seizures, if appropriate.
14. Reinforce need to take medications as prescribed.
15. Explain rationale and measures to maintain hydration and nutritional status.
16. Discuss respite care with family.
17. Teach caregiver to refocus patient's attention to stop behavioral outburst, if necessary.

SUGGESTED READINGS

Ahena, D.N.: Cancer Care Protocols for Hospital and Home Care Use. New York, Springer, 1981.

Aspinall, M.J., and Tanner, C.A.: Decision-Making for Patient Care—Applying the Nursing Process. New York, Appleton-Century-Crofts, 1981.

Bouchard-Kurtz, E., and Speese-Owens, N.: Nursing Care of the Cancer Patient. St. Louis, C.V. Mosby, 1981.

Burns, N.: Nursing and Cancer. Philadelphia, W.B. Saunders. 1982.

Carnevali, D., and Breuckmer, S.: Immobilization: Reassessment of a concept. American Journal of Nursing 70:1502–1507, 1970.

Cox, J.D., Komake, R., and Eierst, D.R.: Irradiation for inoperable carcinoma of the lung and high performance status. Journal of the American Medical Association 244:1931–1933, 1980.

Creason, N.S., Poque, N.J., Nelson, A.A., and Hoyt, C.A.: Validating the nursing diagnosis of impaired mobility. Nursing Clinics of North America 20:669–683, 1985.

Gehrke, M.: Identifying brain tumors. Journal of Neurosurgical Nursing 12:203–205, 1980.

Gordon, M.: Manual of Nursing Diagnosis. New York, McGraw-Hill, 1982.

Lengel, N.L.: Handbook of Nursing Diagnosis. Bowie, MD, Robert J. Brady, 1982.

Lenox, A.C.: When motor nerves die. American Journal of Nursing 83:540–546, 1983.

Martin, N., Holt, N.B., and Hicks, D.: Comprehensive Rehabilitation Nursing. New York, McGraw-Hill, 1980.

Milde, F.K.: Impaired physical mobility. Journal of Gerontological Nursing 14(3):20–24;38–40, 1988.

Mitchell, P.M., and Loustau, A.: Concepts Basic to Nursing. New York, McGraw-Hill, 1981.

Murray, R.B., Huelskoetter, M.N., and O'Driscoll, D.L.: Nursing Process in Later Maturity. Englewood Cliffs, NJ, Prentice-Hall, 1980.

Ryan, L.S.: Nursing assessment of the ambulatory patient with brain metastases. Cancer Nursing 4:281–291, 1981.

Simpson, J.F., and Magie, K.R.: Clinical Evaluation of the Nervous System. Boston, Little, Brown & Co., 1970.

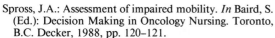

Spross, J.A.: Assessment of impaired mobility. *In* Baird, S. (Ed.): Decision Making in Oncology Nursing. Toronto, B.C. Decker, 1988, pp. 120–121.

Taylor, J.W., and Ballinger, S.: Neurological Dysfunctions and Nursing Intervention. New York, McGraw-Hill, 1980.

Walleck, C.A.: A neurologic assessment procedure that won't make you nervous. Nursing *12:*50–58, 1982.

Wilson, C.V., Fulton, D.S., and Seager, M.L.: Supportive management of the patient with malignant brain tumor. Journal of the American Medical Association *244:*1249–1251, 1980.

Yurick, A.G., Robb, S.F., Spier, B.E., et al.: A Primer of Brain Tumors. Chicago, IL, Association for Brain Tumor Research, 1980.

PATIENT EDUCATION MATERIALS AND COMMUNITY RESOURCES

Association for Brain Tumor Research, 3725 N. Talman Avenue, Chicago, IL 60618, ph. 312-286-5571.

Contact the rehabilitation department of your local hospital.

Mobility, Impaired Physical, Related to Spinal Cord Compression

Pamela Gentzsch

42

Population at Risk

- Individuals with primary or metastatic spinal tumors
- Individuals with lymphoma, multiple myeloma, and primary malignancies of breast, lung, kidney, gastrointestinal tract, thyroid (at high risk for vertebral metastasis and cord compression)
- Individuals with benign bone and neural tumors (e.g., neuroma, ependymoma, meningioma, hemangioma)

LEVEL 1: Potential

EXPECTED OUTCOME

1. Patient demonstrates knowledge related to potential impairment in mobility:
   - verbalizes signs and symptoms of spinal cord compression to report to health care team.
   - identifies risk factors.
2. Patient maintains current level of mobility:
   - absence of neurologic defects.
   - ability to perform activities of daily living independently.

NURSING MANAGEMENT

Assessment

1. Examine patient's risk factors.
2. Assess mobility status (gait, coordination, range of motion).
3. Assess ability to perform activities of daily living.
4. Determine neurologic status (sensation in extremities, deep tendon reflexes).
5. Assess bowel function (do baseline abdominal examination including listening for bowel sounds).
6. Assess bladder function.
7. Assess sexual function.
8. Observe for evidence of back pain (usually a presenting symptom; pain is present over involved vertebrae and may be radicular in nature).

Patient Teaching

1. Teach relationship between cancer and impaired mobility related to spinal cord compression.

2. Teach need to observe and report early symptoms:
   - altered gait.
   - sensory loss (decreased sensation, numbness, paresthesia, increased feeling of cold).
   - motor loss (weakness and paraplegia).
   - changes in bowel, bladder, sexual function.
   - back pain.
   - teach need to obtain medical intervention before onset of paralysis for favorable prognosis (retention of ambulation).

LEVEL 2: Mild to Moderate

EXPECTED OUTCOME

1. Patient demonstrates knowledge related to impairment in mobility:
   - verbalizes degree of impairment.
   - identifies factors that influence maintenance or disruption in mobility.
   - identifies potential sequelae/complications.
2. Patient demonstrates measures to maintain optimal mobility and prevent complications:
   - performs necessary treatment and procedures.
   - demonstrates necessary life style adaptations.
   - demonstrates proper knowledge and administration of medications.
   - demonstrates safety measures.
   - demonstrates measures to achieve bowel and bladder function.
   - identifies signs and symptoms to report to health care team.
3. Patient achieves or maintains optimal mobility consistent with disease process as evidenced by:
   - mobility sufficient to manage activities of daily living.
   - independent transfers.
   - ambulation with assistance.

NURSING MANAGEMENT

Assessment

1. See Assessment, Level 1.
2. Determine changes in musculoskeletal system:
   - serum calcium abnormalities.
   - sensory paresthesia or loss.
   - fibrotic changes in muscles.
   - motor weakness or dysfunction.
3. Assess for changes in patterns of elimination:
   - constipation.
   - abdominal distention.
   - decreased bowel sounds.
   - decreased urinary output in relationship to oral or IV input.
   - distended bladder.
4. Check for evidence of venous thrombosis resulting from immobilization:
   - redness.
   - warmth.
   - edema (measure both calves daily).
   - red streaking up vein.
   - positive Homans' sign.
5. Assess for changes in sexual function (e.g., impotence); include sexual partner.

6. Identify patient's/significant other's response to psychological issues of impaired mobility.

Nursing Interventions

1. If ordered, immobilize patient.
2. Turn patient q2h by log rolling technique.
3. Maintain extremities in functional position.
4. Use antiembolic stockings as ordered.
5. Provide range-of-motion exercises as ordered.
6. Establish bowel program:
   - schedule use of suppositories, stool softeners, laxatives, bulk products, lubricants.
   - diet high in bulk and fiber.
   - high fluid intake.
7. Implement urinary elimination program:
   - maintain accurate intake and output.
8. Administer prescribed analgesic within prescribed schedule; titrate medication dosage/frequency based on patient's response.
9. Arrange for physical therapy consult for rehabilitation program including conditioning and strengthening plan.
10. Obtain occupational therapy consult for rehabilitation program including use of adaptive equipment and techniques for resumption of independent activities of daily living.
11. If radiation therapy is indicated, provide appropriate care and teaching.
12. If surgery is indicated, provide pre- and postoperative care.
13. Encourage patient/significant other to express feelings and concerns.
14. Obtain consult for counseling, if appropriate.

Patient Teaching

1. See Patient Teaching, Level 1.
2. Teach signs and symptoms of potential complications.
3. Teach and involve family in caregiving.
4. Communicate need to report any evidence of decreased sensation; muscle weakness; bowel, bladder, sexual dysfunction; pain; or decreased ability to perform activities of daily living to health care team.
5. Teach pre- and postoperative procedures.
6. If steroids are prescribed, teach side effects, and risk of abruptly stopping medication.
7. Teach procedures for and side effects of radiation therapy.
8. Teach use of assistive and supportive devices collaboratively with physical therapy and occupational therapy.
9. Explain rationale and measures for appropriate bowel and bladder program.
10. Refer to home health agency for continuation of physical therapy and occupational therapy at home.
11. Refer to appropriate community support group in keeping with disease process/limitations.

LEVEL 3: Severe

EXPECTED OUTCOME

1. Patient/caregiver demonstrate knowledge related to severely impaired mobility:
   - verbalize signs and symptoms to report to health care team.
   - identify factors that influence maintenance or disruption in mobility.
   - identify potential sequelae/complications.

2. Patient/caregiver demonstrate measures to manage impaired mobility and minimize complications:
   - perform necessary treatments and procedures.
   - demonstrate necessary life style adaptations.
   - demonstrate safety measures.
   - demonstrate measures to maintain bowel and bladder function.
   - demonstrate use of assistive devices.
   - verbalize support from community agencies.
   - use alternative methods to express and fulfill sexual needs.
3. Patient demonstrates absence of complications of impaired mobility:
   - respiratory status within normal limits.
   - vital signs within normal limits.
   - skin integrity intact.
4. Patient achieves or maintains optimal mobility consistent with spinal cord compression as evidenced by:
   - mobility sufficient to manage activities of daily living with assistance.
   - proper transfer techniques.
   - improved or stable range of motion.
5. Patient/caregiver demonstrate psychological adaptation to impaired mobility as evidenced by:
   - intact coping mechanism.
   - referrals to appropriate community services.

NURSING MANAGEMENT

Assessment

1. See Assessment, Levels 1 and 2.
2. Determine respiratory status:
   - chest excursion.
   - arterial blood gas.
   - breath sounds.
   - chest x-ray.
   - vital signs.
   - pulmonary function tests.
3. Assess for autonomic hyperreflexia, if cord compression is above T6 level:
   - pounding headache.
   - vasodilation.
   - flushing.
   - profuse sweating.
   - nausea.
   - chest pain.
   - bradycardia.
4. Note and record changes in blood pressure.
5. Examine for evidence of dermal ulcers.
6. Assess nutritional status (e.g., laboratory data, anthropometric measurements).
7. Observe for evidence of spasticity.
8. Determine level of patient's injury in relationship to sexual functioning (sexual functioning is controlled at spinal levels S2, S3, S4; T11 to L2 contain fibers for seminal emission).
9. Determine level of patient's pain and efficacy of prescribed medication.
10. Assess psychological reaction to change in body image.

Nursing Interventions

1. See Nursing Interventions, Level 2.
2. Reposition patient using log rolling technique q2h.
3. Implement measures to improve respiratory function.

4. Implement effective bowel and bladder program.
5. Implement measures to provide skin integrity:
   - massage pressure points every 2 hours.
   - modify bed surface with therapeutic mattress.
   - attach Gelfoam pad to chair when patient is sitting up.
6. Administer muscle relaxants per physician order.
7. Refer to a sexual counselor, if appropriate.
8. Inform patient that sexual experience will probably be altered, if appropriate.
9. Refer for penile implant, if appropriate.
10. Suggest use of tilt table if patient is experiencing autonomic hyperreflexia.
11. Assist with rehabilitative program established by physical and occupational therapy.
12. Assist patient in performing self-care activities.
13. Refer to supportive groups as indicated (e.g., Wellness Community, Make Today Count, I Can Cope).
14. Refer to rehabilitative center, either for outpatient therapy or inpatient care, as appropriate.

Patient Teaching

1. See Patient Teaching, Levels 1 and 2.
2. Discuss rationale and measures to prevent respiratory complications.
3. Describe signs and symptoms of respiratory complications to report.
4. Explain rationale and measures to prevent thrombophlebitis.
5. Outline signs and symptoms of thrombophlebitis to report:
   - pain.
   - erythema.
   - warmth.
   - edema.
6. Teach rationale and measures to prevent orthostatic hypotension:
   - gradual change in position.
   - use of elastic bandages or elastic stockings.
   - use of abdominal binder.
7. Describe rationale and measures to prevent dermal ulcers:
   - change position every 2 hours.
   - need for adequate dietary intake of protein.
   - good hygiene measures.
   - necessity of massage to bony prominences.
8. Explain rationale to prevent or minimize musculoskeletal complications:
   - range-of-motion exercises.
   - proper body alignment.
   - high fluid intake.
   - assistive devices.
9. Teach transfer techniques.
10. Teach use of assistive devices (e.g., overbed trapeze, transfer board, Hoyer lift).
11. State rationale and measures to prevent spasticity:
    - range-of-motion exercises.
    - relationship of triggering mechanism.
    - need for compliance with drug program.
12. Give rationale and measures to prevent neurogenic bladder:
    - high fluid intake.
    - catheter care.
    - techniques of catheterization.
13. Encourage compliance with bladder and bowel program.
14. Explain rationale and measures to prevent constipation.
15. Discuss relationship between spinal cord injury and sexual functioning.
16. Discuss rationale for appropriate pain medication program.
17. Discuss rationale for appropriate community referrals.
18. Discuss coping mechanisms and alteration in body image and family life style.

Mobility, Impaired Physical, Related to Spinal Cord Compression

SUGGESTED READINGS

Adams, R.: Principles of Neurology. New York, McGraw-Hill, 1977.

Baldwin, P.: Epidural spinal cord compression secondary to metastatic disease: A review of the literature. Cancer Nursing 6:441, 1983.

Couillard-Getrever, D.: Obstructive emergencies: Spinal cord compression. *In* Johnson, B.L., and Gross, J. (Eds.): Handbook of Oncology Nursing. New York, John Wiley & Sons, 1985, p. 416.

Mayer, D.: Spinal cord compression. *In* Baird, S. (Ed.): Decision in Oncology Nursing. Toronto, B.C. Decker, Inc., 1988, p. 212.

Posner, J.: Neurological complications of systemic cancer. Medical Clinics of North America 63(4):783, 1979.

Yasko, J.M.: Guidelines for Cancer Care: Symptom Management. Reston, VA, Reston Publishing, 1982.

Mobility, Impaired Physical, Related to Amputation

43

Patricia Manda Collins

Population at Risk

- Individuals with soft-tissue sarcomas, bone sarcomas, resectable miscellaneous tumors, and severe tissue damage from necrotizing drugs

LEVEL 1: Anticipated (Preoperative Care)

EXPECTED OUTCOME

1. Patient demonstrates knowledge related to anticipated alteration in physical mobility:
   - identifies signs and symptoms of anticipated limits in mobility.
   - identifies factors that influence mobility.
2. Patient identifies factors to prevent or correct impairment of mobility:
   - demonstrates active participation in therapy and treatment.
   - demonstrates self-direction and self-management of health maintenance and activities of daily living.
3. Patient maintains physical mobility:
   - performs activities of daily living without assistance.
   - performs independent ambulation.

NURSING MANAGEMENT

Assessment

1. Determine intellectual and emotional status.
2. Evaluate orthopedic status:
   - range of motion of joints.
   - position and appearance of extremities and trunk.
   - growth and development for age.
   - gait, balance, coordination.
   - sensation and circulation.
   - posture.
   - muscle strength, reflexes.
3. Determine perceptions and expectations related to potential loss of body part.

Nursing Interventions

1. Obtain doctor's order for physical and occupational therapy.
2. Assist patient with strengthening exercises.
3. Encourage patient to practice proper positioning and range-of-motion exercises.
4. Arrange for contact with rehabilitated amputee if appropriate.

273

5. Assign same nursing personnel as much as possible.
6. Encourage expression of feelings related to the surgery and cancer.

Patient Teaching

1. Discuss importance of mobility and methods to increase mobility.

2. Teach range-of-motion exercises.
3. Describe proper anatomic positioning.
4. Relate importance of proper nutrition and hydration.
5. Note signs and symptoms to relate to health care team (e.g., increased pain, decreased or change in sensations at stump site).
6. Discuss anticipated procedures and activities.

LEVEL 2: Moderate (Postoperative Care)

EXPECTED OUTCOME

1. Patient demonstrates knowledge related to impaired mobility:
   - identifies signs and symptoms of limits in mobility.
   - identifies factors that influence mobility.
   - identifies potential sequelae/complications of impaired mobility.
2. Patient identifies/demonstrates measures to correct or improve impaired mobility:
   - demonstrates proper knowledge and administration of medications.
   - performs necessary treatments and procedures.
   - identifies/utilizes appropriate community resources.
   - verbalizes/demonstrates necessary life style adaptations.
   - manipulates environment to minimize joint and limb stress and provide for home safety.
3. Patient achieves or maintains optimal mobility:
   - full or moderately decreased range of motion.
   - mobility sufficient to manage activities of daily living.
   - independent transfers.

NURSING MANAGEMENT

Assessment

1. See Assessment, Level 1.
2. Perform postoperative assessments:
   - circulatory status of stump (color, blanching).
   - status of incision, flaps, drains.
   - vital signs.
   - ability to perform range-of-motion exercises.
   - ability to assume proper body positioning.
   - general physical status.
   - emotional status.
   - signs and symptoms of possible complications:
     - hemorrhage.
     - infection.
     - severe, unrelenting pain related to possible compartment syndrome (in-

274

creased pressure within muscle tissue that compresses blood vessels and decreases blood supply to limb).
- pulmonary embolus.
- skin breakdown.
- comfort level: if discomfort present, differentiate between phantom limb sensations, incisional pain, compartment syndrome, edema, infection, skin breakdown, phlebitis, restrictive dressings or improperly wrapped elastic bandage.
- patient's/family's response to care.
3. Perform rehabilitative assessments:
   - ability to use assistive devices (crutches, wheelchair, prosthesis).
   - ability to care for stump and related articles.
   - ability to care for prosthesis.
4. Observe for signs and symptoms of complications of impaired mobility:
   - skin breakdown.
   - phlebitis.
   - embolism.
   - atelectasis.
   - pneumonia.
   - urinary retention, urinary tract infection.
   - renal calculi.
   - constipation.
   - anorexia.
5. Assess patient's/family's ability to integrate mobility changes into life style.
6. Refer to vocational rehabilitation counselor, if appropriate.

Nursing Interventions

1. See Nursing Interventions, Level 1.
2. Perform postoperative nursing actions:
   - use comfort measures as well as analgesics to reduce discomfort.
   - supervise ambulation if lower limb has been amputated, as patient may inadvertently attempt to use phantom leg and lose balance.
   - provide firm support for bed.

- elevate stump on plastic-covered pillow first 12 to 24 hours only.
- while patient is supine, place pillow under head only, except in instance previously noted.
- initiate immediate and frequent range-of-motion exercises in consultation with physician, physical therapist.
- if lower limb amputation, position stump to ensure hip extension and neutral rotation; avoid abduction. Use trochanter rolls along outer aspect of affected limb, if necessary.
- place patient in prone position at specific intervals and duration (e.g., q4h for 30 to 60 min).
- implement measures to maintain proper nutrition and hydration.
- if patient has rigid plaster dressing, keep cast exposed to air to dry; check cast for fit.
- if patient has elastic bandages and wrap changes are prescribed:
  - remove and reapply bid.
  - wash, dry, expose stump to air before wrap is reapplied.
  - use clean, dry wrap each time.
  - wrap stump firmly but without impairing circulation using figure-eight technique.
  - wraps must be wrinkle-free.
- apply antiembolism stocking to unaffected lower extremity.
- follow principles of routine postoperative care.
- perform circulation checks.
3. Perform rehabilitative nursing actions:
   - coordinate care with rehabilitation team.
   - with aid of photograph, home visit, discussions, evaluate home environment and advise patient/family of structural alterations that may be needed:
     - type of surface leading to entrance of home and in home.
     - presence of hazards (e.g., throw rugs).
     - presence of steps.

○ width of doorways.
○ bathroom setup (are light switches within easy reach; safety rails, raised toilet seats, shower bench needed?)
○ kitchen setup (appliances, cupboards within reach?)
○ location of telephones.
- encourage independence.
- refer patient/family to appropriate resources for additional help and information as needed, such as social services, amputee groups, amputee clinic, prosthetist and physical and occupational therapists.
- advise patient/family of organizations involved in recreation for the disabled.

Patient Teaching

1. See Patient Teaching, Level 1.
2. Teach postoperative procedures:
   - nature of phantom limb sensations (e.g., common experience, possible reasons for sensations, methods of dealing with them).
   - one-handed self-care for upper extremity amputation (consult with occupational therapist for assistive devices).
   - signs and symptoms of complications to report to health care team.
   - purposes of interventions.
   - if lower limb amputation, caution patient/family to avoid the following:
     ○ hanging stump over bed.
     ○ sitting in wheelchair or chair with stump flexed.
     ○ placing pillows under hips or knees.
     ○ placing pillow under back of curving spine.
     ○ lying with knees flexed.
     ○ resting stump on crutch handle.
     ○ placing pillow between thighs.
     ○ abducting stump.
3. Ensure that patient/caregiver have adequate information about treatment and rehabilitation, as this is vital to development of functional coping style.

4. Rehabilitative teaching is as follows:
   - reinforce importance of general health maintenance activities such as proper nutrition and hydration.
   - explain medications, administration schedules, potential side effects.
   - review exercises.
   - instruct patient/family that if slightest irritation is noted, if cast becomes too loose or too tight, or any mechanical parts break, prosthesis should not be worn and health care team should be notified immediately.
   - instruct patient/family on stump care, conditioning, and strengthening after sutures have been removed:
     ○ wash stump daily as any other part of body. Use mild soap and water, rinse and dry well. Expose stump to air daily and prn.
     ○ do not use lotions, creams, disinfectants on skin; cornstarch may be recommended.
     ○ bathing in evening is recommended, as morning baths may cause swelling of stump and subsequent problems with prosthetic fit.
     ○ shaving stump may cause irritation, itchy rash.
     ○ massage stump daily.
     ○ for stump conditioning and desensitization, push stump against pillow; progress to pushing against firmer surfaces.
     ○ prone positioning, daily exercise recommended.
   - Instruct about rationale and circumstances for stump wrapping:
     ○ if prosthesis is not worn daily.
     ○ if normally fitting prosthesis does not fit because of swelling.
     ○ if patient has stump pain or phantom sensations, especially at night.
   - Instruct patient/family on care and use of elastic wraps, stump shrinker, stump sheaths, socks, prosthesis:
     ○ wash and dry wraps by hand.
     ○ use appropriate number and ply of stump socks for good prosthetic fit.

- change stump sheath and socks daily. Do not use if damp, torn, patched, or roughened. Sheath and socks must be wrinkle-free.
- reinforce prosthetist's and physical therapist's instructions in care of prosthesis.
- inspect prosthesis periodically to determine if parts need repair or replacement. Signs of malfunction include joint clicks, foot creaking, changes in way stump looks or feels.

LEVEL 3: Severe

EXPECTED OUTCOME

1. Patient/caregiver demonstrate knowledge related to complications of amputation and effect on mobility:
   - identify signs and symptoms of impaired mobility and complications of amputation.
   - identify factors that influence mobility/complications.
   - identify potential sequelae/complications of impaired mobility.
2. Patient/caregiver minimize mobility impairment:
   - demonstrate proper administration of medications.
   - perform necessary treatment procedures.
   - identify signs and symptoms to report to health care team.
   - identify/utilize appropriate community resources.
   - verbalize/demonstrate necessary life style adaptations.
   - seek assistance for activities beyond capabilities or that aggravate condition.
   - manipulate environment to minimize joint and limb stress, provide for home/institutional safety.
3. Patient/caregiver demonstrate behaviors to prevent or minimize complications of impaired mobility:
   - demonstrate measures to prevent or manage skin breakdown.
   - demonstrate measures to prevent or manage respiratory dysfunction.
   - demonstrate measures to maintain bowel and bladder function.
   - demonstrate measures to promote adequate circulation to tissues.
4. Patient achieves/maintains optimal mobility, as evidenced by:
   - improved or stable range of motion.
   - transfers independently or with assistance.
   - mobility sufficient to manage activities of daily living independently or with assistance.

NURSING MANAGEMENT

Assessment

1. See Assessment, Levels 1 and 2.
2. Observe for postoperative complications:
   - improper wound healing.
   - infection.
   - hemorrhage.
   - decreased circulation.
   - compartment syndrome.
3. Determine if prosthesis fits properly.

4. Evaluate patient's psychological and physical ability to wear prosthesis.
5. Observe for complications of impaired mobility:
   - pneumonia.
   - atelectasis.
   - renal calculi.
   - urinary tract infection.
   - constipation.
   - skin breakdown.
   - contractures.
   - thrombophlebitis.
6. Assess patient's/family's psychological response to loss of body part, complications, and impaired mobility.

Nursing Interventions

1. See Nursing Interventions, Levels 1 and 2.
2. Implement medical treatment plan.
3. Encourage patient/family to express feelings and concerns and to seek counseling if needed.
4. Promote patient's feelings of self-worth, self-esteem, and independence (see Chapter 19).
5. Provide nursing care to alleviate complications of impaired mobility.
6. Implement measures to promote or improve respiratory function (see Chapter 57).
7. Implement measures to prevent constipation (see Chapter 45).
8. Implement measures to promote proper bladder function (see Chapter 50).
9. Implement measures to prevent skin breakdown.

Patient Teaching

1. See Patient Teaching, Levels 1 and 2.
2. Explain treatments (e.g., wound care).
3. Discuss rationale for treatment measures to alleviate complications.
4. Emphasize importance of open communication.

5. Note availability of group support for patient/family.
6. Outline measures to prevent further complications of impaired mobility (skin care, pulmonary hygiene, prevention of constipation, promotion of renal function).

SUGGESTED READINGS

Brunner, L., and Suddarth, D.: Textbook of Medical-Surgical Nursing (6th ed.). Philadelphia, J.B. Lippincott, 1988.

Ceccio, C.M., and Horosz, J.E.: Teaching the elderly amputee to meet the world. RN 51:70–77, 1988.

Donahoo, C., and Spicker, L.: Core curriculum of orthopedic nursing. Atlanta, GA, Orthopedic Nursing Association, Inc, 1980.

Dunlop, J.G.: Critical problems facing young adults with cancer. Oncology Nursing Forum 9:33–35, 1982.

Farrell, J.: Illustrated Guide to Orthopedic Nursing (3rd ed.). Philadelphia, J.B. Lippincott, 1986.

Getz, P.A.; and Blossom, B.M.: Preventing contractures: The little "extras" that help so much. RN 45:45–48, 1982.

Kenner, C.V., Guzzetta, C.E., and Dossey, B.M.: Critical Care Nursing: Body-Mind-Spirit. Boston, Little, Brown & Co., 1981.

Lavin, R.J.: The high-pressure demands of compartment syndrome. RN 52:22–25, 1989.

Livingstone, O.P.: The D–Z stump protection. Journal of Occupational Therapy 42:185–187, 1988.

Luckmann, J., and Sorensen, K.: Medical-Surgical Nursing (3rd ed.). Philadelphia, W.B. Saunders, 1987.

Marvin, N., Holt, N., and Hicks, D.: Comprehensive Rehabilitation Nursing. New York, McGraw-Hill, 1981.

Tucker, S.M., Breeding, M.A., Canobbio, M.M., et al.: Patient Care Standards. St. Louis, C.V. Mosby, 1988.

Turek, S.L.: Orthopedics, Principles and Their Application (4th ed.). Philadelphia, J.B. Lippincott, 1984.

Working with Orthopedic Patients. Springhouse, PA, Nursing '82 Books, Intermed Communications, 1982.

PATIENT EDUCATION MATERIALS AND COMMUNITY RESOURCES

Access for the Handicapped, 1012 14th Street NW, Washington, DC 20005.

American Running and Fitness Association, 2420 K Street NW, Washington, DC 20037.

Amputee in Motion, 5900 Sepulveda Boulevard, Sherman Oaks, CA 91411.

Amputee Shoe and Glove Exchange, 1635 Warwickshire Drive, Houston, TX 77077.

52 Association (Sport Program for Amputees), 441 Lexington Avenue, New York, NY 10017.

Canadian Association for Disabled Skiing, Box 307, Kimberly, BC, Canada VIA2Y9.

Canadian Federation of Sport Organizations for the Disabled, 1600 James Naismith Drive, Gloucester, Ontario, Canada K1B5N4.

National Amputation Foundation, 12–45 150th Street, Whitestone, NY 11357.

National Easter Seal Society, 2023 W Ogden Avenue, Chicago, IL 60612.

National Inconvenienced Sportsman's Association, 5928 Illinois Avenue, Orangevale, CA 95662.

National Institute of Arthritis and Musculoskeletal and Skin Diseases, National Institutes of Health, Bethesda, MD 20892.

National Odd Shoe Exchange, RR 1, Indianola, IA 50125.

Self-Care Deficit, Related to Disease Process and Treatment

Debrynda Brewer Davey

Population at Risk

- Individuals who experience loss of body part as a result of disease process or treatment
- Individuals who are fatigued, anemic, dyspneic, or in pain as a result of disease process or treatment
- Individuals at level of psychosocial development in which self-care deficit may precipitate crisis
- Individuals who experience potential or actual impairment of self-care abilities resulting from loss or impairment of motor function, cognitive ability, attention span, judgment ability, or sensation
- Individuals receiving radiation therapy to CNS or chemotherapeutic agents with neurotoxicity
- Unconscious individuals
- Individuals with CNS infections

LEVEL 1: Potential

EXPECTED OUTCOME

1. Patient demonstrates knowledge related to potential self-care deficit:
    - correctly describes mechanisms in which disease or treatment may compromise self-care abilities.
    - identifies factors that promote or hinder self-care.
    - identifies social support available.
    - names persons/agencies able to assist in both routine and emergency situations.
2. Patient performs self-care activities free of impairment:
    - performs activities of daily living independently.
    - performs health-related tasks.
    - performs normal roles and functions.
3. Patient demonstrates measures to prevent self-care deficits:
    - follows treatment plan for malignancy.
    - makes necessary environmental changes.
    - eats well-balanced diet.
    - participates in exercise program.
    - performs activities designed to prevent deficits.

- verbalizes signs and symptoms of self-care impairment to report to health care team.

NURSING MANAGEMENT

Assessment

1. Make subjective assessments:
   - impaired sensation.
   - easily fatigued.
   - impaired memory.
   - headache, pain.
   - self-concept and coping skills.
   - perception of patient by family members.
   - sexual identity
2. Make objective assessments:
   - history of malignancy.
   - current/planned therapy.
   - patient's understanding of disease, treatment, potential loss of self-care abilities.
   - usual patterns and methods of self-care.
   - change in physical ability to perform self-care.
   - neurologic examination including:
     - history.
     - mental status examination.
     - motor function (muscle strength and tone, coordination, gait).
     - sensory function (reflexes).
     - cranial nerve function.
     - speech and language function.
     - sexual function.
     - usual methods of coping.
   - nature and availability of support systems: family, friends, facility, community.
   - environmental conditions at home.
   - patient/family readiness to learn.
   - financial status.
   - employment relative to potential self-care deficits.
   - family structure and potential changes:
     - roles.
     - power.
     - communication.
   - each family member's stage in grief process.
   - response to crisis.

Patient Teaching

1. Focus teaching on wellness behaviors to encourage self-responsibility and health-promoting behaviors.
2. Teach effective use of present self-care abilities.
3. Explain nature, extent, cause, and duration of disease and potential disability.
4. Give rationale for preventive measures:
   - importance of following treatment plan for malignancy.
   - well-balanced diet.
   - daily exercise program.
5. Explain rationale for early detection of self-care impairment.
6. Discuss signs and symptoms of self-care impairment to report (motor or sensory function disturbance, increasing fatigue, personality change).
7. Discuss community agencies offering rehabilitative support and programs designed to help patients and families cope with cancer such as: I Can Cope, Reach to Recovery, Can Surmount, Ostomy Rehabilitation, Make Today Count, ChemoCare, We Can Weekend, Coma Recovery Association.
8. Discuss employment considerations:
   - setting.
   - sharing information about diagnosis with coworkers.
   - identifying potential problems and solutions related to disease- and treatment-related disabilities.

LEVEL 2: Minimal to Moderate (Paresis/Paralysis, Mental Status Change)

EXPECTED OUTCOME

1. Patient demonstrates knowledge related to self-care deficits:
   - describes realistic prognosis for self-care deficits, accurately reflecting medical diagnosis, prognosis, physical condition.
2. Patient demonstrates measures to manage self-care deficits:
   - uses support systems effectively.
   - makes necessary environmental changes.
   - demonstrates correct use of assistive devices.
   - directs or assists caretakers in performance of care.
   - sets reachable goals.
   - alerts health care team if problems in recovery arise.
   - relinquishes help as improvements in condition allow.
   - lists achievements.
   - performs self-care tasks according to physical capacity.
   - incorporates new self-care skills into daily routine.
   - follows medical regimen designed to minimize deficits and promote recovery.
3. Family members will maintain or develop a functional family system:
   - exhibit improved methods of communication.
   - express increased feelings of control over family's situation.
   - identify changes in family roles and responsibilities related to patient's illness.

NURSING MANAGEMENT

Assessment

1. See Assessment, Level 1.
2. Make subjective assessment:
   - loss of sensation or strength in upper or lower extremities.
   - patient's motivation, emotional status.
3. Make objective assessment:
   - upper extremities:
     - muscle strength.
     - mobility.
     - coordination.
     - opposition of thumb and fingers.
     - handgrasp.
   - mental status.
   - perceptual deficits.
4. Monitor laboratory tests:
   - total protein.
   - albumin.
   - lymphocytes.
   - serum osmolality.
   - hematocrit.
   - urinalysis.
   - urine culture.
   - electrolytes (especially calcium).
5. Check for body weight change.
6. Note skin turgor.
7. Observe for slow or negative vein filling.
8. Determine nature and extent of self-care deficits, probable duration.
9. Assess patient's willingness to allow family to assist.
10. Assess family members' readiness to assist patient, if needed.

Nursing Interventions

1. Involve patient/significant others in planning, implementation, and evaluation of patient care and teaching program.
2. Provide extended supervision to patient, when needed.
3. Start with easy, familiar tasks such as eating and grooming.
4. Encourage patient to perform self-care tasks.
5. Make referral to occupational and physical therapy to evaluate deficit and plan care.
6. Provide proper assistive devices for each activity.
7. Choose setting where patient will not be interrupted. Allow sufficient time to accomplish activity. Observe for fatigue.
8. Encourage patient to use affected extremity to restore more normal posture, tone, movement, and function.
9. Refer for financial planning and assistance as needed.
10. Suggest or arrange contacts with home care services, community agencies, and self-help groups as needed.
11. Serve as case manager for other members of health care team, within and across institutions.
12. Support effective coping mechanisms of patient/family.

Patient Teaching

1. Inform all persons involved with patient care of the rehabilitative procedures.
2. Teach use of assistive devices.
3. Explore environmental alterations that will assist patient.
4. Provide written materials that may be obtained from organizations without cost.
5. Reinforce teaching by other therapists (e.g., occupational, respiratory, physical therapists).
6. Focus on the patient's progress and praise attempts to perform an activity.

LEVEL 2A: Impairment of Ability to Feed Self

EXPECTED OUTCOME

1. Patient maintains adequate fluid and nutritional status, as evidenced by
   - laboratory values within normal limits.
   - body weight remaining within 4 kg of baseline weight.
   - vital signs within normal limits.
   - mucous membranes moist and glistening.
   - normal skin turgor and vein filling.
2. Patient demonstrates ability to adequately feed self with minimal assistance:
   - demonstrates adequate nutritional intake.
   - accepts assistance only when needed.
   - uses adaptive equipment or utensils if needed.
3. Patient demonstrates knowledge related to adequate fluid and nutritional status:
   - verbalizes components of adequate fluid and food intake.
   - identifies signs and symptoms of inadequate hydration and nutrition.

Self-Care Deficit, Related to Disease Process and Treatment

NURSING MANAGEMENT

Assessment

1. See Assessment, Level 2.
2. Monitor caloric intake.
3. Assess change in self-feeding ability.

Nursing Interventions

1. See Nursing Interventions, Level 2.
2. Keep patient in comfortable sitting position throughout meal.
3. Have patient wear dentures at meals, if applicable.
4. Allow sufficient time for meal (e.g., 1 hr).
5. Assist patient by opening containers, cutting meat, buttering bread, and so on.
6. When possible, serve meals attractively, in a form that is easy for patient to handle, and is within patient's reach and field of vision.
7. If patient has difficulty swallowing, offer semisolids and thick fluids.
8. Provide assistive devices such as rocker knife, utensils with fat handles, weighted utensils, and plate rims.

Patient Teaching

1. Discuss adequate food and fluid intake.
2. Explain technique for cutting soft foods: hold fork in unaffected hand, insert tines in food, rock handle back and forth until bite-sized piece of food is broken off.
3. Describe cutting food of firm consistency with a knife: hold knife in unaffected hand, insert blade into food, rock handle back and forth until bite-sized piece of food is broken off.
4. For safety, instruct the patient to eat only small, bite-sized pieces of food and teach the family the Heimlich maneuver.
5. Teach use of small, light pitchers with wide base of support for beverages.
6. Review signs and symptoms of impaired nutrition and hydration.

LEVEL 2B: Impairment of Ability to Bathe Self

EXPECTED OUTCOME

1. Patient demonstrates adequate personal hygiene, as evidenced by:
   - skin clean, dry, intact.
   - absence of body odor.
2. Patient demonstrates ability to adequately bathe self with minimal assistance.
3. Patient demonstrates knowledge related to personal hygiene:
   - verbalizes rationale for actions.
   - verbalizes signs and symptoms to report to health care team (e.g., skin breakdown, rashes).

NURSING MANAGEMENT

Assessment

1. See Assessment, Level 2.
2. Assess change in self-bathing ability.

3. Note impairment of skin integrity or body odor.

Nursing Interventions

1. See Nursing Interventions, Level 2.
2. Encourage patient to complete major portion of bath gradually.
3. Provide assistive devices:
   - small hand brush attached to inside of basin with suction cups.
   - long-handled bath brush and soap, each tied to a piece of rope suspended from faucet.

Patient Teaching

1. Discuss rationale for maintaining personal hygiene.

2. Explain use of long-handled bath brush to wash hard-to-reach areas.
3. Teach patient to wash hands by soaping and rubbing unaffected hand over brush, then soaping and washing affected hand with unaffected hand.
4. Teach patient to dry unaffected hand and arm by holding towel taut and placing the end of the towel under the affected arm or tucking in belt. Rub unaffected hand and arm over towel to dry.
5. Teach signs and symptoms of skin breakdown to report to health care team.

LEVEL 2C: Impairment of Ability to Perform Oral Hygiene

EXPECTED OUTCOME

1. Patient demonstrates ability to perform oral hygiene measures adequately:
   - utilizes appropriate equipment.
   - inspects oral cavity as instructed.
   - employs appropriate brushing technique.
2. Patient demonstrates adequate oral hygiene:
   - mucosa pink, moist, intact.
   - no dental caries.
   - absence of food debris.
3. Patient demonstrates knowledge of oral hygiene:
   - verbalizes signs and symptoms of mouth disease to report to health care team.
   - identifies factors that promote healthy oral mucosa.

NURSING MANAGEMENT

Assessment

1. See Assessment, Level 2.
2. Note reports of oral burning or pain after eating seasoned food.
3. Monitor change in ability to perform oral hygiene.

4. Do oral examination daily and note halitosis, bleeding, fungal infection, caries.

Nursing Interventions

1. See Nursing Interventions, Level 2.
2. After eating, patient should check affected

side of mouth for food by feeling with finger.

3. Provide dental floss holder to allow patient to floss independently.
4. Provide wall-hung plastic toothpaste dispenser for patient.
5. Lubricate lips with petrolatum jelly to prevent drying and cracking.

Patient Teaching

1. Review appropriate technique to brush teeth:

- soft nylon brush or electric toothbrush should be used to brush teeth qid.
- denture brush may be attached to side of basin with suction cups, if patient wears dentures.

2. Instruct patient to clean dentures regularly over basin filled with water to prevent breaking if dentures are dropped.
3. Explain signs and symptoms of stomatitis, gingivitis, periodontitis.

LEVEL 2D: Impairment of Grooming Ability

EXPECTED OUTCOME

1. Patient demonstrates ability to safely perform grooming measures:
   - shaves self.
   - manicures nails.
   - shampoos and arranges hair with minimal assistance.
   - applies makeup if desired or appropriate.
   - opens containers of grooming products.
   - verbalizes safety precautions to use in grooming.
   - reports changes in ability to health care team.

NURSING MANAGEMENT

Assessment

1. See Assessment, Level 2.
2. Assess change in ability to groom self:
   - unshaven or poorly shaven.
   - unkempt hair and nails.
   - nonuse of makeup that is normally used.
   - loss of skin integrity.

Nursing Interventions

1. See Nursing Interventions, Level 2.
2. Encourage grooming activities to increase self-esteem and independence.

3. Trim nails of unaffected hand and foot.

Patient Teaching

1. For safety, teach patient to obtain help for manicuring toenails.
2. Instruct patient to use electric razor to eliminate need for handling shaving cream and blades, and to puff out cheeks to pull skin taut.
3. Encourage patient to have hair cut and styled in a manner that will allow combing and brushing to be accomplished with one hand.
4. To file nails, have emery board or nail file

taped to side of a table or counter and instruct patient to run nails across file to shape.
5. To shampoo, instruct patient and family that a protective tray device that fits around patient's neck and slopes down into sink may be used if patient is unable to tilt head. Dry shampoo may be used.
6. Encourage patient to practice opening and closing makeup containers. Contents should be transferred to easily opened plastic containers.

LEVEL 2E: Impairment of Ability to Dress Self

EXPECTED OUTCOME

1. Patient dresses self:
   • puts on and removes jacket, shirt, dress that opens down front.
   • puts on and removes pullover shirt.
   • puts on and removes shorts, pants, underwear.
   • puts on and removes bra, if female.
   • reports change in ability to dress self to health care team.

NURSING MANAGEMENT

Assessment

1. See Assessment, Level 2.
2. Assess change in ability to dress self.

Nursing Interventions

1. See Nursing Interventions, Level 2.
2. Begin training in dressing techniques early in course of illness.
3. If balance is good, have patient dress while sitting on side of bed. If balance is poor, have patient dress while sitting in wheelchair.
4. If patient has perceptual impairment, color-code clothing for easy matching.
5. Teach patients with damage to left hemisphere by example, as verbal instructions will confuse them.

Patient Teaching

1. Instruct patient to start dressing by clothing affected limb first and undressing by removing clothing from affected limb last.
2. Instruct patient to wear clothing that fastens easily in front or on side.
3. Instruct patient that Velcro closures may be substituted for snaps, buttons, zippers, hooks and eyes, or bows.
4. Instruct patient to put on jacket, shirt, or dress that opens in front as follows:
   • position shirt on lap with inside of shirt up, collar toward chest and close to affected hand.
   • using unaffected hand, place affected hand into shirt sleeve opening and work sleeve up over elbow. Put unaffected arm into sleeve, raising arm up to "shake" sleeve into position past elbow.
   • gather garment up middle of back from hemline to collar with unaffected hand, then raise shirt over head.
   • with unaffected hand work shirt down.
   • begin buttoning with bottom button.
5. Instruct patient to remove jacket, shirt, or dress that opens in front as follows:

- unbutton shirt.
- with unaffected arm, gather material up in back of neck and pull material over head.

6. Instruct patient to put on pullover shirt as follows:
   - shirt is positioned on lap, bottom toward chest, label facing down.
   - with unaffected hand, roll up bottom edge of shirt all the way up to sleeve on affected side.
   - using unaffected hand, place affected arm in sleeve opening and pull shirt up onto arm past elbow.
   - insert unaffected arm into sleeve.
   - gather shirt back with unaffected hand and pass shirt over head.

7. Instruct patient to remove pullover shirt by starting at the top back and gathering the shirt up, then passing shirt over head.

8. Instruct patient to put on shorts, pants, or underwear as follows:
   - patient sits in straight chair or in wheelchair. Unaffected leg should be positioned directly in front of midline of body with knee flexed 90 degrees. Using unaffected hand, grasp ankle of involved leg and lift affected leg over unaffected leg to crossed position.
   - slip pants onto affected leg until foot is completely inside of trouser leg; uncross affected leg.
   - unaffected leg is inserted and pants worked up on hips as far as possible.
   - Patient now stands and pulls pants over hips. To prevent pants from dropping as patient stands, affected hand is placed in pocket, or one finger is slipped into belt loop. Patient should sit down to button front.

9. Instruct patient to remove shorts, pants, underwear:
   - in sitting position, patient unfastens pants and works them down.
   - patient stands and pulls pants past hips.
   - pants are removed from unaffected leg.
   - patient crosses affected leg over unaffected leg, removes pants, uncrosses legs.

10. Instruct patient to put on bra by hooking in front and slipping around to the back at waistline level.

LEVEL 2F: Inability to Empty Bladder

EXPECTED OUTCOME

1. Patient maintains adequate urinary control and elimination:
   - expresses desire to void.
   - follows pattern of fluid intake and voiding.
   - voids before activities that are prolonged.
   - checks bladder for overdistention when appropriate.
   - uses appropriate measures to initiate voiding when necessary.
   - takes in enough fluids to keep urine dilute and to avoid cystitis.
   - voids q2–3h during day.
   - maintains socially acceptable bladder emptying program.
2. Patient demonstrates knowledge of urinary control and elimination:
   - verbalizes signs and symptoms of bladder distention.
   - verbalizes need to take in 2000 to 3000 ml of fluid per day.
   - verbalizes knowledge of medications being taken.

NURSING MANAGEMENT

Assessment

1. See Assessment, Level 2.
2. Note signs and symptoms of overdistention:
   - perspiration or restlessness.
   - elevation of blood pressure.
   - palpable bladder wall directly over symphysis pubis.
3. Monitor intake and output including type of fluid, amount, and time taken.
4. Note characteristics of incontinent voiding: including continual, occasional, or only at specific times.
5. Determine if the patient is aware of spontaneous voiding and sensation of a full bladder.
6. Assess residual urine by catheterization after voiding.

Nursing Interventions

1. See Nursing Interventions, Level 2.
2. Establish bladder training program:
   - remove catheter at 7:00 AM daily.
   - establish fluid intake schedule.
   - provide for privacy.
   - use measures to stimulate voiding (e.g., pour warm water over perineum, use warm bedpan, let water run from tap, stroke insides of thighs, pull on pubic hair, use Credé method of applying pressure over suprapubic area, contract abdominal and diaphragmatic muscles).
   - establish voiding schedule for bedpan and urinal use.
   - catheterize for residual each time patient voids until residual is less than 50 ml.
3. If bladder training program is not appropriate, begin intermittent sterile catheterization program.
4. Administer parasympathomimetic drug therapy as ordered.

Patient Teaching

1. Teach signs and symptoms of overdistention of bladder.
2. Discuss need for fluid intake of 2000 to 3000 ml/day unless contraindicated.
3. Discuss need to void q2–3 hr during day.
4. Outline measures to stimulate voiding.
5. Instruct clean self-catheterization technique for home catheterization.
6. Instruct regarding medications being taken and importance of compliance.
7. Teach signs and symptoms of urinary tract infection.

LEVEL 2G: Abnormal Bowel Function

EXPECTED OUTCOME

1. Patient maintains adequate bowel control and elimination:
   - expresses desire to defecate.
   - takes in adequate fluid and bulk to promote defecation.
   - utilizes schedule for defecation.
   - appropriately uses stool softeners, suppositories.
   - shows absence of fecal impaction.

2. Patient exhibits knowledge of bowel control and elimination:
   - verbalizes signs and symptoms of constipation to report to health care team.
   - verbalizes rationale for bowel training program techniques.
   - demonstrates knowledge of bowel training program techniques.

NURSING MANAGEMENT

Assessment

1. See Assessment, Level 2.
2. Make objective assessment:
   - stools (hard, watery, pencil thin).
   - abdominal distention, decreased bowel sounds.
   - bowel incontinence.
   - inability to contract abdominal muscles.
   - food and fluid intake including fiber content.
   - activity level.
   - rectal examination for retained stool.

Nursing Interventions

1. See Nursing Interventions, Level 2.
2. Establish individually designed bowel training program for each patient.

Patient Teaching

1. Teach signs and symptoms of constipation.
2. Instruct in bowel training program.
3. Instruct regarding medications being used (e.g., stood softeners, suppositories).
4. Encourage well-balanced diet with roughage to help stimulate peristalsis and help prevent constipation.
5. Provide daily exercise program.
6. Instruct need to take in 2000 to 3000 ml of fluid per day unless contraindicated. Hot water, prune juice, or hot coffee every morning helps stimulate a bowel movement.

LEVEL 2H: *Impairment of Skin Integrity*

EXPECTED OUTCOME

1. Patient maintains skin integrity:
   - keeps skin clean and dry, especially if incontinence occurs during course of day.
   - repositions self at least q2h while awake.
   - uses range-of-motion exercises to increase circulation in paralyzed limbs.
   - checks skin daily for areas of potential breakdown.
   - avoids neglect of paralyzed limbs.
   - takes in adequate fluid and food.
2. Patient displays knowledge of skin care:
   - verbalizes rationale for skin care program.
   - verbalizes signs and symptoms of skin breakdown to report to health care team.

NURSING MANAGEMENT

Assessment

1. See Assessment, Level 2.
2. Make objective assessment:
   - change in ability to maintain skin integrity.
   - changes in sensorimotor integrity.
   - areas at high risk for breakdown.

Nursing Interventions

1. See Nursing Interventions, Level 2.
2. Establish skin care program with patient.

Patient Teaching

1. Teach rationale for skin care program.
2. Explain signs and symptoms of skin breakdown.
3. Instruct in daily self-assessment of skin (e.g., pulses, erythema, edema, temperature, integrity).
4. Discuss skin care program including bathing, lubricating skin, prevention of pressure, exercises, adequate nutrition and hydration, repositioning self q2h while awake, keeping skin dry.

LEVEL 3: *Severe (Inability to Perform all Self-Care Activities; Loss of Motor and Sensory Function; Altered Mentation; Decreased Level of Consciousness)*

EXPECTED OUTCOME

1. Patient exhibits good hygienic status:
   - no unpleasant body odor.
   - no skin breakdown.
2. Patient maintains adequate urinary output:
   - urine straw-colored.
   - absence of signs and symptoms of urinary tract infection.
3. Patient maintains adequate bowel elimination.
4. Patient maintains adequate nutrition and hydration.
5. Caregiver demonstrates knowledge of principles and measures of caring for patient:
   - verbalizes rationale for thorough meticulous care of patient.
   - gives hygienic care to patient.
   - identifies family and community resources.
   - provides adequate fluid and nutritional intake.
   - facilitates adequate urinary and bowel output.
   - makes necessary environmental changes.
   - demonstrates correct use of assistive devices.
   - alerts health care team of signs and symptoms of progressive loss.
   - solves problems as changes occur.
6. Caregiver adapts to loss of patient's self-care abilities:
   - describes realistic prognosis for self-care deficits.
   - verbalizes adjustment to loss.

- makes mutually agreeable plans for long-term, rehabilitative, terminal care.
- verbalizes sense of personal well-being.
7. Caregiver uses support systems effectively:
  - recognizes when help is needed.
  - seeks help from appropriate persons/agencies.

NURSING MANAGEMENT

Assessment

1. See Assessment, Levels 1 and 2.
2. Assess performance status of patient.
3. Determine change in level of consciousness.
4. Check eyes for equality, size, reaction of pupils to light, signs and symptoms of inflammation or irritation.
5. Assess results of electroencephalogram, computed tomography scan.
6. Assess patient's reactivity to stimulation of each sense.
7. Evaluate intake and output.
8. Ascertain signs and symptoms of underlying problems.
9. Assess caregiver's ability to perform necessary patient care activities.
10. Assess family's resources to meet level of care needed by the patient.
11. Identify and prioritize nurse, patient, family beliefs, expectations, and goals for rehabilitation.

Nursing Interventions

1. See Nursing Interventions, Level 2.
2. Give family written information about measures to care for the patient.
3. Provide orientation with rehabilitation unit to family's primary contact.
4. Encourage family to attend family support groups.
5. Adjust environment to comfortable temperature, ventilation, and absence of odors.
6. Provide for safety with use of equipment (e.g., seizure precautions).

7. Arrange for thorough hygiene of skin, hair, mouth, eyes, and perineum.
8. Enforce proper positioning:
   - head of bed to be elevated if unconscious patient has cuffed tracheostomy tube or endotracheal tube.
   - alternate positioning of joints in flexion and extension.
   - feet supported with footboard to prevent plantar flexion (may have patient wear high-top sneakers).
9. Implement measures to maintain urinary elimination.
10. Implement measures to maintain bowel elimination.
11. Maintain nutritional and hydration status.
12. Assist family in exploring alternatives for long-term nursing care, if needed.
13. Assist family of coma patient to investigate various inpatient or outpatient coma recovery programs. Family should be cautioned not to undertake an intense multisensory stimulation program for a comatose patient without the guidance of specialists in coma recovery.

Patient Teaching

1. Teach family members or significant others principles of caring for patient with severe self-care deficits.

SUGGESTED READINGS

Adelstein, W.M.: Cost containment in spinal cord injuries. Rehabilitative Nursing *13*(1):32–37, 1988.

Anderson, J.L.: The nurse's role in cancer rehabilitation: Review of the literature. Cancer Nursing *12*(2):85–94, 1989.

Brett, G.: Dressing techniques for the severely hemiplegic patient. American Journal of Occupational Therapy *14*:262–263, 1960.

Conway-Rutkowski, B.L.: Neurological and Neurosurgical Nursing. St. Louis, C.V. Mosby, 1982.

DeYoung, S.: The neurological patient: A nursing perspective. Englewood Cliffs, NJ, Prentice-Hall, 1983.

DeYoung, S., and Grass, R.: Coma recovery program. Rehabilitative Nursing *12*(3):121–124, 1987.

Dring, R.: The informal caregiver responsible for home care of the individual with cognitive dysfunction following brain injury. Journal of Neuroscience Nursing *21*(1):42–45, 1989.

Dudas, S., and Carlson, C.E.: Cancer rehabilitation. Oncology Nursing Forum *15*(2):183–188, 1988.

Gillies, D.A.: Family assessment and counseling by the rehabilitation nurse. Rehabilitative Nursing *12*(2):65–69, 1987.

Hanucharurnkul, S.: Predictors of self-care in cancer patients receiving radiotherapy. Cancer Nursing *12*(1):21–27, 1989.

Hegeman, K.M.: A care plan for the family of a brain trauma client. Rehabilitative Nursing *13*(5):254–258, 1988.

Hickey, J.: The Clinical Practice of Neurological and Neurosurgical Nursing. Philadelphia, J.B. Lippincott, 1981.

Johnson, J.R., and Higgins, L.: Integration of family dynamics into rehabilitation of the brain-injured patient. Rehabilitative Nursing *12*(6):320–322, 1982.

Neal, M.C., Cohen, P.F., and Cooper, P.G.: Nursing Care Planning Guides. Pacific Palisades, CA, Neuroseco, Inc., 1982.

O'Brien, M.T., and Pallett, P.J.: Total Care of the Stroke Patient. Boston, Little, Brown, & Co., 1978.

Passarella, P.M., and Lewis, N.: Nursing application of Bobath principles in stroke care. Journal of Neuroscience Nursing *19*(2):106–109, 1987.

Payne, M.B.: Utilizing role therapy to assist the family with sudden disability. Rehabilitative Nursing *13*(4):191–194, 1988.

Voith, A.M.: Alterations in urinary elimination: Concepts, research, and practice. Rehabilitative Nursing *13*(3):122–131, 1988.

Waters, J.D.: Learning needs of spinal cord-injured patients. Rehabilitative Nursing *12*(6):309–312, 1987.

ELIMINATION

The nurse assesses the patient's past and present patterns of elimination and the effects of disease and treatment to formulate actual or potential nursing diagnoses.

Appropriate patient outcomes to consider in planning nursing interventions will specify the patient's ability to:

1. describe appropriate actions when changes in elimination occur (such as fecal and urinary diversions, fistulas, diarrhea, constipation, bladder insufficiencies, incontinence, and fecal or urinary obstruction).
2. describe the relationship between adequate elimination and physiologic integrity.
3. identify and manage factors that may affect elimination, such as diet, stress, physical activity, and neurogenic conditions.
4. develop a plan for managing an altered elimination route within patient's life style.

Evaluation of the patient's responses to nursing care is based on whether the patient manages alterations in elimination in a way that allows him or her to continue the activities of daily living as much as possible.

Excerpted from the ANA/ONS Standards of Cancer Nursing Practice.

Bowel Elimination, Alteration in: Constipation

Marianne French, Marcia Rostad,
and Sheila K. Wroblewski

Population at Risk

- Individuals receiving narcotic analgesics, antidepressants, anticonvulsants, anticholinergics, antacids, iron, neurotoxic chemotherapy (vinca alkaloids, e.g., vincristine and vinblastine)
- Individuals presenting with diseases of the colon, hypercalcemia, hypokalemia, neurogenic causes secondary to disease process (e.g., spinal cord compression), irritation or pressure in bowel related to metastatic disease, immobility
- Individuals with anorexia, change in food intake (small amounts, soft foods), dehydration (taking in less fluids), poor bowel habits such as laxative abuse or misuse
- Individuals demonstrating signs and symptoms of mental status changes or those experiencing stress
- Individuals with intestinal manipulation or trauma from surgery
- Individuals who fail to respond to defecation reflex as a result of pain, weakness, lethargy

LEVEL 1: Potential

EXPECTED OUTCOME

1. Patient demonstrates knowledge related to potential constipation:
   - identifies factors that influence elimination.
   - identifies early signs and symptoms of altered elimination to report to health care team.
2. Patient demonstrates measures to promote adequate bowel elimination:
   - verbalizes/demonstrates adequate fluid and nutritional intake.
   - utilizes prophylactic stool softeners as indicated.
   - maintains appropriate level of physical mobility.
   - shows timely response to elimination (gastrocolic reflex).
3. Patient demonstrates regular pattern of elimination, as evidenced by
   - soft stools.
   - stools passed without difficulty.

NURSING MANAGEMENT

Assessment

1. Assess bowel habits (including use of laxatives).
2. Determine food and fluid intake.
3. Note current medication regimen (e.g., narcotic analgesia, chemotherapy with vinca alkaloids).

297

4. Evaluate factors of current treatment and processes that predispose to constipation (see Population at Risk).
5. Assess mobility status.
6. Conduct baseline abdominal examination (including bowel sounds).
7. Evaluate mental status, including activity, orientation to time and place, stress level, and privacy level.

Nursing Interventions

1. Arrange for diet high in bulk-forming foods (whole-grain breads and cereals: 1 to 2 T bran or wheat germ added to food each day).
2. Maintain fluid intake at 3000 ml/day if not contraindicated.
3. Encourage moderate physical exercise.
4. Administer prophylactic stool softeners for population at risk:
   - bulk-forming laxatives (methylcellulose, psyllium): must be taken with sufficient water to minimize risk of intestinal or esophageal obstruction.
   - emollient (docusate calcium): stool softeners with no laxative action–useful in conditions in which straining is hazardous.
   - lubricants (e.g., mineral oil): useful to maintain soft stools and avoid strain-

ing–good for patients with thrombocytopenia; do not administer with meals.
5. Implement measures to help control stress and promote privacy.

Patient Teaching

1. Explain factors contributing to constipation (e.g., medication, disease process and treatment, immobility, food and fluid intake, bowel habits, inadequate privacy).
2. Discuss need for good fluid and nutrition intake and activity to stimulate bowel activity.
3. Encourage timely response to elimination reflex.
4. Instruct patients with or at risk for bone marrow depression to maintain soft stools and avoid enemas and suppositories.
5. Instruct patient to maintain a high-fiber diet and to eat foods that provide natural bowel stimulation (e.g., prune juice, apple juice, sauerkraut, fresh fruits).
6. Discuss routines to promote bowel elimination (e.g., coffee after breakfast, lemon juice and hot water before breakfast).
7. Teach early signs and symptoms of constipation to report to health care team (e.g., hard, infrequent stools, increased straining with defecation).

LEVEL 2:   *Early or Mild*

EXPECTED OUTCOME

1. Patient demonstrates knowledge related to early or mild constipation:
   - verbalizes factors that influence elimination.
   - identifies signs and symptoms of altered elimination.
   - identifies potential complications of constipation.
2. Patient demonstrates measures to correct mild constipation:
   - demonstrates proper knowledge and administration of medications.
   - performs necessary treatments and procedures.
   - verbalizes/demonstrates adequate fluid and nutritional intake.
   - identifies appropriate long-term plan of care.

- identifies signs and symptoms to report to health care team.
- shows timely response to elimination (gastrocolic reflex).
3. Patient achieves normal pattern of elimination, as evidenced by:
  - stools of normal frequency for patient.
  - stools of normal consistency for patient.
  - soft abdomen.
  - normal bowel sounds.
  - absence of abdominal distension.
  - absence of abdominal discomfort, pain, tenderness.

NURSING MANAGEMENT

Assessment

1. See Assessment, Level 1.
2. Assess current disease process and treatment.
3. Conduct rectal examination (assess for hemorrhoids, pain, bleeding).

Nursing Interventions

1. See Nursing Interventions, Level 1.
2. Provide psychological and physical environment conducive to defecation (e.g., privacy, sitting position).
3. Administer laxatives as prescribed:
   - combination laxatives (e.g., Senokot S, Peri-Colace).
   - saline/osmotic type (lactulose, magnesium citrate, milk of magnesia).
   - stimulants (bisacodyl [Dulcolax], cascara, castor oil, senna) may produce excessive catharsis. Prolonged use can result in habituation and laxative dependency, may be contraindicated in patients with thrombocytopenia.

Patient Teaching

1. See Patient Teaching, Level 1.
2. Explain rationale for scheduled bowel elimination.
3. Discuss rationale for purpose and desired effects of stool softeners, laxatives, enemas.
4. Teach signs and symptoms of constipation to report to health care team (e.g., absence of bowel elimination for 3 or more days, hard stool, abdominal discomfort, sense of incomplete evacuation, headache, distress in rectum.
5. Encourage patient to promptly report signs and symptoms to health care team.

LEVEL 3: Severe

EXPECTED OUTCOME

1. Patient/caregiver demonstrate knowledge related to severe constipation and impaction:
   - identify signs and symptoms of severe constipation.
   - identify factors that influence severe constipation.
   - identify potential sequelae/complications of severe constipation.

2. Patient/caregiver demonstrate measures to correct severe constipation or impaction:
   - demonstrate proper knowledge and administration of medications.
   - perform necessary treatments and procedures.
   - verbalize/demonstrate adequate fluid and nutritional intake.
   - identify appropriate long-term follow-up plan of care.
3. Patient achieves or maintains adequate defecation pattern, as evidenced by:
   - bowel sounds present.
   - stools of stable frequency.
   - stools of stable consistency.
   - soft abdomen.
   - absence of abdominal distension.
   - absence of or minimal abdominal discomfort, pain, tenderness, cramping.

NURSING MANAGEMENT

Assessment

1. See Assessment, Levels 1 and 2.
2. Observe for signs and symptoms of impaction (e.g., abdominal cramping, abdominal distension, pressure in rectum, frequent liquid stools, hard stool in rectum, continuous feeling of need to defecate).
3. Conduct physical assessment: auscultation of bowel sounds, palpation of abdomen, rectal examination (inspection and digital).

Nursing Interventions

1. See Nursing Interventions, Levels 1 and 2.
2. Provide for removal of stool:
   - oil retention or other types of enemas.
   - manual removal with lubrication (contraindicated in thrombocytopenic and leukopenic patients, patients with rectal tumors, hemorrhoids).
   - mineral oil 1 oz bid; if no results, increase to 2 oz bid until results obtained (usually 2 days). Indications: for patients with thrombocytopenia, lubricating rather than cathartic action promotes safety in elimination (e.g., no bleeding) and, in cases of possible small bowel obstruction, eliminates need to inflate colon with enemas; peristalsis is not increased.
   - milk and molasses enema (1 c whole milk, ½ c molasses, 1 T sugar): mix milk with molasses and sugar; administer as enema (contraindicated in leukopenic, thrombocytopenic patients).
3. Establish bowel program (suppositories may be contraindicated in patients with bone marrow depression).
   - stool softeners daily with glycerin or bisacodyl suppository q2d.
   - neostigmine bromide tablets (Prostigmin, 15 mg tid PO) or bethanechol chloride tablets (e.g., Myotonachol, 10 mg PO tid).
   - glycerin suppository, one rectally 1 hour after breakfast daily.

Patient Teaching

1. See Patient Teaching, Levels 1 and 2.
2. Instruct caregiver in removal of impaction.
3. Explain bowel program.
4. Discuss signs and symptoms of complications:
   - impaction: abdomen distended and hard, abdominal cramps, watery stools, hard stool in rectum, pressure in rectum.
   - bowel obstruction: absence of bowel movement for three or more days, fever, possibly vomiting, severe abdominal cramping.

SUGGESTED READINGS

Baines, M.: Control of other symptoms. *In* Sanders, M. (Ed.): The Management of Terminal Disease. Chicago, Year Book Medical Publishers, 1978, p. 105.

Basch, A.: Changes in elimination. Seminars in Oncology Nursing 3(4):287–292, 1987.

Brunner, L.S., and Suddarth, D.S.: Lippincott Manual of Nursing Practice. Philadelphia, J.B. Lippincott, 1986.

Casciato, D., and Lowitz, B.: Supportive care. *In* Casciato, D., and Lowitz, B. (Eds.): Manual of Clinical Oncology (2nd ed.). Boston, Little, Brown, & Co., 1988, p. 63.

Clark, J.: Nursing management of outcomes of disease, psychological response, treatment and complications. *In* Ziegfeld, C. (Ed.): Core Curriculum for Oncology Nursing (1st ed.). Philadelphia, W.B. Saunders, 1987, pp. 276–277.

Culhane, B.: Constipation. *In* Yasko, J. (Ed.): Guidelines for Cancer Care: Symptom Management (1st ed.). Reston, VA, Reston Publishing, 1983, pp. 184–186.

Gaddis, D.: Bowel elimination hints. Oncology Nursing Forum 9:64, 1982.

Luckmann, J., and Sorensen, K.C.: Medical-Surgical Nursing. Philadelphia, W.B. Saunders, 1987.

Malseed, R.: Drug Therapy and Nursing Considerations. Philadelphia, J.B. Lippincott, 1983, pp. 517–526.

McKenry, L.M., and Salerno, E.: Mosby's Pharmacology in Nursing. St. Louis, C.V. Mosby, 1989.

Sanford, A.: Mineral oil. Oncology Nursing Forum 9:65, 1982.

Somerville, E.: Constipation: A side effect of the vinca alkaloids. Oncology Nursing Forum 9:67, 1982.

Vannicola, P.: Constipation and use of cellulose bulk agents. Oncology Nursing Forum 9:66–67, 1982.

PATIENT EDUCATION MATERIALS AND COMMUNITY RESOURCES

Caring for the Cancer Patient at Home. Atlanta, GA, American Cancer Society, 1988.

Eating Hints: Tips for Better Nutrition During Treatment. Bethesda, MD, National Cancer Institute, 1987.

Home Care of the Hospice Patient. Norwalk, CT, Purdue Frederick Co., 1986.

Patient/Family Guide to Constipation. Long Beach Community Hospital, Hospice Nursing Newsletter 2:3, 1982.

Bowel Elimination, Alteration in: Diarrhea

Jennifer S. Webster

Population at Risk:

- Individuals receiving chemotherapy, or radiation therapy to the abdomen and pelvis
- Individuals with tumors that obstruct or impinge upon the digestive tract
- Individuals undergoing abdominal surgical procedures
- Individuals with altered nutritional status
- Individuals who are immunosuppressed
- Individuals undergoing antimicrobial therapy
- Individuals receiving tube feedings

LEVEL 1: *Potential*

EXPECTED OUTCOME

1. Patient demonstrates knowledge related to potential diarrhea:
   - identifies factors that influence elimination and are potential causes of diarrhea.
   - verbalizes early signs and symptoms of diarrhea and importance of reporting to health care team.
   - verbalizes potential sequelae/complications of diarrhea.
2. Patient demonstrates measures to prevent diarrhea:
   - demonstrates adequate nutritional and fluid intake.
   - eliminates foods and over-the-counter medications that increase potential for loose stools.
   - demonstrates proper administration of medications.
   - initiates stress reduction techniques.
3. Patient demonstrates regular and normal pattern of elimination as evidenced by:
   - stools of normal frequency and consistency.
   - normal bowel sounds.
   - absence of abdominal pain and cramping.

NURSING MANAGEMENT

Assessment

1. Obtain nutrition history and record baseline nutritional status, including weight.

2. Obtain bowel elimination history and record baseline elimination status.
3. Perform baseline abdominal examination and record findings.

4. Identify factors of current disease processes and treatments that predispose patient to diarrhea.
5. Identify foods, beverages, and medications that cause loose stools/diarrhea.
6. Identify and evaluate for physical/psychological stressors that may contribute to decreased appetite or potential for diarrhea.

Nursing Interventions

1. Arrange for low-residue, bland high-protein, high-carbohydrate, balanced diet. Avoid foods that are too hot or too cold, as temperature extremes may stimulate peristalsis.
2. Encourage fluid intake, but avoid liquids that may increase bowel motility such as juices high in acid (orange juice, prune juice, lemonade). Avoid milk products to prevent symptoms of lactose intolerance. Avoid caffeinated or alcoholic beverages.
3. Monitor stools for consistency, frequency, color, and amount.
4. Monitor intake, output, and daily weight.
5. Implement and encourage measures to decrease or cope with stress such as counseling, relaxation training, and communication with family members.

Patient Teaching

1. Explain factors that influence elimination and are potential causes of diarrhea.
2. Discuss sequelae/complications of diarrhea.
3. Identify and review signs and symptoms of diarrhea to report to health care team (e.g., sudden increase in frequency and looseness of bowel movements for more than 2 days in a row, blood in stool or around anal area, fever, drop in urine output/urine discoloration, sudden abdominal distension, development of small amount of diarrhea after several days of constipation, suggesting a fecal impaction).
4. Define and describe daily food requirements (e.g., balanced diet including protein, carbohydrates, fats, calories).
5. Identify foods and fluids that may predispose to diarrhea. Provide patient with written list of foods and fluids allowed and those to avoid.
6. Define and discuss daily fluid requirements.
7. Identify medications that may predispose patient to diarrhea.
8. Identify medications that may reduce potential for diarrhea.
9. Inform patient of relationship between stress and alterations in elimination. Demonstrate stress reduction techniques, if appropriate.

LEVEL 2: Mild to Moderate (Four to Six Stools Per Day)

EXPECTED OUTCOME

1. Patient demonstrates knowledge related to mild to moderate diarrhea:
   - identifies factors that influence elimination and are potential causes of diarrhea.
   - verbalizes signs and symptoms of diarrhea and importance of reporting to health care team.
   - verbalizes potential sequelae/complications of diarrhea.
2. Patient demonstrates measures to control or correct diarrhea:
   - maintains adequate nutritional and fluid intake.

- eliminates foods, fluids, and over-the-counter medications that may contribute to diarrhea.
- demonstrates safe administration of medications.
- demonstrates hygiene and appropriate skin care measures.
- initiates stress reduction techniques.
3. Patient achieves control or correction of diarrhea as evidenced by:
   - stools of normal frequency and consistency.
   - normal or intermittently hyperactive bowel sounds.
   - absence or minimal abdominal pain and cramping.
   - absence or minimal skin breakdown.
   - absence or minimal signs and symptoms of dehydration.

NURSING MANAGEMENT

Assessment

1. See Assessment, Level 1.
2. Determine probable etiology of diarrhea (e.g., infections, treatment side effects, tumor pathology, stress, inappropriate diet). Be alert for possible fecal impaction. Obtain a stool sample if appropriate.
3. Evaluate hydration status (skin turgor, mucous membranes, pulse rate, electrolytes, complaints of thirst, color of urine).
4. Assess intake, output, and daily weight.
5. Perform abdominal examination: assess bowel sounds, abdominal rigidity, tympany, distention, flatus, cramping, pain, discomfort.
6. Assess stools for consistency, frequency, volume, odor, color.
7. Assess for skin excoriation and tenderness in perineal/perianal region.
8. Determine effect on life style.

Nursing Interventions

1. See Nursing Interventions, Level 1.
2. Implement appropriate actions related to the etiology (diet change, stress reduction measures, measures to relieve fecal impaction).
3. Promote fluid intake of at least 3000 ml/day if not contraindicated. Arrange for supplemental hydration, electrolyte replacement, and nutrition as necessary.

4. Administer medications that control diarrhea as ordered. These may be bulk-forming agents (methylcellulose, such as Metamucil), antacids (those that contain aluminum rather than magnesium, such as Amphojel and Basaljel), narcotic agents (opium derivatives such as Lomotil, Imodium, or codeine), and antibiotics (such as tetracycline or vancomycin). These medications are just a few examples of the variety of agents available to control diarrhea.
5. Perform skin care measures for dependent patients. Gently cleanse the perianal region with mild soap and water and pat dry after each bowel movement. Apply moisture barrier to protect the skin and promote healing. Apply a topical anesthetic as necessary.
6. Encourage sitz baths at least 3 to 4 times a day.
7. Encourage verbalization of perceived effect on life style. Offer specific interventions to decrease impact of diarrhea on life style, such as obtaining a bedside commode, increasing frequency of rest periods, using absorbent, disposable pads on bedding to reduce soilage.

Patient Teaching

1. See Patient Teaching, Level 1.
2. Discuss complications of diarrhea (e.g.,

electrolyte imbalance, hypoproteinemia, dehydration). Explain rationale for increasing fluid intake and changing to high-calorie, high-protein, high-carbohydrate diet as appropriate.
3. Describe appropriate hygiene and skin care

measures, and explain the use of topical anesthetics and moisture barriers. Explain and encourage the use of sitz baths.
4. Assist patient to identify and reduce the impact of stressful life events through the use of appropriate relaxation techniques.

LEVEL 3: Severe (More Than Eight Stools per Day)

EXPECTED OUTCOME

1. Patient/caregiver demonstrate knowledge related to severe diarrhea:
   - identify factors that influence elimination and diarrhea.
   - verbalize signs and symptoms of severe diarrhea and importance of notifying health care team promptly upon appearance of these symptoms.
   - verbalize potential sequelae/complications of severe diarrhea.
2. Patient/caregiver demonstrate measures to minimize or treat severe diarrhea:
   - patient maintains adequate nutritional and fluid intake.
   - eliminate foods, fluids, medications that contribute to diarrhea.
   - demonstrate safe administration of medications.
   - demonstrate hygiene and appropriate skin care measures.
   - contribute to long-term care plan.
   - utilize appropriate community resources.
3. Patient achieves or maintains defecation pattern normal for age and condition as evidenced by:
   - improved frequency and consistency of stools.
   - decreased hyperactivity of bowel sounds.
   - decreased abdominal pain and cramping.
   - absence or minimal skin breakdown.
   - absence of signs and symptoms of dehydration and malnutrition.

NURSING MANAGEMENT

Assessment

1. See Assessment, Levels 1 and 2.
2. Record number, frequency, volume, and character of bowel movements.
3. Assess laboratory values (CBC, electrolytes, serum protein).

Nursing Interventions

1. See Nursing Interventions, Levels 1 and 2.

2. Institute liquid diet with high-protein and calorie supplements.
3. Implement tube feedings or total parenteral nutrition per physician order if patient is unable to maintain oral feeding.
4. Administer fluid and electrolyte replacements as ordered.
5. Administer antidiarrheals, antispasmodics, or antianxiety agents as ordered.
6. Perform thorough skin care after each bowel movement, as described previously, using topical moisture barriers and

anesthetics as needed. For skin break-down uncontrolled by these measures, refer to skin care literature and a skin care specialist, if available.

7. Check patient q1–2h for elimination of stool if patient is unable to communicate needs.

8. During severe episodes of diarrhea, patient may require a pouch or rectal bag. Refer to literature and an enterostomal therapist, if available.

9. Offer specific interventions to decrease impact of diarrhea on life style, such as obtaining a bedside commode, increasing frequency of rest periods, using absorbent disposable pads on bedding to collect moisture and reduce soilage, using disposable pads in underwear to absorb uncontrolled elimination from rectum.

10. Implement and encourage stress reduction techniques for the caregivers/family members as necessary, providing them with specific interventions to reduce the physical and emotional effort required to care for the patient with severe diarrhea.

11. Coordinate a multidisciplinary team approach to management of the patient's diarrhea that may include physician involvement, nursing, social services, enterostomal therapists, and physical and occupational therapy.

Patient Teaching

1. See Patient Teaching, Levels 1 and 2.
2. Teach administration, schedule, and potential side effects of medications.
3. Explain course and goals of treatment program.

SUGGESTED READINGS

Basch, A.: Changes in elimination. Seminars in Oncology Nursing 3(4):287–292, 1987.

Boyer, J.: Nutrition. *In* Beyers, M., Durburg, S., and Werner, J. (Eds.): Complete Guide to Cancer Nursing. Oradell, NJ, Medical Economics Co., 1984, pp. 199–218.

Culhane, B.: Diarrhea. *In* Yasko, J. (Ed.): Guidelines for Cancer Care: Symptom Management. Reston, VA, Reston Publishing, 1983.

Donoghue, M., Nunnally, C., and Yasko, J.M.: Nutritional Aspects of Cancer Care. Reston, VA, Reston Publishing, 1982.

Hilderley, L.J.: Radiotherapy. *In* Groenwald, S.L., et al. (Eds.): Cancer Nursing Principles and Practice. Boston, Jones & Bartlett Publishers, 1987, pp. 340–341.

Ropka, M.E.: Nutrition. *In* Johnson, B.L., and Gross, J. (Eds.): Handbook of Oncology Nursing. Bethany, CT, Fleschner Publishing, 1985, pp. 209–211.

Trester, A.K.: Nursing management of patients receiving cancer chemotherapy. Cancer Nursing 5:201–210, 1982.

PATIENT EDUCATION MATERIALS AND COMMUNITY RESOURCES

American Cancer Society: Caring for the Patient with Cancer at Home: A Guide for Patients and Families. 1988. pp. 20–21.

Bowel Elimination, Alteration in: Bowel Obstruction

Marcia Rostad

Population at Risk

- Individuals with tumors of colon, rectum, ovary, uterus, or kidney
- Individuals with soft-tissue sarcoma or malignant lymphoma of colon
- Individuals receiving chemotherapy from vinca alkaloid group (vincristine, vinblastine)
- Individuals with history of radiation therapy to abdomen

LEVEL 1: Potential

EXPECTED OUTCOME

1. Patient demonstrates knowledge of potential bowel obstruction:
   - identifies early signs and symptoms of bowel obstruction to report to health care team.
   - states measures to maintain regular bowel elimination.
2. Patient maintains normal bowel elimination as evidenced by:
   - soft, formed, brown stools passed on a regular basis.
   - absence of abnormal cramping with elimination.

NURSING MANAGEMENT

Assessment

1. Assess frequency, color, and consistency of stools.
2. Determine presence of risk factors (e.g., abdominal metastasis from a primary tumor, adhesions around ostomies).
3. Evaluate treatment and disease factors that might affect bowel function (e.g., treatment with vinca alkaloids).

Patient Teaching

1. Teach signs and symptoms of bowel obstruction to report to health care team:
   - cramping.
   - diarrhea or absence of defecation.
   - abdominal distention, pain.
   - nausea.
   - vomiting.
   - absence of flatus and stools.

2. Discuss rationale and measures to maintain adequate bowel elimination:
   - adequate bulk in diet.
   - adequate fluid intake.
   - need for activity—may include passive and active range of motion.

LEVEL 2: *Mild to Moderate (Partial Bowel Obstruction)*

EXPECTED OUTCOME

1. Patient demonstrates knowledge related to bowel obstruction:
   - verbalizes signs and symptoms of obstruction.
   - identifies factors that influence bowel function.
   - identifies potential sequelae/complications.
2. Patient identifies/demonstrates measures to promote bowel elimination:
   - demonstrates proper knowledge and administration of medications.
   - verbalizes/demonstrates adequate food and fluid intake.
   - identifies signs and symptoms necessary to report to health care team.
3. Patient maintains adequate bowel elimination as evidenced by:
   - soft, formed stools.
   - absence of severe cramping with bowel elimination.

NURSING MANAGEMENT

Assessment

1. See Assessment, Level 1.
2. Obtain history of current bowel functioning status:
   - frequency, color, consistency of stools.
   - abdominal distention.
3. Auscultate bowel sounds; note character. Bowel obstruction produces loud, gurgling, wave-like peristaltic sounds usually accompanied by abdominal pain.
4. Note signs and symptoms of obstruction:
   - abdominal distention.
   - absence of stool or diarrhea.
   - discharge of blood or mucus from rectum.
   - presence of nausea and vomiting. Emesis progresses from stomach contents to green bile-like material, to light-brown emesis with fecal odor.
   - wave-like abdominal pain, cramping.
5. Determine nutritional status:
   - food intake.
   - weight.
   - change in biceps measurement.
6. Assess hydrational status:
   - mucous membrane status.
   - skin turgor.
7. Check laboratory studies (e.g., hemoglobin, hematocrit, WBC, platelet count).
8. Check for treatment with drugs that may affect peristalsis (e.g., narcotics, vinca alkaloids).
9. Assess for presence of tenesmus.
10. Do digital rectal examination for presence of fecal mass.

Nursing Interventions

1. Administer medications as prescribed (e.g., analgesics, laxatives, stool softeners, antiemetics).
2. Maintain record of signs and symptoms (e.g., bowel sounds, temperature, abdomi-

nal girth, expulsion of flatus or stool). Report changes to physician.
3. Increase fluid intake. If patient is unable to ingest sufficient oral fluids, obtain order for IV fluids.
4. Monitor intake and output.

Patient Teaching

1. See Patient Teaching, Level 1.
2. Encourage patient to notify health care team promptly of any signs and symptoms.

3. Emphasize need to maintain adequate nutritional and fluid intake, suggesting ways to achieve this (e.g., eat small, frequent meals, drink small amounts of fluids frequently).
4. Instruct patient on measurement of intake and output.
5. Explain purpose and side effects of medications.
6. Discuss diagnostic studies to be performed and rationale for same.

LEVEL 3:   Severe (Complete Bowel Obstruction)

EXPECTED OUTCOME

1. Patient/caregiver demonstrate knowledge of bowel obstruction:
   - identify signs and symptoms of bowel obstruction.
   - identify complications of bowel obstruction.
   - identify medical/surgical treatment for bowel obstruction and rationale for same.
2. Patient/caregiver demonstrate measures to control or manage bowel obstruction:
   - perform necessary treatments and procedures.
   - demonstrate proper knowledge and administration of medication.
   - verbalize/demonstrate adequate nutritional and fluid intake.
3. Patient demonstrates optimal level of comfort as evidenced by:
   - absent or tolerable pain.
   - absence of nausea and vomiting.
   - absence of cramping.

NURSING MANAGEMENT

Assessment

1. See Assessment, Levels 1 and 2.
2. Obtain history of rectal bleeding.
3. Determine patient's knowledge of seriousness of bowel obstruction, treatments, and possibility of a colostomy.
4. Assess patient's ability to cope.

Nursing Interventions

1. See Nursing Interventions, Levels 1 and 2.
2. Administer medications, IV fluids, and blood as ordered.
3. Care for nasogastric intubation following usual nursing procedure:

- anchor tubing.
- allow to drain or attach suction as ordered.
- provide oral hygiene frequently.
- provide emollient for lips and nostrils to prevent crusting.
- monitor output.

4. If colon drainage tube is used, follow procedures for nasogastric intubation, except anchor permanently. Advance tube periodically as ordered.
5. Record and report changes in patient status.
6. Provide measures to promote comfort (e.g., position change, oral hygiene, back rubs).
7. Monitor for electrolyte imbalance (serum sodium, potassium chloride, carbon dioxide, and arterial blood gases).
8. Prepare patient for surgery to relieve obstruction (see Chapter 15).
9. Provide postoperative care to colostomy patients (see Chapter 48).
10. Provide emotional support to patient/family.

Patient Teaching

1. See Patient Teaching, Level 2.
2. Discuss medical/surgical treatments for bowel obstruction and rationale for the same:
   - intestinal intubation to decompress intestine.
   - IV fluids to maintain fluid and electrolyte balance, colostomy to relieve obstruction.
3. Teach measures to manage colostomy (see Chapter 48).

SUGGESTED READINGS

Beaton, H.L.: Abdominal surgerical emergencies in patients with cancer. Topics in Emergency Medicine *8*(2):45–52, 1986.

Bullock, B.L.: Normal function of the gastrointestinal system. *In* Bullock, B.L., and Rosendahl, P.P. (Eds.): Pathophysiology: Adaptations and Alterations in Function. Boston, Little, Brown & Co., 1984.

Cargill, N.D.: Buying time when you face a bowel obstruction. RN *48*(8):40–44, 58, 1985.

Chernecky, C.C., and Ramsey P.W.: Critical Nursing Care of the Client with Cancer. Norwalk, CT, Appleton-Century-Crofts, 1984.

Davis, L.S.: Bowel obstruction. *In* Johnson, B.L., and Gross, J. (Eds.): Handbook of Oncology Nursing. Bethany, CT, Fleshner Publishing Co., 1985.

Given, B.A., and Simmons, S.J.: Gastroenterology in Clinical Nursing. St. Louis, C.V. Mosby, 1984.

Luckman, J., and Sorensen, K.C. (Eds.): Medical-Surgical Nursing. Philadelphia, W.B. Saunders, 1987, pp. 1317–1326.

Mayer, D.K.: Diagnosis and management of intestinal obstruction in individuals with cancer. Nurse Practitioner *11*(2):35,38,41, 1986.

McConnell, E.A.: Meeting the challenge of intestinal obstruction. Nursing *17*(7):34–42, 1987.

McCormick, A., Itkin, J., and Cloud, C.: RN master care plans: the patient with intestinal blockage. RN *48*(8):45–46, 1985.

Rottenberg, R.: Acute abdomen: When you suspect intestinal obstruction. Patient Care *18*(18):72–77, 80–82, 84–87, 1984.

Spiro, H.M.: Clinical Gastroenterology, New York, Macmillan, 1989.

Bowel Elimination, Alteration in: Diversional Methods

Mary McCarty Spencer

48

Population at Risk

- Individuals with colon cancer, ovarian cancer, uterine cancer, abdominal metastases, bowel obstruction

LEVEL 1: Potential

EXPECTED OUTCOME

Patient demonstrates knowledge related to potential diversional method of bowel elimination:
- verbalizes understanding of planned surgical procedure.
- verbalizes understanding of stoma appearance and function.
- verbalizes plans of stoma care as part of daily routine.

NURSING MANAGEMENT

Assessment

1. Do complete preoperative assessment, as for all major surgery.
2. Evaluate patient's knowledge of:
   - surgical procedure.
   - stoma appearance, location, function.
   - stoma care as part of activities of daily living.
3. Determine physical ability to do independent ostomy care (eyesight, physical strength, ability to use hands and fingers).
4. Gauge patient's reaction to prospect of ostomy.

Nursing Interventions

1. Consult enterostomal therapist if available.
2. Allow patient to ventilate fears, including previous experience regarding ostomies.
3. Reassure patient that fears are normal and that enterostomal therapist and nursing staff will assist patient/significant other to learn independent ostomy care.
4. Ensure that enterostomal therapist or surgeon has marked stoma site before surgery.
5. Provide opportunity for patient to meet well-adjusted ostomate.

Patient Teaching

1. Provide preoperative information regarding:
   - surgical procedure.
   - normal/ostomy anatomy and physiology, of gastrointestinal tract.
   - location of stoma.
   - appearance of stoma:
     ◦ color (pink).
     ◦ texture (mucous membrane—like inside of lips).
     ◦ absence of sensation in stoma.
2. Provide brief demonstration of pouch system.

LEVEL 2: Normal Postoperative

EXPECTED OUTCOME

1. Patient demonstrates knowledge related to diversional method of bowel elimination:
   - identifies changes in bowel habits.
   - verbalizes signs and symptoms of malfunctioning ostomy to report to health care team.
   - identifies potential complications of surgical intervention.
2. Patient identifies/demonstrates measures to manage alteration in bowel elimination:
   - independently performs ostomy care.
   - identifies/demonstrates measures that promote maintenance of peristomal skin.
   - identifies appropriate food and fluid intake.
   - verbalizes/demonstrates necessary life style adaptations.
   - identifies/utilizes appropriate community resources.
   - identifies appropriate long-term care plan.
3. Patient demonstrates bowel elimination within normal limits for patient:
   - stool consistency appropriate.
   - stool quantity adequate.
   - return of peristalsis within 5 days.

NURSING MANAGEMENT

Assessment

1. See Assessment, Level 1.
2. Check for viable stoma:
   - stoma should be pink (darkened stoma indicates necrosis from inadequate vascular supply).
   - peristomal skin should be intact and not irritated.
3. Assess bowel sounds.
4. Check for appropriate output from ostomy:
   - ileostomy: thin effluent (drainage) immediately.

- cecostomy: thin effluent (drainage).
- ascending colostomy (right): paste-like fecal output.
- transverse: paste-like thin fecal output.
- descending/sigmoid (left): thick, solid fecal output.

5. Assess if ostomy pouch is appropriate:
   - drainable pouch.
   - opening around stoma ⅛ to ¹⁄₁₆ inch larger than stoma.
   - no leakage under pouch.
   - optional features–gas filters, odor proofing, color and material of pouch.
6. Evaluate peristomal skin care practices of patient.
7. Determine nutritional and fluid status.
8. Ascertain occupational, recreational, social, and spiritual activities.
9. Evaluate support system.
10. Assess financial needs.

Nursing Interventions

1. Measure and apply appropriate size and type of pouch (should open and have clamp at bottom for drainage).
2. Gently change pouch every 3 to 5 days (otherwise can empty or drain flatus or feces) as appropriate for individual patient.
3. Record amount and type of output.
4. Consult enterostomal therapist, if available, for discharge planning.
5. Provide peristomal skin care:
   - clean skin gently with warm water (mild soap may be used, but should be thoroughly rinsed off).
   - allow skin to air-dry (gauze may be used to retain liquid contents from stoma during skin care).
   - apply pouch with appropriate adhesive:
     - ileostomy and cecostomy: skin barrier (e.g., Stomahesive, Hollihesive), or plasticized skin covering (e.g., Skin Prep Skin Gel).
     - transverse colostomy: same as for ileostomy.
     - sigmoid/descending colostomy: possible to wear closed pouch or stoma covering if regulated with irrigation.
6. Consult enterostomal therapist, if available, for complications of peristomal skin, stoma, or difficulty with pouch adherence.
7. Make referral for visit from well-adjusted ostomate.

Patient Teaching

1. See Patient Teaching, Level 1.
2. Implement ostomy teaching as soon as patient is alert and has physical strength to actively participate.
3. Refer to home health nurse or outpatient consultation with enterostomal therapist if patient cannot perform ostomy care independently before discharge.
4. Provide patient with written information.
5. Consult with clinical dietitian or enterostomal therapist for patient's dietary considerations:
   - foods that cause blockage in ileostomy (e.g., popcorn, nuts, spinach, lettuce).
   - foods that cause odor or flatus (e.g., beans, cabbage, carbonated beverages).
6. Provide printed information on ostomy appliance and place of purchase, along with how to measure for appropriate size.
7. Ensure that patient has printed information with names and phone numbers of enterostomal therapist and physician for consultation.
8. Describe helpful hints for social, sexual, or professional activities. If appropriate, include significant other in discussion.
9. Give information concerning future radiation or chemotherapy, if indicated (see chapters 11 and 12).
10. Provide reassurance, instruction, positive feedback, and supervision during learning process.
11. Discuss community resources (e.g., American Cancer Society, United Ostomy Association, and vocational rehabilitation service support).

LEVEL 3: Problems and Complications

EXPECTED OUTCOME

1. Patient/caregiver demonstrate knowledge related to problems and complications of diversional method:
   - identify signs and symptoms of complications.
   - verbalize factors influencing problem(s).
   - identify potential sequelae.
2. Patient/caregiver identify/demonstrate measures to manage or resolve identified problem(s):
   - perform necessary treatments and procedures.
   - demonstrate proper knowledge and administration of medications.
   - identify signs and symptoms to report to health care team.
   - identify/utilize appropriate community resources.
   - verbalize/demonstrate necessary life style adaptations.
   - identify appropriate long-term follow-up plan of care.
3. Patient achieves/maintains adequate functioning of diversional method with resolution or control of associated problems:
   - adequate bowel elimination.
   - absence or control of skin breakdown.
   - stoma that remains viable.

NURSING MANAGEMENT

Assessment

1. See Assessment, Levels 1 and 2.
2. Determine area causing pain or discomfort (e.g., peristomal skin, stomal function).
3. Assess stomal output (type, amount, odor).
4. Take patient's vital signs.
5. Evaluate laboratory studies (electrolytes, CBC).
6. Obtain history of problem:
   - onset.
   - symptoms.
   - factors that relieve or worsen symptoms.
   - course of symptoms.
   - actions of patient preceding symptoms (diet, exercise, travel, exposure to illness, medication, chemotherapy, radiation therapy).
7. Observe stoma appearance.
8. Check peristomal skin.
9. Check pouch fit and size.
10. Assess patient's hygiene and routine of ostomy care.
11. Assess nutritional and hydrational status.

Nursing Interventions

1. See Nursing Interventions, Levels 1 and 2.
2. For excoriated peristomal skin, proceed as follows:
   - remove pouch.
   - clean gently with warm water only.
   - allow skin to air-dry.
   - apply skin barrier to skin—should be cut with opening for stoma. Do not use alcohol, Skin Prep, or any product with alcohol.
   - if peristomal skin is erythematous or maculopapular rash is present, patient may have candidal infection. Notify

physician and obtain order for nystatin (Mycostatin) powder. Apply thin layer of powder before applying pouch.
- apply pouch to skin barrier.
- change gently and record appearance.
- consult enterostomal therapist or physician.
3. For obstruction of output, proceed as follows:
- consult physician.
- if patient usually irrigates sigmoid or descending colostomy, may irrigate with 30 ml warm water. Teach colostomy patient to eat more fiber and drink more fluids.
- if ileostomy stoma obstruction, consult physician. Do not irrigate (physician or enterostomal therapist may use gentle lavage).
- teach or reinforce dietary considerations of food that may cause blockage; instruct patient to increase fluid intake.
4. For stoma prolapse (elongation), proceed as follows:
- inform physician immediately.
- place patient in prone position.
- remove pouch, apply saline soaked gauze; may need larger opening of pouch around stoma.
- assess color of stoma, output, subjective pain, retraction when in prone position.
5. For stoma retraction, proceed as follows:
- consult/inform physician and enterostomal therapy nurse.
- assess pouch adherence.
- apply adhesive paste or barrier in crease or retracted area; apply pouch; patient may need to wear belt with pouch.
6. For change in effluence (e.g., diarrhea from radiation, enteritis), proceed as follows:
- contact physician if change lasts more than 24 hours.
- monitor intake and output.
- monitor hydrational status.
- encourage fluids.
- arrange for low-residue diet.
- administer antidiarrheal medications as ordered.
- consult enterostomal therapy nurse.

Patient Teaching

1. See Patient Teaching, Level 2.
2. Outline measures to maintain fluid and electrolyte balance:
- encourage patient to drink 4 to 6 glasses of fluid per day.
- ileostomy patients are more prone to fluid loss and electrolyte imbalance.
- Gatorade is excellent replacement if patient has diarrhea or perspiration.
3. See Nursing Interventions for care of peristomal skin.
4. Teach signs and symptoms to report to health care team.

SUGGESTED READINGS

Broadwell, D., and Jackson, B.: Principles of Ostomy Care. St. Louis, C.V. Mosby, 1982.

Burns, N.: Nursing and Cancer. Philadelphia, W.B. Saunders, 1982.

Given, B.A., and Simmons, S.J.: Gastroenterology in Clinical Nursing (ed. 3). St. Louis, C.V. Mosby, 1979.

Groenwald, S.: Cancer Nursing: Principles and Practices. Boston, Jones & Bartlett, 1987.

Jensen, V.: Better Techniques for Bagging Stomas, Part 3: Ileostomies. Nursing 4:60–63, 1974.

Kneisl, C.R., and Ames S.A.: Adult Health Nursing: A Biophysical Social Approach. Reading, PA, Addison-Wesley. 1986.

Simmons, K.N.: Sexuality and the female ostomate. American Journal of Nursing 83:409–411, 1983.

Traverso, C.: SOAP noting common stomal problems. Journal of Enterostomy Therapy 7:(1,2,3), 1980.

PATIENT EDUCATION MATERIALS AND COMMUNITY RESOURCES

American Cancer Society; 1599 Clifton Road NE, Atlanta GA 30329, or contact local chapter.

International Association of Enterostomal Therapy, 2081 Business Center Drive, Suite 290, Irvine, CA 92715 (literature available from distributors/representatives of ostomy products).

United Ostomy Association, Inc., 36 Executive Park, Suite 120, Irvine, CA 92714 (Phone 714–660–8624).

49 Urinary Elimination, Alteration in: Diversional Methods

Mary McCarty Spencer

Population at Risk

- Individuals with bladder cancer, ovarian cancer, uterine cancer, or pelvic metastases of colorectal cancer

LEVEL 1: Potential

EXPECTED OUTCOME

Patient demonstrates knowledge related to potential diversional methods of urinary elimination:
- verbalizes understanding of planned surgical procedure.
- verbalizes understanding of stoma appearance and function.
- verbalizes necessity of stoma care as part of activities of daily living.

NURSING MANAGEMENT

Assessment

1. Do complete preoperative physical as for all major surgery.
2. Evaluate patient's knowledge of:
   - surgical procedure.
   - stoma appearance, location, function.
   - stoma care as part of activities of daily living.
3. Determine physical ability (eyesight, fine motor skills) to perform ostomy care.
4. Assess coping mechanisms.

Nursing Interventions

1. Consult enterostomal therapist, if available.
2. Allow patient to ventilate fears, including previous experience regarding ostomies.
3. Reassure patient that fears are normal and that enterostomal therapist and nursing staff will assist patient/significant other to learn independent ostomy care.
4. Ensure that enterostomal therapist or surgeon has marked stoma site before surgery.
5. Provide opportunity for patient to meet well-adjusted ostomate.

Patient Teaching

1. Provide preoperative information regarding surgical procedure to be performed.
2. Explain normal and ostomy anatomy and physiology of genitourinary tract.

3. Describe stoma appearance:
   - color (pink).
   - texture (mucous membrane—like inside of lips).
   - absence of sensation in stoma.
4. Provide brief demonstration of pouch system.

LEVEL 2: Normal Postoperative

EXPECTED OUTCOME

1. Patient demonstrates knowledge related to diversional method of urinary elimination:
   - identifies changes in urinary habits.
   - verbalizes signs and symptoms of malfunctioning ostomy to report to health care team.
   - identifies potential complications of surgical intervention.
2. Patient identifies/demonstrates measures to manage urinary alteration:
   - demonstrates bag emptying and changing.
   - identifies/demonstrates measures to promote maintenance of peristomal skin.
   - verbalizes/demonstrates necessary life style adaptations.
   - identifies/utilizes appropriate community resources.
   - identifies appropriate long-term care plan.
3. Patient demonstrates adequate urinary elimination:
   - clear urine (may have whitish mucus).
   - absence of foul odor.
   - absence of concentrated, dark urine.
   - absence of blood in urine (after first 24 hours after surgery).
   - intake and output within normal limits.

NURSING MANAGEMENT

Assessment

1. See Assessment, Level 1.
2. Check for viable stoma:
   - stoma should be pink (darkened stoma indicates necrosis from inadequate vascular supply)
   - ideal stoma protrudes ½ to ¾ inch above skin to allow urine to drain into pouch.
   - peristomal skin should be intact and not irritated.
3. See that output is appropriate (>60 ml/ hr, mucus in urine, hematuria normal only 24 hours after surgery).
4. Do not pull on stents, if present.
5. Check presence and patency of nephrostomy tubes, if appropriate.
6. Examine for appropriate pouch for stoma:
   - drainable urostomy pouch with connector for bedside container.
   - no karaya seal (urine dissolves karaya, seal is lost).
   - no leakage under pouch.

- opening around stoma same size and shape as stoma.
7. Evaluate peristomal skin and patient's skin care practices.
8. Determine nutritional and fluid status.
9. Ascertain occupational, recreational, social, and spiritual activities.
10. Evaluate support systems.
11. Assess financial needs.

Nursing Interventions

1. Measure and apply appropriate size and type of pouch (see Assessment, Level 2).
2. Gently change pouch q3–5d.
3. Provide peristomal skin care:
   - clean skin gently with warm water (mild soap may be used but should be thoroughly washed off).
   - allow skin to air-dry (may use gauze over stoma or tampon in stoma to prevent urine from draining on skin).
   - apply pouch with appropriate adhesive (may use Stomahesive, Reliaseal, Hollihesive wafer for skin protection).
4. Consult enterostomal therapist for fitting patient with appropriate pouch system (may use permanent pouch system with reusable faceplate and pouches or a 2-piece disposable system).
5. Consult physician and enterostomal therapist for complications of peristomal skin and stoma, or difficulty with pouch adherence, foul-smelling or bloody urine.
6. Maintain strict aseptic technique when caring for nephrostomy.
7. Make referral for visit from well-adjusted ostomate.

Patient Teaching

1. See Patient Teaching, Level 1.
2. Implement ostomy teaching as soon as patient is alert and has the physical strength to participate.
3. Refer to home health nurse or outpatient enterostomal therapist if patient can not perform ostomy care independently.
4. Provide patient with written information regarding ostomy care before discharge from hospital.
5. Consult with clinical dietitian or enterostomal therapist regarding dietary needs.
   - explain need for increased fluid intake.
   - cranberry juice and vitamin C tablets help prevent infection in urine.
   - asparagus may give urine a pungent odor.
6. Provide printed information on ostomy appliance and place of purchase, along with how to measure for appropriate size.
7. Ensure that patient has printed information with names and phone numbers of enterostomal therapist, home health nurse, and physician for consultation.
8. Give information concerning future radiation or chemotherapy, if indicated (see Chapters 11 and 12).
9. Provide reassurance, instruction, positive feedback, and supervision during learning process.
10. Consult enterostomal therapist to plan discharge teaching.
11. Instruct patient to use bedside drainage or larger pouch at night. Some patients prefer to get up during night and empty pouch. This prevents pouch from becoming too full and leaking or pulling off.
12. Discuss community resources (e.g., American Cancer Society, United Ostomy Association, vocational rehabilitation service).
13. Describe care of nephrostomy.
14. If sexual dysfunction is anticipated (erectile impotence) provide information on penile prosthesis.
15. Provide suggestions for social, professional, or sexual activities (if appropriate, include significant other in discussion).

EXPECTED OUTCOME

1. Patient/caregiver demonstrate knowledge related to problems and complications of diversional method:
   * identify signs and symptoms of complications.
   * verbalize factors influencing problem(s).
2. Patient/caregiver identify/demonstrate measures to manage or resolve identified problem(s):
   * perform necessary treatments and procedures.
   * demonstrate proper knowledge and administration of medications.
   * identify signs and symptoms to report to health care team.
   * identify/utilize appropriate community resources.
   * verbalize/demonstrate necessary life style adaptations.
   * identify appropriate long-term follow-up plan of care.
3. Patient achieves/maintains adequate functioning of diversional method with resolution or control of associated problems:
   * establishes adequate urinary elimination.
   * maintains intake and output within normal limits.
   * shows absence or control of signs and symptoms of urinary tract infection.
   * shows absence or control of skin breakdown.

NURSING MANAGEMENT

Assessment

1. See Assessment, Level 2.
2. Assess area causing pain or discomfort (e.g., peristomal skin, stomal function).
3. Check patient's vital signs.
4. Evaluate laboratory studies: electrolytes, urinalysis, blood urea nitrogen, creatinine, CBC.
5. Obtain history of problem:
   * onset.
   * symptoms.
   * factors that relieve or worsen symptoms.
   * actions of patient preceding symptoms (diet, exercise, travel, exposure to illness, medications).
6. Assess patient's hygiene and routine of ostomy care.

Nursing Interventions

1. See Nursing Interventions, Levels 1 and 2.
2. For excoriated peristomal skin, proceed as follows:
   * remove pouch.
   * clean gently with warm water only.
   * apply Stomahesive, Reliaseal, or Hollihesive to skin to act as barrier—should be cut with opening for stoma; do not use alcohol, Skin Prep, or any product containing alcohol.
   * apply pouch to skin barrier.
   * change gently, record appearance.
3. For urinary tract infection, proceed as follows:
   * encourage fluids.
   * administer medications.
   * monitor intake and output.

- check temperature.
- observe output (color, odor).
4. Treat obstruction of nephrostomy tubes:
   - irrigate per physician order.
   - use strict aseptic technique in providing care.

Patient Teaching

1. See Patient Teaching, Level 2.
2. Instruct patient to have urinalysis done q6mo or if signs of infection develop (change in color or odor of urine).
3. Instruct patient to drink 6 to 8 glasses of fluid per day, more in hot weather or when exercising.
4. Ensure that patient has names and phone numbers of physician, enterostomal therapist, and home health nurse, as appropriate.
5. Instruct patient to take 500–1000 mg/day of vitamin C (consult with physician).
6. Encourage patient to consult physician or enterostomal therapist if:
   - urine is foul-smelling (may indicate infection).
   - stoma becomes retracted (urine may leak around appliance).
   - crystals form on peristomal skin (may need vinegar soaks on peristomal skin and faceplate, or appliance opening around stoma may be too large).
7. Instruct patient to periodically check pouch opening around stoma (stoma size may have decreased since surgery).
8. Instruct that some foods (such as asparagus) may give urine a pungent odor; and some medications may alter the color of urine.
9. Tell patient to change pouch (with 2-piece system) or add ostomy deodorant to pouch to decrease odor.
10. Instruct patient/caregiver regarding need for and methods of good handwashing.

SUGGESTED READINGS

Broadwell, D., and Jackson, B.: Principles of Ostomy Care. St. Louis, C.V. Mosby, 1982.

Burns, N.: Nursing and Cancer. Philadelphia, W.B. Saunders, 1982.

Given, B.A., and Simmons, S.J.: Gastroenterology in Clinical Nursing (ed. 3). St. Louis, C.V. Mosby, 1979.

Groenwald, S.: Cancer Nursing: Principles and Practices. Boston, Jones & Bartlett, 1987.

Kneisl, C.R., and Ames, S.A.: Adult Health Nursing: A Biopsychosocial Approach. Reading, MA, Addison-Wesley. 1986.

Simmons, K.N.: Sexuality and the female ostomate. American Journal of Nursing 83:409–411, 1983.

Traverso, C.: SOAP noting common stomal problems. Journal of Enterostomy Therapy 7:(1,2,3), 1980.

PATIENT EDUCATION MATERIALS AND COMMUNITY RESOURCES

American Cancer Society, 1599 Clifton Road NE, Atlanta, GA 30329, or contact local chapter.

International Association of Enterostomal Therapy, 1081 Business Center Drive, Suite 290, Irvine, CA 92715 (literature available from distributors/representatives of ostomy products).

United Ostomy Association, Inc., 36 Executive Park, Suite 120, Irvine, CA 92714 (Phone 714–660-8624).

Urinary Elimination, Alteration in: Bladder Irritation

Haidee F. Waters and Patricia A. Stuckey

50

Population at Risk

- Individuals receiving cyclophosphamide, ifosfamide, bleomycin, busulfan, nitrogen mustard, penicillins, doxorubicin HCl with prior administration of cyclophosphamide/pelvic irradiation causing urotoxicity (other reported potential urotoxic drug combinations include vinblastine and bleomycin and vincristine and nitrogen mustard)
- Individuals with bladder cancer

LEVEL 1: Potential Bladder Irritation/Cystitis/Hematuria

EXPECTED OUTCOME

1. Patient demonstrates knowledge related to potential bladder irritation:
   - verbalizes signs and symptoms of bladder irritation.
   - identifies potential causes of bladder irritation.
2. Patient maintains urinary elimination within normal limits:
   - absence of signs and symptoms of cystitis and hematuria.
   - laboratory tests within normal limits.
   - intake and output with normal limits.
3. Patient identifies/demonstrates measures to prevent or minimize urotoxicity:
   - verbalizes/demonstrates adequate fluid intake.
   - demonstrates proper knowledge and administration of medications.
   - demonstrates appropriate voiding habits.
   - identifies signs and symptoms to report to health care team.

NURSING MANAGEMENT

Assessment

1. Assess pattern of fluid intake.
2. Determine pattern of urination.
3. Identify factors associated with increased risk of urotoxicity:
   - internal or external pelvic irradiation.
   - cyclophosphamide (unrelated to dosage, long-term oral therapy, IV administration).
   - ifosfamide (single high dose given without uroprotective agent).
   - busulfan.
   - nitrogen mustard.
   - penicillins (penicillinase-resistant and penicillin G).

321

- administration of doxorubicin HCl following previous treatment with cyclophosphamide.
- combination of cyclophosphamide and pelvic irradiation.
- history of bladder cancer.
4. Assess for other causes of urinary signs and symptoms:
   - evidence of infection (fever, flank pain, positive urine culture).
   - platelet count $< 50,000/mm^3$.
5. Observe and report:
   - signs and symptoms of urotoxicity:
   - dysuria, frequency, urgency, burning (cystitis), mild incontinence, enuresis.
   - characteristics of urine (color, odor).
   - blood in urine (by dipstick or > 5 RBCs/high power field).
   - inappropriately concentrated urine (specific gravity > 1.030).

Nursing Interventions

1. Minimize effects of internal or external pelvic irradiation/contact of toxic metabolites of alkylating agents (cyclophosphamide, ifosfamide, nitrogen mustard, busulfan) with bladder wall:
   - record accurate intake and output for 48 hours after drug administration.
   - encourage high fluid intake (3 to 4 l/24 hr) before and 48 hours after drug administration (unless contraindicated).
   - encourage frequent voiding (q2–4h). Patient should not hold urine.
   - bladder should be emptied before retiring and if awakened at night.
   - administer cyclophosphamide and ifosfamide early in day to prevent urine pooling in bladder overnight.
   - administer mesna (uroprotective agent) as ordered before ifosfamide administration and then either intermittently or continuously according to protocol thereafter.
   - observe for decrease in urine output 4 to 12 hours after cyclophosphamide administration (syndrome of inappropri-

ate antidiuretic hormone secondary to cyclophosphamide).
   - consult with physician regarding possible need for diuretics and desirability of alkalinization of urine with sodium bicarbonate.
   - check pH of urine as appropriate.
2. If nausea or vomiting prevents adequate oral intake of fluids, IV fluids should be administered (consult physician).
3. Test urine with a dipstick for blood daily or at each clinic, office, or home visit (as per assessment).

Patient Teaching

1. Teach relationship between contact of metabolites of alkylating agents in the urine and the bladder wall:
   - need for high fluid volume (3 to 4 l/day or 12 to 16 glasses of liquid) beginning 24 hours before drug administration and continuing for 48 hours after administration.
   - frequent voiding or empty bladder before retiring.
   - oral dosage of cyclophosphamide or busulfan taken in morning after eating/ early evening, not later than 6 PM with increased fluid intake.
2. Explain relationship between pelvic irradiation and cystitis.
3. Encourage foods contributing to an alkaline urine (e.g., all vegetables, fruit juices, milk).
4. Encourage avoidance of foods and other substances that may be irritating to epithelial lining of bladder (coffee or tea, alcoholic beverages, spices, tobacco products).
5. Teach signs and symptoms of urotoxicity.
6. Explain relationship between pelvic irradiation and cyclophosphamide administration and secondary bladder cancer and measures to manage:
   - need for long-term follow-up.
   - signs and symptoms of bladder cancer:
     ○ hematuria.

- ○ frequency, dysuria, burning, urgency.
- ○ difficulty starting stream; incomplete emptying of bladder.

LEVEL 2: *Cystitis/Hematuria*

EXPECTED OUTCOME

1. Patient demonstrates knowledge related to bladder irritation:
   - identifies signs and symptoms of cystitis, hematuria.
   - identifies causative factors pertinent to patient.
   - identifies potential sequelae/complications.
2. Patient demonstrates measures to prevent, correct, or manage bladder irritation:
   - verbalizes/demonstrates nutritional and fluid intake.
   - demonstrates proper knowledge and administration of medications.
   - demonstrates appropriate voiding patterns.
   - identifies signs and symptoms to report to health care team.
   - identifies plan for long-term follow-up care.
3. Patient achieves urinary elimination within normal limits:
   - absence of signs and symptoms of cystitis/hematuria.
   - intake and output within normal limits.
   - laboratory tests within normal limits.

NURSING MANAGEMENT

Assessment

1. See Assessment, Level 1.
2. Check intake and output.
3. Observe and record signs and symptoms of cystitis (dysuria, frequency, urgency, burning).
4. Analyze urine daily:
   - inspect for blood and shreds of mucus.
   - dipstick for occult blood.
5. Assess contributing factors:
   - thrombocytopenia.
   - bladder tumors.
   - coagulopathies.
   - drugs (e.g., aspirin).
6. Assess for alteration in hemoglobin and hematocrit.
   - hemoglobin < 10 g/100 ml.
   - hematocrit < 30%.
7. Observe for signs and symptoms of anemia:
   - fatigue (chronic).
   - dyspnea.
   - palpitations.
   - weakness.
   - dizziness.
   - syncope.
   - headache.
   - pallor.
8. Gauge impact on patient's life style.
9. Identify need for referrals to social services, home care, counseling, and other community resources.

Nursing Interventions

1. See Nursing Interventions, Level 1.
2. Measure and record vital signs.

323

3. Ensure minimum fluid intake of 1000 ml/8 hr (if not contraindicated).
4. Measure urine output and report output if less than 60 ml/hr.
5. Consult with physician regarding order for:
   - forced diuresis with diuretics.
   - alkalinization of urine with sodium bicarbonate.
   - stool softeners (straining at stool aggravates bladder hemorrhage).
   - discontinuing causative/other contributing drugs.
   - withholding ifosfamide and increasing mesna infusion rate until hematuria resolves (<10 RBCs/high power field).
6. Consult with physician regarding possible use of investigational uroprotective therapies (other than mesna):
   - intravesical instillation of N-acetylcysteine, prostaglandin E_2, and sucralfate.
   - oral sodium pentosanpolysulfate.
7. Administer pain medication (narcotics) as ordered.
8. Administer bladder antispasmodics/analgesics as ordered:
   - phenazopyridine (Pyridium).
   - flavoxate HCl (Uripas)
9. Report changes in level of bleeding and symptoms.
10. Provide for continuous bladder irrigation if ordered.
11. Implement identified referral needs as noted in assessment.

Patient Teaching

1. See Patient Teaching, Level 1.
2. Discuss rationale for long-term follow-up:
   - without history of hemorrhagic cystitis:
     - regular urine cytologies.
     - cystoscopies as indicated.
     - ultrasound of urinary tract (biannual or annual)
   - with history of hemorrhagic cystitis:
     - periodic excretory urography (IVP) every few years.
     - annual urinalysis, cytology, cystoscopy (with biopsy as needed).
3. Discuss relationship between bladder cancer and smoking and other possible carcinogenic agents.
4. Teach signs and symptoms of bladder fibrosis (decreased bladder capacity) and bladder cancer.
5. If patient receives phenazopyridine for pain, tell patient that drug will color urine red or orange.
6. Explain rationale and procedure for bladder irrigation or investigational uroprotective therapies, if ordered.

LEVEL 3: *Intractable Hemorrhage/Chronic Cystitis/Hematuria*

EXPECTED OUTCOME

1. Patient/caregiver demonstrate knowledge related to severe impairment in urinary elimination:
   - identify signs and symptoms of severe impairment.
   - identify factors that influence severe impairment in urinary elimination.
   - identify potential sequelae/complications of severe impairment in urinary elimination.

2. Patient/caregiver identify/demonstrate measures to control, manage, or improve severe impairment in urinary eliminations:
   - demonstrate proper knowledge and administration of medications.
   - perform necessary treatments and procedures.
   - identify signs and symptoms to report to health care team.
   - identify/demonstrate appropriate fluid and dietary modifications.
   - identify appropriate long-term follow-up care.
3. Patient maintains or achieves optimal level of urinary elimination consistent with disease process:
   - vital signs stable or improved for patient.
   - stable input and output.
   - decreased or stable signs and symptoms of impairment.
   - laboratory tests stable for patient.
   - decreased discomfort or pain.

NURSING MANAGEMENT

Assessment

1. See Assessment, Levels 1 and 2.
2. Observe urine for blood or clots at each voiding.
3. Observe for signs and symptoms of hypovolemic shock:
   - decreasing blood pressure, decreasing pulse pressure.
   - pulse less than 60 or more than 120.
   - respirations greater than 30 or less than 10.
   - decreasing urine output less than 30 ml/hr.
   - pallor.
   - cold, clammy skin.
4. Evaluate patient's/caregiver's coping abilities in response to life-threatening event and chronic disease process.

Nursing Interventions

1. See Nursing Interventions, Levels 1 and 2.
2. Take actions related to restoration or maintenance of adequate circulatory blood volume:
   - administer blood transfusions as required.
   - observe, record, report to physician changes in vital signs.
3. Perform bladder irrigations as ordered to decrease clots in urine.
4. Take actions related to definitive treatment to restore hemostasis:
   - check for underlying bone marrow depression and coagulopathies.
   - administer IV vasopressin if ordered and observe for complications (e.g., abdominal pain, hypertension, bradycardia, fluid retention).
   - administer intravesical instillation of alum, silver nitrate, formalin or prostaglandin F_2 alpha to bladder:
     - prepare patient for cystoscopy before treatment (to rule out ureterovesical reflux).
     - after instillation, observe for complications (e.g., dysuria, urgency, suprapubic pain, obstruction with hydronephrosis secondary to reflux).
   - prepare patient for corrective surgery, if required:
     - cystoscopy with fulguration of bleeding points.
     - hypogastric artery diversion.
     - cystectomy.
5. For patients with a urinary diversion, see

Chapter 49 for further actions and rehabilitative interventions.

6. Provide emotional support for patient and family.

Patient Teaching

1. See Patient Teaching, Levels 1 and 2.
2. Discuss relationship between dietary intake (iron-rich food) and hematopoiesis. Explain need for iron supplements.
3. Do further teaching specific to definitive treatment.
4. Reemphasize need for adequate fluid intake and long-term follow-up.
5. Discuss potential for recurrence of hemorrhagic cystitis and development of bladder cancer.
6. Discuss relationship between smoking and bladder cancer.
7. Refer to related Chapters 16 and 17 for specific teaching needs that are pertinent to optimal adjustment to chronic process.

SUGGESTED READINGS

Cantwell, B.M.J., Harris, A.L., Patrick, D., and Hall, R.R.: Hemorrhagic cystitis after IV bleomycin, vinblastine, cisplatin and etoposide for testicular cancer. Cancer Treatment Reports 70:548–549, 1986.

Ershler, W.B., Gilchrist, K.W., and Citrin, D.L.: Adriamycin enhancement of cyclophosphamide-induced bladder injury. Journal of Urology 123:121–122, 1980.

Goodman, M.: Managing the side effects of chemotherapy. Seminars in Oncology Nursing 5(Suppl. 1):29–52, 1989.

Groenwald, S.L. (Ed.): Cancer Nursing Principles and Practice. Boston, Jones & Bartlett, 1987.

Higgs, D., Nagy, C., and Einhorn, L.H.: Ifosfamide: A clinical review. Seminars in Oncology Nursing 5(Suppl. 1):70–77, 1989.

Jenkins, G., Noe, H., and Hill, D.: Treatment of complications of cyclophosphamide cystitis. Journal of Urology 139:923–925, 1988.

Karch, A., and Boyd, E.: Handbook of Drugs and the Nursing Process. Philadelphia, J.B. Lippincott, 1989.

Millard, R.J.: Busulfan-induced hemorrhagic cystitis. Urology 18:143–144, 1981.

Parsons, C.L.: Successful management of radiation cystitis with sodium pentosanpolysulfate. Journal of Urology 136:813–817, 1986.

Pyeritz, R.E., Droller, M.J., Bender, W.L., et al.: An approach to the control of massive hemorrhage in cyclophosphamide-induced hemorrhagic cystitis by intravenous vasopressin: A case report. Journal of Urology 120:153–154, 1978.

Relling, M.V., and Schunk, J.E.: Drug-induced hemorrhagic cystitis. Clinical Pharmacy 5:590–597, 1986.

Shrom, S.H., Donaldson, M.H., Duckett, J.W., et al.: Formalin treatment for intractable hemorrhagic cystitis. A review of the literature with 16 additional cases. Cancer 38:1785–1789, 1976.

Shurafa, M., Shumaker, E., and Cronin, S.: Prostaglandin F_2-Alpha bladder irrigation for control of intractable cyclophosphamide-induced hemorrhagic cystitis. Journal of Urology 137:1230–1231, 1987.

Stillwell, T.J., and Benson, R.C.: Cyclophosphamide-induced hemorrhagic cystitis. A review of 100 patients. Cancer 61:451–457, 1988.

Stillwell, T.J., Benson, R.C., and Burgert, E.O.: Cyclophosphamide-induced hemorrhagic cystitis in Ewing's sarcoma. Journal of Clinical Oncology 6:76–82, 1988.

Stillwell, T.J., Benson, R.C., DeRemee, R.A., et al.: Cyclophosphamide-induced bladder toxicity in Wegener granulomatosis. Arthritis and Rheumatism 31:465–470, 1988.

Tenenbaum, L.: Cancer Chemotherapy. A Reference Guide. Philadelphia, W.B. Saunders, 1989.

Yasko, J.M.: Care of the client receiving external radiation therapy. Reston, VA, Reston Publishing, 1982.

Ziegfeld, C.R. (Ed.): Core Curriculum for Oncology Nursing. Philadelphia, W.B. Saunders, 1987.

Elimination, Alteration in: Enterocutaneous Fistula Formation

51

Susan Jane Hagan and Patricia McFarland

Population at Risk

- Individuals who have undergone surgery
- Individuals who have received or are presently receiving chemotherapy or radiation therapy to abdomen, those presently receiving steroids or other antiinflammatory therapy
- Individuals with inflammatory bowel disease, intraabdominal sepsis, mesenteric vascular disease, bowel obstruction, necrosis or an area of the gastrointestinal tract, or unresected carcinoma

LEVEL 1: Potential

EXPECTED OUTCOME

1. Patient demonstrates knowledge related to potential for fistula formation:
   - identifies factors that predispose to fistula formation.
   - verbalizes signs and symptoms of fistula.
2. Patient identifies/demonstrates measures to prevent fistula formation:
   - identifies/demonstrates measures to promote wound healing.
3. Patient remains free of fistula:
   - intact skin.
   - no evidence of fecal or digestive material drainage.

NURSING MANAGEMENT

Assessment

1. Evaluate factors affecting wound healing:
   - protein balance (e.g., serum protein, albumin, blood urea nitrogen, albumin-globulin ratio).
   - oxygenation (e.g., anemia, hematoma at incision, hypovolemia, decreased circulation to area).
   - nutritional status (height, weight, anthropometric measurements, serum albumin, total iron-binding capacity).
   - medications decreasing healing (steroids, chemotherapeutic drugs).
   - diseases affecting wound healing (diabetes, cancer in surgical area, inflammatory bowel diseases, multiple operations to intestinal tract, postradiation to abdomen or pelvis).
   - sepsis (hypotension, fever, mental confusion).
2. Inspect skin for:
   - redness, pain, swelling, increased temperature.
   - drainage from abdominal area.

Nursing Interventions

1. Use sterile wound care to prevent sepsis.
2. Assess need for prophylactic use of antibiotic agents and request physician order if indicated.
3. Encourage high-protein, high-carbohydrate diet with adequate intake of vitamins C and A and iron.
4. Arrange dietary consult.

Patient Teaching

1. Teach signs and symptoms of early fistula formation necessary to report to health care team (e.g., localized pain, inflamma-

tion, possible decreased fecal output from rectum or colostomy, opening in skin, dehiscence of incision, evidence of fecal or digestive material drainage on external abdomen).
2. Explain rationale and measures to promote wound healing:
   - maintain adequate fluid and nutritional status (diet high in vitamin C, iron, protein, carbohydrates, and fat).
   - maintain oxygenation (stop or decrease smoking).
   - decrease risk of infection with aseptic wound care.
3. Discuss factors that predispose patient to fistula formation.

LEVEL 2: Small or Moderate

EXPECTED OUTCOME

1. Patient demonstrates knowledge of altered elimination related to fistula formation:
   - verbalizes signs and symptoms of fistula formation.
   - identifies complications of fistula formation.
2. Patient identifies/demonstrates measures to promote wound healing:
   - performs necessary treatments and procedures.
   - demonstrates proper knowledge and administration of medications.
   - identifies/demonstrates adequate nutritional intake.
   - identifies signs and symptoms necessary to report to health care team.
3. Patient exhibits healing or control of fistula:
   - decreased size of fistula stoma.
   - decreased amount of drainage.
   - absence of infection.
   - development of granulation or scar tissue around fistula site.

NURSING MANAGEMENT

Assessment

1. See Assessment, Level 1.
2. Observe fistula size, location, and amount, type, and odor of drainage.
3. Assess skin surrounding fistula for excoriation.
4. Check for fluid and electrolyte imbalance.
5. Evaluate signs and symptoms of local or

systemic infection (elevated temperature, redness, inflammation).

6. Assess nutritional depletion resulting from fistula drainage (e.g., protein, vitamins).
7. Determine mental status (anxiety or depression).

Nursing Interventions

1. See Nursing Interventions, Level 1.
2. Culture initial drainage.
3. Prevent dehydration with increased oral fluid intake or IV fluids (per physician order).
4. Administer systemic antibiotics per physician order.
5. Implement hyperalimentation per order for gastric, duodenal, or small-bowel fistulae, to provide bowel rest.
6. Implement hyperalimentation or elemental or low-residue diet for patients with colonic fistulae.
7. Provide diet high in protein to promote wound healing.
8. Maintain skin integrity and contain effluent:
   - cleanse gently around stoma with tepid water and very mild soap or cleansing agent, such as Uniwash, Peri-Wash, Cara-Klenz, or Biolex.
   - dry skin with heat lamp or hair dryer set on warm (only by nurse if skin is very moist).
   - antacids such as Amphojel may be applied before drying skin.
   - apply thin layer of cream such as Skin Care, Unicare, Hollister Skin to correct excoriation resulting from auto-digestion around fistula site.
   - apply skin protector such as Skin Prep, Skin Gel around stoma to maintain protective seal over skin if skin is not reddened.
   - apply Hollister or Squibb wound management system—if not available then follow next four steps:
     - apply skin barrier such as Stomahesive or Premium Skin Barrier

that has been cut to conform to fistula stoma.
- fill in areas of exposed skin around fistula with karaya or Stomahesive paste or equivalent product, being certain not to occlude passage of (effluent) drainage.
- apply open-ended pouch over skin barrier (urinary ostomy pouch may facilitate collection with loose effluent).
- affix with paper tape, if necessary, over layer of skin, observing for possible allergic reaction or skin excoriation.
- empty pouch frequently (at least q4h) to prevent leakage of pouch and to prevent increased risk of infection.
- attach pouch to suction or dependent drainage bag for high output.
- should other drains be present, alternate methods of pouching may be necessary.
- maintain sterile technique if fistula originates at site other than colon.
- measure fistula output when emptying pouch.

9. Perform measures to control odors:
   - clean wound and change pouch prn.
   - apply antiodor agents to pouch (baking soda, fentichlor, vanilla extract, Banish, Dignity).
10. Support patient who may be depressed as a result of setback in recovery.

Patient Teaching

1. Teach signs and symptoms of fistula formation and drainage complications (fluid and electrolyte imbalance, infection, skin excoriation).
2. Explain effects and side effects of medications.
3. Discuss rationale and measures to maintain adequate nutrition (bowel rest and elemental diets for colon fistula, hyperalimentation for other fistulae).

4. Describe rationale and measures to promote skin integrity.
5. Explain rationale and measures for fistula pouching.
6. Teach signs and symptoms to report to health care team.
7. Outline measures to control pain if necessary (analgesics, relaxation, hypnosis).
8. Discuss rationale for potential surgical intervention (e.g., closure, drainage of abscess, diversion of drainage).
9. Describe measures to control odor.

LEVEL 3: Severe and Complications

EXPECTED OUTCOME

1. Patient/caregiver demonstrate knowledge related to severe alteration in elimination:
   - identify factors that influence impairment or maintenance of wound healing.
   - identify signs and symptoms necessary to report to health care team.
2. Patient/caregiver identify/demonstrate measures to manage severe alterations in elimination:
   - perform necessary treatments and procedures.
   - demonstrate proper knowledge and administration of medications.
   - verbalize/demonstrate adequate nutritional and fluid intake.
3. Patient exhibits stabilization of severe alteration in elimination:
   - no increase in size of fistula.
   - decreased amount of drainage from fistula.
   - maintenance of electrolyte balance.
   - maintenance of hydration and nutritional status.
   - control of infection.
   - decrease in skin excoriation.
4. Patients will resume activities of daily living as energy and well-being increase and as fistula decreases in size.

NURSING MANAGEMENT

Assessment

1. See Assessment, Levels 1 and 2.
2. Determine fluid and electrolyte balance, skin turgor, intake and output, physical examination, lung sounds, blood chemistry.

Nursing Interventions

1. See Nursing Interventions, Level 2.
2. Diphenoxylate HCl, Kaopectate, or opiates may be necessary to control fistula drainage from intestines.
3. Replace electrolytes parenterally or enterally as ordered.
4. Employ hyperalimentation or elemental diet to prevent malnutrition, promote wound healing, return patient to state of anabolism, and provide complete bowel rest.
5. Alternative feeding routes to bypass fistula may be necessary: jejunostomy tube may be placed distal to fistula.

6. Apply nystatin powder around fistula if candidal infection is present.
7. Control pain by use of narcotics as appropriate.
8. Provide support and encouragement to patient/family.
9. Refer to home health care nurse to continue post-discharge care until patient is independent in care.

Patient Teaching

1. See Patient Teaching, Level 2.
2. Discuss rationale to promote fistula healing by surgical intervention:
   - excision of fistulous tract.
   - fecal diversion with ostomy to provide complete bowel rest.

SUGGESTED READINGS

Boarini, J.H., Bryant, R.A., and Irrgang, S.J.: Fistula management. Seminars in Oncology Nursing 2(4):287–292, 1986.

Dunavent, H.: Wound and fistula management. In Broadwell, D. (Ed.): Principles of Ostomy Care. St. Louis, C.V. Mosby, 1982.

Dyer, S., Clark, P., and Wilkins, L.: Ileostomy and fistula appliances. Professional Nurse 3(11):462–463, 1988.

Fowler, E., Jeter, K., and Schwartz, A.: How to cope when your patient has an enterocutaneous fistula. American Journal of Nursing 80:426–429, 1980.

Geels, W., Bagley, K., and Vander, L.: The enterocutaneous fistula: Supplanting surgery with meticulous nursing care. Nursing 8:52–55, 1978.

Jackson, B.S., Powers, M.I., Rush-Martin, et al.: A case control clinical trial of two wound drainage collection systems. Journal of Enterostomal Therapy 15(5):191–195, 1988.

Manson, H.: Exorcising excoriation from fistulae and other draining wounds. Nursing 6:57–60, 1976.

Pollack, S.: Wound healing: A review (parts I, II, III). Journal of Dermatologic Surgical Oncology 5:389–393, 477–481, 615–619, 1979.

Sage, S.J.: An unusual challenge: Oral-cutaneous fistula. Journal of Enterostomal Therapy 15(2):91–92, 1988.

Schauder, J., and Jaffrey, I.: Better management of fecal fistulas with stoma bags. RN 37:56–59, 1974.

Schumann, D.: How to help wound healing. Nursing 10:34–40, 1980.

Stuver, L., Kirkpatrick, S., Smiley, K., et al.: Wound management: How teamwork and innovation met a dying patient's needs. Nursing 9:30–42, 1979.

Taylor, V.: Meeting the challenge of fistulae and draining wounds. Nursing 10:45–51, 1980.

Tonn, J.: Management of fistula care with a wound drainage collector. Journal of Enterostomal Therapy 15(2):51–98, 1988.

Wessel, L.: Management of a wound with multiple drains. Journal of Enterostomal Therapy 16(1):26–28, 1989.

PATIENT EDUCATION MATERIALS AND COMMUNITY RESOURCES

No specific publications are available for fistula care; however, several publications are available through United Ostomy Association, 36 Executive Park, Suite 120, Irvine, CA 92714, phone 714–660–8624.

Elimination, Alteration in: Nonenterocutaneous Fistula Formation

Susan Jane Hagan and Patricia McFarland

Population at Risk

- Individuals who have undergone pelvic surgery affecting genitourinary/gastrointestinal systems
- Individuals with gynecologic or urologic malignancies
- Individuals who have received or are presently receiving chemotherapy; radiation therapy (external or internal) to pelvic area
- Individuals who are presently receiving steroids or other antiinflammatory therapy
- Individuals with pelvic sepsis or unresected carcinoma in pelvic area

LEVEL 1: Potential

EXPECTED OUTCOME

1. Patient demonstrates knowledge related to potential for fistula formation:
   - identifies factors that predispose to fistula formation.
   - verbalizes signs and symptoms of fistulae.
2. Patient identifies/demonstrates measures to prevent fistula formation:
   - identifies/demonstrates measures to promote wound healing.
3. Patient remains free of fistula:
   - no abnormal drainage from vagina, urethra, rectum.

NURSING MANAGEMENT

Assessment

1. Evaluate factors affecting wound healing:
   - protein balance (e.g., serum protein, albumin, blood urea nitrogen, albumin-globulin ratio).
   - oxygenation (e.g., anemia, hematoma at incision, hypovolemia, decreased circulation to area).
   - nutritional status (height, weight, anthropometric measurements, serum albumin, total iron-binding capacity).
   - medications decreasing healing (steroids, chemotherapeutic drugs).
   - diseases affecting wound healing (diabetes, cancer in surgical area, multiple surgical procedures to pelvic area, postradiation to pelvis).
   - sepsis (hypotension, fever, mental confusion).

2. Assess unusual drainage from vagina, urethra, or rectum.

Nursing Interventions

1. Assess need for prophylactic use of antibiotic agents and request physician order if indicated.
2. Encourage high-protein, high-carbohydrate diet with adequate intake of vitamins C and A and iron.
3. Arrange dietary consult.
4. Perform invasive techniques carefully (enemas, catheterization, douches, rectal temperatures); avoid, if possible.

Patient Teaching

1. Teach signs and symptoms of early fistula formation necessary to report to health care team:

- vesicovaginal: urinary tract infection, urine from vagina, pain, drainage of pus or mucus.
- enterovaginal: foul-smelling vaginal drainage (tan or brown-tinged), pain, drainage of pus or mucus.
- enterovesical: urinary tract infection, urine from rectum, pain, drainage of pus or mucus.
2. Discuss rationale and measures to promote wound healing:
- maintain adequate fluid and nutritional status (diet high in vitamin C, iron, protein, carbohydrates, fat).
- maintain oxygenation (stop or decrease smoking).
- decrease risk of infection with aseptic wound care.
- avoid mechanical irritation (enemas, douches, rectal temperature).
3. Explain factors that predispose patient to fistula formation.

LEVEL 2:   Small or Moderate

EXPECTED OUTCOME

1. Patient demonstrates knowledge of altered elimination related to fistula formation:
   - verbalizes signs and symptoms of fistula formation.
   - identifies complications of fistula formation necessary to report to health care team.
2. Patient identifies/demonstrates measures to promote wound healing:
   - performs necessary treatments and procedures.
   - identifies signs and symptoms necessary to report to health care team.
   - identifies/demonstrates adequate nutritional intake.
   - demonstrates proper knowledge and administration of medications.
3. Patient exhibits healing or control of fistula as evidenced by:
   - decreased amount of drainage.
   - absence of infection.
   - absence of excoriated perineal skin.

NURSING MANAGEMENT

Assessment

1. See Assessment, Level 1.
2. Observe location, amount, type, and odor of drainage.
3. Check perineal skin for excoriation.
4. Determine fluid and electrolyte imbalance.
5. Note signs and symptoms of infection (elevated temperature).
6. Assess nutritional depletion resulting from fistula drainage (e.g., protein, vitamins).
7. Ascertain mental status (anxiety or depression).
8. Determine factors affecting possible surgical repair of fistula:
   * presence of infection.
   * extent of tissue damage from radiation therapy, cancer, previous surgeries.
   * patient's ability to tolerate surgery.
9. Evaluate impact of fistula on sexuality:
   * perceptions of self.
   * changes in sexual practice.

Nursing Interventions

1. See Nursing Interventions, Level 1.
2. Culture suspicious drainage.
3. Prevent dehydration with increased oral fluid intake or IV fluids (per physician order).
4. Administer systemic antibiotics per physician order.
5. Implement hyperalimentation per order for duodenal or small-bowel fistulae to provide bowel rest.
6. Provide hyperalimentation or elemental or low-residue diet for patients with colonic fistulae.
7. Provide diet high in protein to promote wound healing.
8. Maintain skin integrity and contain effluent:
   * cleanse gently around perineum with water and very mild cleansing agent (e.g., Uniwash, Peri-Wash, Cara-Klenz, or Biolex) after each void.
   * dry area with heat lamp or hair dryer set on warm (only by nurse if skin is very moist).
   * apply thin layer of cream such as Skin Care, Unicare, or Hollister Skin Conditioning cream to correct excoriation.
   * apply skin barrier such as Stomahesive, Premium Skin Barrier, Op Site, Tegaderm, or equivalent product to excoriated skin.
   * if not using barrier, apply thick layer of water repellent salve (e.g., petrolatum jelly or Unisalve) over Skin Care Cream or apply Bard Incontinent Spray directly to skin. Reapply after each voiding.
   * position patient to allow exposure of perineum to air.
9. Control effluent:
   * urine: use Foley catheter, nephrostomy, suprapubic catheter, incontinent pads.
   * fecal: use incontinent pads.
   * vaginal: may use diaphragm with catheter inserted, large balloon Foley to tamponade, drainage tubes to suction, perineal pads, incontinent pads, diapers, tampons.
10. Maintain odor control:
    * frequent cleansing.
    * activated charcoal in drainage bottles.
    * buttermilk douches for vaginal fistulae.
    * oral yogurt for enteral fistulae.
    * clean wound and change dressing as frequently as necessary.
    * apply antiodor agents to outer dressing (e.g., baking soda, fentichlor, Banish, Hex-On, Dignity).
11. Provide support to patient who may be depressed as a result of setback in recovery.

Patient Teaching

1. See Patient Teaching, Level 1.
2. Teach signs and symptoms of:
   - fistula formation and drainage.
   - complications (fluid/electrolyte imbalance, infection, perineal skin excoriation).
   - effects and side effects of medications.
3. Explain rationale and measures to maintain adequate nutrition (hyperalimentation if appropriate).
4. Discuss rationale and measures to promote skin integrity.
5. Describe signs and symptoms to report to health care team.
6. Outline measures to control pain (analgesics, relaxation, hypnosis) if necessary.
7. Discuss rationale for potential surgical intervention (e.g., closure, drainage of abscess, diversion of drainage).

8. Teach rationale and measures to control odor.
9. Explain rationale and measures to divert secretions from fistula site:
   - urinary: suprapubic catheter, Foley catheter, nephrostomy, ileal conduit (dependent on fistula location).
   - fecal: bowel rest (elemental diet for colon fistula and npo for other enteral fistula).
10. Describe rationale and measures to control drainage:
    - urinary: Foley catheter.
    - vaginal: diaphragm tamponade via catheter with large balloon, placement of other drainage tubes to suction.
    - fecal: incontinent pads.
11. Discuss measures to promote sexuality (see Chapter 53).

LEVEL 3: Severe Alteration and Complications

EXPECTED OUTCOME

1. Patient/caregiver demonstrate knowledge related to severe alteration in elimination:
   - identify factors that influence impairment or maintenance of wound healing.
   - identify signs and symptoms necessary to report to health care team.
2. Patient/caregiver identify/demonstrate measures to manage severe alterations in eliminations:
   - perform necessary treatment and procedures.
   - demonstrate proper knowledge and administration of medications.
   - verbalize/demonstrate adequate fluid and nutritional intake.
3. Patient exhibits stabilization of severe alteration in elimination.
   - no increase in amount of drainage from fistula.
   - maintenance of electrolyte balance.
   - maintenance of hydration and nutritional status.
   - control of infection.
   - decrease in excoriation of perineal skin.
4. Patients will resume activities of daily living as energy and well-being increase and fistula decreases in size.

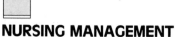

NURSING MANAGEMENT

Assessment

1. See Assessment, Levels 1 and 2.
2. Determine fluid and electrolyte balance, skin turgor, intake and output, lung sounds, blood chemistry.
3. Evaluate factors affecting wound healing:
   - nutritional factors.
   - sepsis.
   - adequate circulation.

Nursing Interventions

1. See Nursing Interventions, Level 2.
2. Replace electrolytes parenterally or enterally as ordered.
3. Provide hyperalimentation or elemental diet to prevent malnutrition, promote wound healing, return patient to state of anabolism, and provide complete bowel rest.
4. Apply nystatin powder around fistula if Candida is present.
5. Control pain by use of narcotics as appropriate.
6. Provide support and encouragement to patient/family.
7. Instruct regarding ostomy care if indicated (see Chapters 51 and 52).
8. Refer patient for home care to continue nursing management until patient is independent in care.

Patient Teaching

1. See Patient Teaching, Level 2.
2. Discuss rationale to promote fistula healing by surgical intervention:

- excision of fistulous tract.
- ostomy to provide complete bowel rest.
- excision of additional pockets of sepsis.

SUGGESTED READINGS

Boarini, J.H., Bryant, R.A., and Irrgang, S.J.: Fistula management. Seminars in Oncology Nursing 24:287–292, 1986.

Dunvent, M.: Wound and fistula management. *In* Broadwell, D. (Ed.): Principles of Ostomy Care. St. Louis, C.V. Mosby, 1982.

Fitzgerald, J.: Vaginal fistulas: One management method. Journal of Enterostomal Therapy 9:25–26, 1982.

Givel, J., Hawker, P., Allan, R., et al.: Enterovaginal fistulas associated with Crohn's disease. Surgery, Gynecology and Obstetrics 155:494–496, 1982.

Manson, H.: Exorcising excoriation from fistulae and other draining wounds. Nursing 6:57–60, 1976.

Pollak, S.: Wound healing: A review (parts I, II, III). Journal of Dermatologic Surgical Oncology 5:389–393, 477–481, 615–619, 1979.

Schauder, M., and Jaffrey, I.: Better management of fecal fistulas with stoma bags. RN 37:56–59, 1974.

Schumann, D.: How to help wound healing. Nursing 10:34–40, 1980.

Stuver, L., Kirkpatrick, D., Smiley, K., et al.: Wound management: How teamwork and innovation met a dying patient's needs. Nursing 9:30–42, 1979.

Taylor, V.: Meeting the challenge of fistulae and draining wounds. Nursing 10:45–51, 1980.

Thompson, J., Engen, D., Beart, R., et al.: The management of acquired rectourinary fistula. Diseases of the Colon and Rectum 25:689–692, 1982.

PATIENT EDUCATION MATERIALS AND COMMUNITY RESOURCES

American Cancer Society–contact local chapters.

United Ostomy Association, 36 Executive Park, Suite 120, Irvine, CA 92714, phone 714–660–9624.

SEXUALITY

The nurse assesses the patient's physical and psychological response to disease and treatment and past and present sexual patterns and functioning to formulate actual or potential nursing diagnoses.

Appropriate patient outcomes to consider in planning nursing interventions will specify the patient's ability to:

1. identify potential or actual alterations in perception of sexuality or sexual function.
2. identify satisfactory alternative methods for expressing sexuality.

Evaluation of the patient's responses to nursing care is based on whether the patient identifies aspects of sexuality that may be threatened by disease or treatment and identifies ways to maintain his or her sexual identity.

Excerpted from the ANA/ONS Standards of Cancer Nursing Practice.

Sexual Dysfunction Related to Disease Process and Treatment

53

Catherine M. Hogan

Population at Risk

- Individuals with cancer, particularly patients undergoing treatment, including surgery, chemotherapy, radiation therapy, or biotherapy
- Individuals who are survivors of cancer and cancer therapies

LEVEL 1: Potential

EXPECTED OUTCOME

1. Patient demonstrates knowledge related to potential alteration in sexuality:
   - states potential impact of disease/treatment on sexuality.
   - identifies factors that influence sexual identity.
   - identifies manifestations of alteration in sexuality.
2. Patient maintains satisfying sexual role and concept:
   - verbalizes/demonstrates awareness and acceptance of self as sexual being.
   - states satisfaction with sexual expressions.

NURSING MANAGEMENT

Assessment

1. Assess adult developmental level to determine potential alterations in self-concept, role, and sexual function:
   - role function: student, spouse, parent.
   - living arrangements: independent (apartment, dormitory, own home) vs. dependent (living with family of origin).
   - impact of diagnosis on significant, intimate relationships (e.g., partner(s), spouse).
   - impact of diagnosis on interpersonal relationships (e.g., employer, colleagues, friends, children).
   - impact of diagnosis on developmental activities (e.g., student, establishing career, establishing independence, flourishing in career activities, establishing and supporting "own" nuclear family).
2. Elicit information about previous sexual history as appropriate:
   - sexual activity.
   - reproductive history.
   - desire for children.
   - use of contraceptives.
   - impact of previous therapies (e.g., drugs, previous cancer treatment) on sexuality and sexual function.
   - coping style.

339

- attitudes about sex.
- impact of involved body part on sexuality.

3. Determine if disease and attendant psychophysiologic changes have affected sexual self-image.
4. Allow patient to discuss perception of how disease process/treatment will affect sexuality and sexual function.
5. Upon elicitation of a specific problem, gather data relative to:
   - onset of problem.
   - course of events.
   - patient's perception of problem.

Nursing Interventions

1. Examine own knowledge, attitudes, and skills in area of sexuality, sexual dysfunction, and sexual counseling.
2. Utilize interviewing techniques that demonstrate acceptance of a variety of sexual behaviors as within a normal range in order to increase patient comfort.
3. Structure therapeutic milieu that allows patient to feel comfortable discussing sexual concerns:
   - assure patient that all communications will be kept confidential.
   - ensure privacy.
   - consider use of McPhenbridge and Lamb model that assesses sexual function in a manner from least sensitive to most sensitive issues:
     - Has being ill (receiving chemotherapy, radiation therapy) interfered with your being a mother, father, wife, husband?
     - Has surgery (chemotherapy, radiation therapy, biotherapy) changed the way you see yourself as a man or a woman?
     - Has cancer (chemotherapy, radiation therapy) affected your sexual function?
4. Respect sociocultural factors (religion, culture, peer pressure) that may affect the individual's sexual concept and identity.

5. Utilize Annon's Plissit model to develop nursing interventions. Use levels with which you feel comfortable:
   - P = Permission: convey permission to have (or not have) sexual thoughts, concerns, feelings (assure patient that concerns regarding sexual function after cancer diagnosis are legitimate).
   - LI = Limited Information: provide limited information relative to patient's problem while acknowledging that other individuals experience similar concerns (e.g., many individuals have concerns about type of birth control recommended while receiving chemotherapy).
   - SS = Specific Suggestions: offer specific suggestions relevant to patient's problems (e.g., use of pillows and coital positions that minimize or allay threat of pathologic fractures).
   - IT = Intensive Therapy: refer to appropriate resource for longer-term therapy or rehabilitation (e.g., sex therapist for continued erectile dysfunction, surgeon for reconstructive surgery).
6. Focus all information on the individual meaning of the questions that are raised.
7. Stress that all concerns, orientations, and behaviors (celibacy, heterosexuality, homosexuality) are legitimate and are not judged by caregivers.

Patient Teaching

1. Discuss potential impact of disease process/treatment on sexuality as appropriate:
   - process of cancer (includes feelings of being ill and fatigued, alterations in body functions).
   - personal process of accepting cancer diagnosis.
   - treatment effects:
     - surgical interventions.
     - radiation therapy.
     - chemotherapy.
     - biotherapy.
     - side effect of therapies.

- results of disease or treatment on physical appearance, self-image.
- impact of diagnosis of cancer on family and uncertain future that accompanies it (e.g., anticipatory grief, role changes).

2. Clarify terms relative to sexuality to ensure understanding.
3. Clarify myths and misconceptions about normal sexual responses to provide basis for understanding potential changes.
4. Identify major areas of sexuality that cancer may potentially affect.

5. Identify measures to assist patient/partner to prevent or cope with possible change:
   - methods to prevent fatigue.
   - proper use of medications (e.g., analgesics, antiemetics).
   - signs and symptoms that may signal need for intervention (e.g., "low mood," avoidance of intimacy).
6. Describe available community resources and groups.

LEVEL 2: Moderate or Possible Permanent Alterations in Sexual Activity

EXPECTED OUTCOME

1. Patient demonstrates knowledge related to alteration in sexuality:
   - identifies alterations in sexuality and sexual function resulting from disease process/treatment.
   - identifies factors that influence sexual identity.
   - identifies manifestations of alteration in sexuality.
2. Patient identifies/demonstrates strategies to manage or correct alteration in sexuality:
   - demonstrates proper knowledge and administration of medications.
   - performs necessary treatments and procedures.
   - identifies/demonstrates behaviors and measures to promote acceptance of self as sexual being.
   - identifies appropriate long-term care plan.
3. Patient achieves improving or satisfying sexual role and concept:
   - verbalizes/demonstrates awareness and acceptance of self as sexual being.
   - states satisfaction with sexual expressions.

NURSING MANAGEMENT

Assessment

1. See Assessment, Level 1.
2. Ask specific questions relative to altered sexual function in order to identify problems early.
3. Integrate knowledge of disease process and treatment plan to identify problem areas.

Nursing Interventions

1. See Nursing Interventions, Level 1.
2. Maintain open, nonjudgmental communication pattern with patient/partner to facilitate verbalization of sexual concerns.
3. Refer to community agencies that offer support programs.

341

Sexual Dysfunction Related to Disease Process and Treatment

Patient Teaching

1. See Patient Teaching, Level 1.
2. Identify expected duration of sexual alteration highlighting timeframe within which alteration is expected to normalize (e.g., sexual activity may be resumed at specific time following surgery).
3. Provide information appropriate to specific problem exhibited by patient.
4. General considerations:
   - dyspnea:
     - use of oxygen, bronchodilators, altered positions, waterbed;
     - suction before sexual activity, avoiding sexual activity when cough pattern is at its worst.
   - fatigue: scheduling sexual activity after rest periods, before large meals, before exercise.
   - pain:
     - administration of analgesics so that peak of action coincides with sexual activity (if drugs interfere with arousal, sexual activity may be scheduled when analgesic effect is decreased);
     - warm baths and soaks, pillows, position changes, other noninvasive methods of pain management may be appropriate to make patient more comfortable during sexual activity.
   - erectile dysfunction:
     - may be related to fatigue, stress, anxiety, depression, neurotoxic effects of chemotherapy, surgical interventions;
     - in certain cases, penile prosthesis may be an option.
   - dyspareunia:
     - may be secondary to radiation therapy or chemotherapy-induced vaginitis or fibrosis, decreased vaginal lubrication; water-soluble lubrication (e.g., KY Jelly, Ortho Personal Lubricant) can be used to ameliorate vaginal dryness;
     - when appropriate, use of vaginal dilator in conjunction with adequate lubrication may prevent further fibrosis and vaginal tightening;
     - hormonal replacement therapy may be appropriate for female patients experiencing premature menopausal symptoms; however, hormone replacement is contraindicated with hormonally dependent tumors.
   - decreased libido:
     - reassure individual that decreased libido is normal and may be secondary to disease, treatment, medications;
     - encourage sexual activities such as fondling, hugging, kissing, which may increase desire, strongly encouraging individual not to consider genital intercourse as the only option in sexual expression during episodes of decreased libido.
   - alopecia:
     - Kold Kaps may prevent further scalp hair loss if not medically contraindicated;
     - prepare individual for loss of non-scalp hair (mustache, eyebrows, pubic hair, chest hair);
     - wigs, scarves, head coverings, additional makeup, jewelry may assist individual to feel more normal.
   - changes in normal body weight: encourage individual to express feelings regarding changes from normal weight:
     - weight gain: assure individual of temporary nature if result of steroid or hormonal therapy;
     - weight loss: suggest use of nontailored clothes, makeup, jewelry to draw attention away from torso.
5. Surgical considerations:
   - head and neck surgery:
     - encourage prosthetic follow-up to facilitate rehabilitation, minimize concerns regarding physical appearance;
     - provide information related to specific coital positions that minimize fear of air hunger or suffocation;
     - females may wish to wear high-necked nightgowns;

342

- provide information related to tracheostomy care to avoid unpleasant odors.
- mastectomy:
  - elicit meaning of breast loss to patient/partner, allowing opportunity for discussion;
  - breast prostheses, camouflaging clothes, reconstructive surgery, support groups such as Reach to Recovery are approaches that may facilitate rehabilitation;
  - encouraging patient/partner to view mastectomy scar and discuss feelings is important, as acknowledgment of loss and frank discussion of feelings are first steps toward acceptance of alteration in body image.
- lumpectomy/segmental resection: provide information regarding prosthesis that may be needed by the large-breasted woman who has undergone either procedure or who has experienced extensive changes from radiotherapy.
- hysterectomy:
  - advise whether hormonal effects should be expected (as in oophorectomy);
  - prepare individuals for anticipated menopausal symptoms;
  - advise individual when normal sexual activity may be resumed.
- vaginectomy:
  - may be partial or complete–those undergoing partial vaginectomies usually can engage in normal intercourse with use of large amounts of lubricant and modified positioning;
  - provide information illustrating positions that increase perceived length of vaginal barrel as well as to minimize discomfort associated with penile thrusting.
- retrograde ejaculation:
  - may follow transurethral resection of prostate and retroperitoneal lymph node dissection;
  - nerve-sparing procedures are now available, depending upon extent of surgical intervention;
  - sympathetic-mimicking agents such as imipramine HCl and pseudo-ephedrine may be helpful in some cases in restoring antegrade ejaculation.
- indwelling catheters:
  - genital intercourse may still be performed with indwelling catheter in place;
  - catheter may be folded back along penis or taped on abdomen;
  - instruct patient to empty drainage bag before intercourse.
- ostomies: encourage patient to empty appliance before sexual activity, use pouch coverings if desired, and use odor-minimizing foods such as yogurt and buttermilk.

LEVEL 3: Severe (Permanent Inability to Engage in Genital Intercourse)

EXPECTED OUTCOME

1. Patient/partner demonstrate knowledge related to severe alterations in sexuality:
   - identify impact of disease/treatment on sexuality.
   - identify factors that influence sexual identity.
   - identify manifestations of alteration in sexuality.

2. Patient/partner identify/demonstrate strategies to manage severe alterations in sexuality:
   - identify alternate methods of sexual expression and intimacy.
   - identify/demonstrate behaviors and measures to promote acceptance of self as sexual being.
   - identify/utilize appropriate community resources.

NURSING MANAGEMENT

Assessment

1. See Assessment, Levels 1 and 2.
2. Utilize assessment process to further clarify long-term alterations in sexuality and sexual function.

Nursing Interventions

1. See Nursing Interventions, Levels 1 and 2.
2. Make referrals to appropriate agencies for sexual counseling to maximize rehabilitation.

Patient Teaching

1. See Patient Teaching, Levels 1 and 2.
2. Provide information specific to alterations in sexuality and sexual function. Individuals who are unable to engage in genital intercourse may wish to explore alternate methods as appropriate. Manual stimulation, oral-genital stimulation, anal intercourse, and mutual masturbation may all be successful alternatives if such methods are congruent with the individual's social, cultural, and religious belief systems.

SUGGESTED READINGS

Annon, J.: The Behavioral Treatment of Sexual Problems, vol. I. Honolulu, HI, Enabling Systems, Inc., 1974.

Chapman, R.M.: Effect of cytoxic therapy on sexuality and gonadal function. Seminars in Oncology 9(1):84–94, 1984.

Daiter, S., Larson, R., Weedington, W., and Ultman, J.: Psychosocial symptomatology, personal growth and development among young adult patients following the diagnosis of leukemia or lymphoma. Journal of Clinical Oncology 6(4):613–617, 1988.

Feldman, J.: Ovarian failure and cancer treatment: Incidence and interventions for the premenopausal woman. Oncology Nursing Forum 16(5):651–657, 1989.

Henrick-Rynning, T.: Prostatic cancer treatments and their effects on sexual functioning. Oncology Nursing Forum 14(6):37–41, 1989.

Lamb, M., and Wood, N.: Sexuality and the cancer patient. Cancer Nursing 4(2):137–148, 1981.

Loescher, L., Welch-McCaffery, D., Leigh, S., et al.: Surviving adult concerns. Part I: Physiologic effects. Annals of Internal Medicine 111(5):411–432, 1989.

Richards, S., and Hiratzka, S.: Vaginal dilatation post pelvic irradiation: A patient education tool. Oncology Nursing Forum 13(4):89–91, 1987.

Rozary, M.: How to take a sexual history. American Journal of Nursing 76:1279–1282, 1976.

Schover, L.R.: Sexuality and Cancer for the Man Who has Cancer and his Partner. American Cancer Society, 1988.

Shell, J.: Sexuality and the person with cancer (Clinical Practice Corner). Oncology Nursing Forum 13(2):86–89, 1986.

Welch-McCaffery, D., Hoffman, B., Leigh, S., et al.: Surviving adult cancers. Part II: Psychological implications. Annals of Internal Medicine 111(6):517–529, 1989.

Yarbo, C. (Ed.): Sexuality and cancer. In Seminars in Oncology Nursing 1(1), 1985 (entire issue).

Sexual Dysfunction: Infertility

Joy Stair

Population at Risk

Individuals in childbearing years undergoing cancer treatment:

- chemotherapy, especially alkylating agents (chlorambucil, cyclophosphamide), doxorubicin HCl, cytarabine, procarbazine, vinblastine, busulfan, and antiestrogen therapy
- radiation therapy to lower abdomen, pelvis, gonads
- surgical procedures to reproductive organs (hysterectomy, bilateral oophorectomy, bilateral orchiectomy)

LEVEL 1: Potential

EXPECTED OUTCOME

Patient demonstrates knowledge related to potential infertility:
- states definitions of terms used in discussion of potential infertility.
- identifies effects of cancer treatment(s) on reproductive functioning.
- identifies personal factors impacting on reproductive functioning.
- identifies potential effects of treatment(s) on future offspring.
- identifies modalities to promote future childbearing/conception.
- identifies methods of contraception during treatment.

NURSING MANAGEMENT

Assessment

1. Obtain brief sexual history:
   - current sexual practices.
   - sex education and attitudes (e.g., importance of sexual activity to relationship).
   - effect of disease/treatment on sexual function.
2. Obtain reproductive and contraceptive history of patient/partner.
3. Assess knowledge level of patient/partner related to:
   - terminology (fertility, infertility, sterility, gonads).
   - effects of cancer treatment(s) on reproductive function.
4. Evaluate gonadal function:
   - males:
     - serum follicle-stimulating hormone (FSH): elevation of FSH level after chemotherapy or radiation therapy may serve as marker of testicular germinal aplasia; testosterone levels may be normal.
     - decrease in testicular volume.
     - sperm count.
   - females:
     - serum FSH, luteinizing hormone

345

(LH): elevation associated with decreased serum estradiol.

- presence or absence of menses.
- symptoms of estrogen deficiency (e.g., "hot flashes," vaginal dryness, dyspareunia).

5. Determine current or planned cancer treatment:
   - chemotherapy: drug(s), dosage (individual and total), duration of treatment.
   - radiation therapy (external beam): location, dosage (one dose or fractionated).

6. Note plans to salvage gonadal function:
   - oophoropexy (surgical movement of ovaries out of treatment field of radiation–therapy done at time of staging laparotomy).
   - sperm banking.
   - storing ova.

Patient Teaching

1. Patient teaching must be individualized and based on type of treatment, age, gender, and desire for future family.
2. Teach terminology related to reproductive functioning (e.g., gonads, fertility, infertility, sterility).
3. Explain effects of chemotherapy on gonadal functioning:
   - drugs commonly causing oligospermia and azoospermia, amenorrhea (e.g., alkylating agents [chlorambucil, cyclophosphamide], doxorubicin HCl, procarbazine, vinblastine, cytarabine).
   - males:
     - infertility in men receiving single alkylating agent therapy is dose-related; within 2 to 3 months of therapy, a decrease in sperm count progressing to azoospermia is seen.
     - methotrexate causes rapid decrease in sperm count within 2 to 3 weeks of onset of chemotherapy.
     - combination chemotherapy regimens that include alkylating agents

have profound effects on spermatogenesis.
- Hodgkin's patients on MVPP or MOPP experience azoospermia after 1 to 2 cycles of chemotherapy with poor outlook for recovery of spermatogenesis.
- sex drive and capability are not usually affected (testosterone is still produced).
- azoospermia may be transient; however, recovery is slow and prolonged (years) and often incomplete.
- some male patients on chemotherapy have impregnated females.
- treatment with combination chemotherapy may produce more long-lasting azoospermia than does therapy with single agents.
- studies of survivors of childhood cancers generally report long-term impairment of spermatogenesis and fertility deficit of 50 to 60 per cent depending on drug, dosage, duration of treatment.

- females:
  - long-term cyclophosphamide treatment causes ovarian failure including destruction of oocytes; irregular menses or amenorrhea tend to be permanent; drug dosage is major variable in gonadal effect.
  - amenorrhea is a commonly noted side effect with busulfan; patients become amenorrheic within 6 months of starting therapy.
  - onset of amenorrhea and resumption of menses in patients on adjuvant therapy is related to age during chemotherapy and total dose administered (permanent amenorrhea is more common in women older than 40 years of age).
  - alkylating agent chemotherapy accelerates onset of menopause, particularly in older patients, while younger patients may tolerate higher total dosages before amenorrhea becomes irreversible.

- nearly every anticancer drug has potential to cause teratogenic and mutagenic changes in exposed eggs and sperm; however, current studies show that normal offspring may be conceived and delivered following chemotherapy.
4. Discuss effects of radiation therapy on gonadal functioning:
   - males:
     - may produce partial or permanent sterility in males, depending on dosage and fractionation used.
     - single dose of 15 to 400 rads produces temporary sterility.
     - dosages of 500 to 950 rads or greater causes permanent sterility.
     - decreased sperm count begins 60 to 80 days after exposure; duration depends on dosage given.
     - mature sperm present in ejaculate for 60 to 80 days after irradiation contain chromosomal damage, which may manifest as dominant first-generation abnormalities.
     - higher single doses cause more rapid onset of oligospermia and azoospermia.
     - with single-dose exposures, complete recovery of sperm production occurs within 9 to 18 months after 200 to 300 rads; in 5 or more years, after 400 to 600 rads.
     - if both testes are included in single-dose field (e.g., one-half body irradiation to 600 to 800 rads), permanent sterility or prolonged azoospermia (5 years or longer) is common.
     - testes that receive standard fractionated dosages greater than 1000 rads total dosage will be sterile.
     - lower abdominal fields (e.g., inverted Y) expose gonads to a significant dosage; despite shielding of testes, inverted Y causes 70 to 100 per cent azoospermia within 6 weeks of irradiation.
   - females:
     - ovaries are less sensitive to radiation than testes.
     - size of radiation dosage required to induce complete and permanent sterility is related to age at time of radiation therapy (more precisely, to number of oocytes that remain).
     - in females 40 years of age or older, 600 rads may be associated with subsequent menopause.
     - in young females, 2000 rads fractionated over 5 to 6 weeks has 95 per cent likelihood of producing permanent sterility.
     - females may suffer some loss of libido if ovarian tissue is destroyed.
5. Methods to promote salvage of gonadal function include:
   - oophoropexy: surgical movement out of treatment field before initiation of radiation therapy, done at time of staging laparotomy (consult physician).
   - shielding for radiation therapy (consult physician).
   - if option is available, female patients may want to consider salvage and storage of eggs.
6. Explain availability and considerations regarding sperm banking:
   - ultimate conception rates using preserved semen remain only 50 to 60 per cent.
   - results depend upon sperm counts/motility before receiving therapy (e.g., males with Hodgkin's disease may have decreased sperm counts/motility before treatment).
   - recommend that more than one specimen of sperm be stored before first cancer treatment.
   - encourage teenage and young adult patients to consider sperm banking.
7. Discuss rationale for and methods of contraception during and after treatment (see Chapter 17).
8. Describe effects of treatment on future offspring:
   - there is no increased incidence of spontaneous abortion or fetal abnormalities in individuals treated with chemotherapy compared with general population.

- some studies show that females previously treated with both chemotherapy and radiation therapy have a greater chance of pregnancy ending in abortion or with delivery of an abnormal offspring than do sibling control subjects.
- latent genetic damage to progeny of individuals undergoing irradiation has not been evaluated.

LEVEL 2:   Oligospermia/Azoospermia, Anovulation, Amenorrhea

EXPECTED OUTCOME

Patient demonstrates knowledge related to actual infertility:
- states individual causative factors of infertility.
- identifies potential effects of treatment on future offspring.
- identifies methods of contraception during treatment.
- identifies realistic expectations regarding return to fertility.
- identifies potential duration of infertility.

NURSING MANAGEMENT

Assessment

1. See Assessment, Level 1.
2. Evaluate patient's/partner's coping skills and response to infertility.
3. Determine patient's/partner's expectations related to return of reproductive function.

Nursing Interventions

1. Initiate discussion related to infertility.
2. Refer patient for counseling if appropriate.
3. Encourage ventilation of feelings.
4. Offer options of contraception.

Patient Teaching

1. See Patient Teaching, Level 1.
2. Place special attention on teaching regarding potential duration of infertility and realistic expectations regarding return of reproductive function.
3. Teach patient about signs and symptoms of premature menopause (gonadal dysfunction): decreased libido, hot flashes, insomnia, irritability; may be treated with cyclic estrogen replacement, calcium supplements, Benadryl, clonidine.

LEVEL 3:   Castration Surgery/Long-Term (Years) Azoospermia or Anovulation

Patient/partner demonstrate knowledge related to permanent sterility:
- state understanding of reproductive status (sterile).
- identify realistic option regarding future reproductivity.
- identify long-term follow-up plan of care.

Assessment

1. See Assessment, Levels 1 and 2.
2. Evaluate patient's/partner's understanding of reproductive status.

Nursing Interventions

1. See Nursing Interventions, Level 2.

Patient Teaching

1. See Patient Teaching, Levels 1 and 2.
2. Discuss options regarding future reproductivity (e.g., foster parenthood, adoption); these may not be realistic, depending upon patient's disease status and prognosis.

REFERENCES

Accola, K.M., and Sommerfeld, D.P.: Helping people with cancer consider parenthood. American Journal of Nursing 79:1580–1583, 1979.

Blatt, J., Mulvihill, J.J., and Ziegler, J.L.: Pregnancy outcome following chemotherapy. American Journal of Medicine 69:828–832, 1980.

Byrne, J., Mulvihill, J.J., et al.: Effects of treatment on fertility in long term survivors of childhood or adolescent cancer. New England Journal of Medicine 317(21):1315–1321, 1987.

Carroll, P.R., Morse, M.J., Whitmore, W.F., et al.: Fertility status of patients with clinical state I testis tumors on a surveillance protocol. Journal of Urology 138(7):70–72, 1987.

Chapman, R.: Effect of cytotoxic therapy on sexuality and gonadal function. Seminars in Oncology 14:84–92, 1982.

Damewood, M.D., and Grochow, L.B.: Prospects for fertility after chemotherapy or radiation for neoplastic disease. Fertility and Sterility 45(4):443–459, 1986.

Gershenson, D.M.: Menstrual and reproductive function after treatment with combination chemotherapy for malignant ovarian germ cell tumors. Journal of Clinical Oncology 6(2):270–275, 1988.

Heiney, S.P.: Adolescents with cancer: Sexual and reproductive issues. Cancer Nursing 12(2):95–101, 1989.

Itri, L.M.: The effects of chemotherapy on gonadal function. Your Patient and Cancer 3:45–49, 1983.

Kaempfer, S.H., and Major, P.: Fertility considerations in the gynecologic oncology patient. Oncology Nursing Forum 13(1):23–27, 1986.

Kaempfer, S.H.: The effects of cancer chemotherapy on reproduction: A review of the literature. Oncology Nursing Forum 8:11–18, 1981.

Kaempfer, S.H., Hoffman, D.J., and Wiley, F.M.: Sperm banking: A reproductive option in cancer therapy. Cancer Nursing 6:31–38, 1983.

Kreuser, E.D., Hetzel, W.D., Heit, W., et al.: Reproductive and endocrine gonadal functions in adults following multidrug chemotherapy for acute lymphoblastic or undifferentiated leukemia. Journal of Clinical Oncology 6(4):588–595, 1988.

Meadows, A.T., and Silber, J.: Delayed consequences of therapy for childhood cancer. CA: A Cancer Journal for Clinicians 35(5):271–283, 1985.

Schilsky, R.L., Lewis, B.J., and Sherins, R.J.: Gonadal dysfunction in patients receiving chemotherapy for cancer. Annals of Internal Medicine 93:109–114, 1980.

VENTILATION

The nurse assesses the patient's level of respiratory status, alterations in gas exchange, and history of exposure to respiratory contaminants to formulate actual or potential nursing diagnoses.

Appropriate patient outcomes to consider in planning nursing interventions will specify the patient's ability to:

1. describe plans for daily activity that demonstrate maximum conservation of energy.
2. list measures to reduce or modify pulmonary irritants in the environment, such as smoke, dry air, powders, and aerosols.
3. describe the effect of environmental extremes on ventilatory function and oxygen utilization.
4. describe effective measures to maintain a patent airway.
5. identify reasons for altered ventilation, such as decreased hemoglobin, infection, anxiety, effusion, and an obstructed airway.
6. identify an appropriate plan of action to follow if ventilation becomes altered.
7. develop a plan for managing an altered airway.

Evaluation of the patient's responses to nursing care is based on whether the patient recognizes factors that may impair ventilatory function and knows how to intervene with measures that may enhance optimum ventilatory capacity.

Excerpted from the ANA/ONS Standards of Cancer Nursing Practice.

Ineffective Airway Clearance

Maureen Larkin and Laura M. Benson

55

Population at Risk

- Individuals with abdominothoracic muscles neuromuscularly impaired by disease, treatment, or debilitation, and respirator-assisted patients
- Individuals with history of chronic obstructive pulmonary disease, smoking, narcotics use, tumors of the respiratory tract, exposure to air pollutants (e.g., asbestos, sulfur dioxide)
- Individuals with suppressed immunity predisposing to respiratory infection
- Individuals with history of treatments with chemotherapeutic agents with pulmonary toxicity (bleomycin, mitomycin) or radiation therapy to head, neck, thorax, upper abdomen
- Individuals with superior vena cava syndrome
- Individuals with history of drug use that may cause respiratory depression or bronchospasm
- Individuals with prior pleuroadesis, pleural effusion, or mediastinal tumors

LEVEL 1: Potential

EXPECTED OUTCOME

1. Patient demonstrates knowledge related to potentially ineffective airway clearance:
   - identifies changes in respiratory system that may occur in smokers, individuals with allergies, individuals exposed to inhalation of irritating chemicals.
   - identifies early signs and symptoms to report to health team.
2. Patient demonstrates knowledge of necessary measures to promote respiratory function:
   - reports pertinent signs and symptoms to health care team.
   - performs routine oral and respiratory hygiene.
   - adjusts fluids and nutritional intake as necessary.
   - maintains normal mobility and rest.
   - identifies measures to avoid harmful effects of smoking and other potential occupational and environmental carcinogens.
   - demonstrates adequate techniques in coughing, deep breathing, and postural drainage.
3. Patient maintains effective clearance of airway as evidenced by:
   - respirations within normal limits.
   - ability to cough effectively.
   - clear breath sounds.
   - activity tolerance within normal limits for patient.

NURSING MANAGEMENT

Assessment

1. Assess status of cough:
   - frequency.
   - ability.
   - depth.
   - force.
   - productivity.
2. Assess sputum:
   - odor.
   - color.
   - amount.
   - consistency.
   - time of day produced.
3. Observe respiratory status:
   - rate, depth, breathing pattern.
   - lung sounds (normal or adventitious, increased or decreased).
   - color of skin, mucous membranes, nail beds.
   - capillary refill.
   - dyspnea on exertion.
   - chest x-ray results.
4. Evaluate protective mechanisms, including immunocompetence and integrity of oral mucosa.
5. Determine present level and activity tolerance.
6. Obtain history of:
   - chronic obstructive pulmonary disease.
   - pulmonary infections.
   - allergies.
   - exposure to air pollutants (e.g., asbestos, sulfur dioxide).
   - chemotherapy (bleomycin, mitomycin).
   - radiation therapy to neck, head, thorax, upper abdomen.
   - narcotic use.
   - smoking (how much, how long).
7. Monitor vital signs.
8. Monitor any pulmonary toilet that patient currently receives for preexisting or chronic condition.
9. Perform nutritional assessment.

Nursing Interventions

1. Collect sputum and blood samples as ordered.
2. Encourage frequent turning and repositioning of immobile patients.
3. Encourage frequent coughing, deep breathing (up to 6 times a day), and use of incentive spirometer.
4. Implement hygienic measures to protect patient from infection:
   - handwashing by visitors and health care professionals before patient contact.
   - prohibition of visitors and health care professionals with infection.
   - encourage oral hygiene routine.
   - aseptic technique when delivering respiratory treatments.
5. Implement isolation precautions as needed (do not place immunosuppressed patients in the same room as patient with respiratory infection).
6. Have preoperative respiratory therapy consultation.
7. Encourage non-vigorous or passive range of motion.
8. Allow patient to ventilate feelings.

Patient Teaching

1. Teach coughing and deep breathing.
2. Teach breathing exercises.
3. Teach postural drainage positions.
4. Instruct patient in oral hygiene.
5. Tell patient to report signs and symptoms of early respiratory dysfunction to health care team:
   - increasing shortness of breath on exertion or at rest.
   - green, yellow, or brown sputum.
   - persistent nonproductive cough.
   - feeling of increased congestion.
   - persistent fever, diaphoresis, chills.

6. Explain rationale for and measures to promote respiratory function:
   - avoid smoking.
   - avoid exposure to harmful chemicals that could irritate respiratory tract.
   - maintain appropriate level of physical activity (avoid high level of physical exertion).
   - maintain adequate hydration and nutritional intake (offer high-calorie supplements if needed).
   - avoid exposure to individuals with respiratory infections.
   - describe common seasons for exacerbation of chronic obstructive lung disease (winter, summer, ozone alert days).
7. Include family members in all aspects of patient teaching.
8. Provide forum for family members to ventilate feelings (e.g., support group, social worker).

LEVEL 2: *Moderate*

EXPECTED OUTCOME

1. Patient demonstrates knowledge related to ineffective airway clearance:
   - identifies changes in respiratory status associated with bronchitis, pneumonia, other upper respiratory infections.
   - identifies signs and symptoms to report to health care team.
   - identifies long- and short-term complications of ineffective airway clearance.
2. Patient demonstrates/identifies measures to maintain patent airway and eliminate secretions:
   - performs necessary treatments and procedures.
   - demonstrates knowledge related to administration and side effects of medication.
   - demonstrates measures to promote lung expansion and expectoration of secretions.
   - states need to maintain hydration and adequate nutritional status.
   - demonstrates measures that may prevent further or future lung damage and disease.
   - demonstrates self-positioning techniques to facilitate maximum respiratory aeration.
   - states need for vigorous pulmonary hygiene.
3. Patient achieves or maintains adequate respiratory function:
   - respirations within normal limits for patient.
   - breath sounds clear.
   - production of thin, clear secretions.
   - laboratory values within normal limits for patient.

NURSING MANAGEMENT

Assessment

1. See Assessment, Level 1.
2. Assess chest pain (quality, location, duration, activities that exacerbate pain).
3. Note results of laboratory tests (WBC, hemoglobin, hematocrit, blood gases, sputum, blood cultures, electrolytes).
4. Monitor diagnostic studies (e.g., chest x-ray, pulmonary function tests, CT scan).

Nursing Interventions

1. See Nursing Interventions, Level 1.
2. Implement hygienic measures to protect patient from further infection (e.g., handwashing by visitors and health care professionals before contact with patient, aseptic techniques in delivery of respiratory treatments).
3. Assist with collection of blood.
4. Administer medications as ordered and note any adverse reactions:
   - bronchodilators: tachycardia, anxiety, nausea or vomiting, diaphoresis, syncope, flushing of skin.
   - steroids: personality changes, increased weight gain secondary to increased appetite, increased water retention, Cushingoid syndrome, nausea, vomiting, diarrhea, abdominal cramping.
   - oxygen: respiratory depression in hypercapnic patients, direct lung damage with high concentration.
5. Encourage oral fluid intake for adequate hydration and maintain record.
6. Encourage coughing and deep breathing exercises.
7. Administer oxygen as ordered.
8. Control pain with lowest effective dosage of narcotics.
9. Teach relaxation techniques.
10. Provide adequate rest periods.
11. Assist in and evaluate effectiveness of any treatment received (e.g., intermittent positive pressure breathing, aerosol, or ultrasonic therapy).
12. Assist with expectoration:
    - suction as needed.
    - position patient for postural drainage.
    - perform chest physical therapy as prescribed.
13. Elevate head of bed for patient comfort unless contraindicated.
14. Humidify air as appropriate.
15. Provide oral hygiene.

Patient Teaching

1. See Patient Teaching, Level 1.
2. Teach pulmonary hygiene and breathing techniques:
   - diaphragmatic breathing.
   - pursed-lip breathing.
   - segmental breathing.
3. Explain positions for maximum pulmonary aeration:
   - elevate upper body to 45 degrees or greater with shoulders tilted forward.
   - sit with arms resting on bedside table.
4. Discuss prescribed treatments:
   - importance of being seated comfortably and being relaxed before undergoing any type of treatment (intermittent positive pressure breathing, aerosol, ultrasonic).
   - importance of attempting to cough and expectorate after treatment.
5. Note usual duration of present illness (in adults with pneumonia, chest x-ray takes 6 weeks or more to return to normal).
6. Emphasize importance of and maintain hydration and adequate nutritional status.
7. Discuss avoiding irritants to respiratory tract (smoke, chemicals).
8. Explain side effects and actions of medications, note expiration dates and individual storage instructions for bronchodilators (some require refrigeration).

9. Describe care and cleaning of any respiratory equipment at home.
10. Note need to space periods of rest between activities.

11. Teach importance of proper disposal of secretions.
12. Instruct on appropriate suctioning techniques and care of equipment.

LEVEL 3: Severe

EXPECTED OUTCOME

1. Patient/caregiver identify/demonstrate knowledge related to severe inability to clear airway:
   - identify signs and symptoms to report to health care team.
   - identify factors influencing respiratory function.
   - identify potential sequelae/complications of ineffective airway clearance.
2. Patient/caregiver demonstrate measures to maintain patent airway:
   - demonstrate knowledge related to administration and side effects of medication.
   - perform treatments and procedures.
   - identify safety measures in using oxygen and other types of respiratory equipment in home.
   - identify necessity of adequate hydration and nutritional intake.
   - identify/demonstrate pulmonary hygiene measures.
   - demonstrate measures for promoting lung expansion and expectoration of secretions.
   - pace activities to promote optimal functioning.
3. Patient maintains adequate respiratory function:
   - vital signs stable.
   - respirations stable for age and condition.
   - breath sounds stable or improved.
   - sputum clear.
   - activity tolerance stable for age and condition.

NURSING MANAGEMENT

Assessment

See Assessment, Levels 1 and 2.

Nursing Interventions

1. See Nursing Interventions, Levels 1 and 2.
2. Employ vigorous suctioning, using aseptic technique.

Patient Teaching

1. See Patient Teaching, Levels 1 and 2.
2. Emphasize prevention of infection and good handwashing technique.
3. Discuss need for pulmonary rehabilitation:
   - official programs available locally (e.g., breathers' clubs, American Lung Association, support groups, smoking

cessation groups [if applicable], hospital-based pulmonary rehabilitation programs).

4. Discuss measures to promote respiratory function:
   - necessity of adhering to prescribed oxygen liter flow.
   - performance of pulmonary hygiene as prescribed.
   - acceptance of disease state as lifelong, chronic condition.
   - adjustments of activities to level of fatigue.
   - immunizations for influenza.
   - avoidance of individuals with upper respiratory infections.
   - use of humidifiers at home (avoid when patients are immunosuppressed, receiving chemotherapy, or have low WBC).
   - use of air conditioning on high-humidity days.

5. Teach energy-saving techniques:
   - restful positions.
   - use of stool in shower.
   - rest period between activities.
   - prevent constipation.
   - use of bedside commode if bathroom is on another level.
   - eating soft, chopped, easily digested foods.
   - aid for ambulation (e.g., cane, wheelchair).

6. Initiate visiting nurse, social service referral to provide home health assistance as needed.

7. Provide assistance in home adaptation (move bed to first floor of home if patient can not negotiate stairs; use hospital bed if needed).

8. Refer for employment counseling if patient is no longer able to maintain present position.

9. Utilize portable oxygen to increase patient's level of sociability.

10. Offer sexual counseling to provide techniques to be used to minimize overexertion and dyspnea.

11. Encourage patient and family to continue family activities and traditions.

SUGGESTED READINGS

Chernecky, C.C., and Ramsey, P.W.: Critical Nursing Care of the Client with Cancer. Norwalk, CT, Appleton-Century-Crofts, 1984, pp. 114–117.

Dietz, H.J. Jr.: Rehabilitation Oncology. New York, John Wiley & Sons, 1981.

Groenwald, S. (Ed.): Cancer Nursing: Principles and Practices. Monterey, CA, Jones & Bartlett, 1987, pp. 634–653.

Johnson, B., and Gross, J. (Eds.): Handbook of Oncology Nursing. New York, John Wiley & Sons, 1985.

Lareau, S., and Larson, J.L.: Ineffective breathing pattern related to airflow limitation. Nursing Clinics of North America 22(1):179–191, 1987.

Yarbro, C.H. (Ed.): Head and neck cancer. Seminars in Oncology Nursing 5(3):1–219, 1989.

PATIENT EDUCATION MATERIALS AND COMMUNITY RESOURCES

American Lung Association (Smoking Cessation).

American Cancer Society (I Can Cope Support Groups) (Smoking Cessation).

Alcoholics Anonymous.

International Association of Laryngectomies.

State Offices of Vocational Rehabilitation (Cancer Information Service) Call 1–800–4–CANCER.

"Talking Time" (Support for people with cancer and the people who care about them) provided by National Cancer Institute (no charge).

"Eating Hints" (Recipes and tips for better nutrition during cancer treatment) provided by National Cancer Institute (no charge).

When Cancer Recurs–Meeting the Challenge Again, provided by National Cancer Institute (no charge).

Progress Against Cancer of the Lungs, provided by National Cancer Institute (no charge).

What We Need To Know About Cancer of Larynx.

Copies of:
  –National Cancer Act 1971.
  –Rehabilitation Act 1973.

Ineffective Breathing Pattern

Hilary Ann Wood and Jan M. Ellerhorst-Ryan

Population at Risk

- Individuals with primary malignancies: Hodgkin's and non-Hodgkin's lymphomas; head/neck, breast, thyroid, lung cancers; thymoma; acute leukemias
- Individuals with metastatic malignancies that affect the respiratory system
- Individuals with superior vena cava syndrome, malignant pleural effusion, pulmonary fibrosis, pneumonitis, history of tuberculosis
- Individuals with neuromuscular impairment, musculoskeletal impairment, pain, decreased energy
- Individuals receiving chemotherapeutic agents that are known to have pulmonary toxicity
- Individuals who have received radiation therapy to middle or upper thorax, head, or neck
- Individuals receiving drugs that cause respiratory depression or bronchospasm
- Individuals with acquired immunodeficiency syndrome
- Individuals with pulmonary infections and infiltrates

LEVEL 1: Potential

EXPECTED OUTCOME

1. Patient demonstrates knowledge related to potential impairment of breathing pattern:
   - identifies signs and symptoms of respiratory impairment.
   - verbalizes importance of promptly communicating signs and symptoms to health care professionals.
2. Patient demonstrates knowledge of measures to prevent respiratory impairment:
   - identifies strategies to promote general well-being, thereby reducing potential for respiratory infection.
   - maintains activities within limits imposed by disease process.
   - performs respiratory toilet measures.
3. Patient maintains effective breathing pattern:
   - chest clear by auscultation.
   - laboratory data within normal limits.
   - respirations regular and nonlabored.
   - absence of tenacious sputum or secretions.

359

NURSING MANAGEMENT

Assessment

1. Assess patient's understanding of disease process and individual therapy.
2. Determine current pulmonary status:
   - auscultate chest, noting absence or presence of rales, rhonchi, or friction rubs.
   - note character and ease of respirations (e.g., intercostal retractions, sub- or supracostal retractions).
3. Obtain history of chest or neck radiation therapy:
   - total (cumulative dosage).
   - length of treatment.
   - area irradiated.
4. Obtain history of chemotherapy:
   - agents given.
   - cumulative dosages (where applicable).
   - other medications that may potentiate toxic pulmonary effects.
5. Obtain history of past or coexisting pulmonary disease (e.g., tuberculosis, chronic obstructive pulmonary disease, respiratory infection, smoking).
6. Monitor diagnostic data:
   - purified protein derivative.
   - chest x-rays.
   - pulmonary function studies.
   - CBC.
   - arterial blood gases.
   - sputums for acid-fast bacillus.
   - routine cultures: bacteria, viral, fungal.
   - biopsy for *Pneumocystis carinii*.
7. Obtain baseline data:
   - vital signs.
   - mental status.
   - activity level.
   - respiratory status.

Patient Teaching

1. Teach signs and symptoms of respiratory impairment to report to health care team:
   - air hunger.
   - dyspnea on exertion.
   - dry cough.
   - temperature elevation.
   - hoarseness.
   - altered breath sounds (stridor).
   - productive cough.
   - pain or discomfort associated with breathing.
2. Outline rationale and measures to promote respiratory function. Encourage mobility, smoking cessation, fluid restriction where applicable.
3. Teach coughing and deep-breathing exercises as indicated.
4. Discuss optimal hydration and nutritional status.
5. Describe measures to prevent infection:
   - avoid crowds and exposure to individuals with infection.
   - maintain nutritional status.
6. Make available resource materials from American Cancer Society, National Cancer Institute, and American Lung Association including telephone numbers of the local branches.

LEVEL 2: Mild to Moderate

EXPECTED OUTCOME

1. Patient demonstrates knowledge related to ineffective breathing pattern:
   - identifies signs and symptoms of altered respiratory status.
   - identifies factors that influence respiratory function.
   - identifies potential sequelae/complications of ineffective breathing pattern.

2. Patient demonstrates measures to promote optimal breathing patterns:
   - demonstrates proper knowledge and administration of medications.
   - performs necessary treatments and procedures.
   - identifies signs and symptoms to report to health care team.
   - demonstrates measures to control or correct edema related to disease.
   - identifies/demonstrates measures to prevent or minimize anxiety and apprehension.
3. Patient exhibits effective breathing pattern:
   - chest clear by auscultation.
   - laboratory values within normal limits.
   - respirations regular and nonlabored.
   - vital signs within normal limits.

NURSING MANAGEMENT

Assessment

1. See Assessment, Level 1.
2. Assess for:
   - pallor, cool and clammy skin.
   - history of dyspnea on exertion, cough, presence and character of sputum.
   - edema in head, neck, extremities that may suggest disease-related pulmonary complications.
   - cyanosis.
3. Monitor for temperature elevation with or without chills.
4. Evaluate level of anxiety and apprehension.
5. Assess need for home care equipment (e.g., commode, wheelchair, and the like).

Nursing Interventions

1. Initiate oxygen therapy as indicated.
2. Assist patient to position of comfort to minimize or reduce respiratory effect.
3. Obtain sputum specimen for culture and sensitivity, acid-fast bacillus, fungus, virus if indicated.
4. Maintain calm, supportive environment to minimize anxiety and apprehension during acute episodes.
5. Prevent exposure to individuals with infections.
6. Administer medications (e.g., analgesics,

antianxiety agents, bronchodilators, expectorants, antimicrobials, steroids, anticholinergics) and other treatments as prescribed. Monitor effects of drug therapy.
7. Encourage optimal hydration and nutritional status.
8. Encourage level of activity consistent with stage of disease.
9. Monitor administration of transfusions and drainage of effusions.
10. Refer to respiratory home care service as needed.

Patient Teaching

1. See Patient Teaching, Level 1.
2. Describe use of oxygen therapy at home when applicable.
3. Explain measures to enhance respiratory function:
   - demonstrate positioning that allows for maximum chest expansion.
   - identify importance of adequate hydration.
   - perform appropriate breathing exercises (e.g., diaphragmatic pursed lip breathing, apical expansion, nasal expansion).
   - fluid restrictions as prescribed by physician.
   - dietary restriction (e.g., limit milk products).
   - positioning and comfort measures.

- relaxation techniques, controlled breathing patterns.
- breathing exercises, including use of abdominal muscles and other accessory muscles of respiration.
- maintaining maximal mobility and activity levels within limitations of disease.
- compliance with medical plan of care

(e.g., administration of medications as prescribed).

4. Discuss rationale for treatment and side effects of drugs and therapies known to have pulmonary toxicity. Discuss the need to assess continuously for signs of toxicity and to report them immediately to health care team.

LEVEL 3: Severe

EXPECTED OUTCOME

1. Patient/caregiver demonstrate knowledge related to respiratory distress:
   - identify signs and symptoms of respiratory distress.
   - verbalize importance of seeking emergency treatment when these signs and symptoms are observed.
2. Patient exhibits improved respiratory status as evidenced by:
   - reduction in abnormal breath sounds.
   - laboratory values approaching normal limits.
   - reduction in signs and symptoms of respiratory impairment.
   - ability to resume self-care activities.
   - maintenance of normal respiratory rate and function.
3. Patient/caregiver demonstrate measures to promote optimal breathing patterns:
   - demonstrate proper knowledge and administration of medications.
   - perform necessary treatments and procedures.
   - demonstrate energy-saving techniques.

NURSING MANAGEMENT

Assessment

1. See Assessment, Levels 1 and 2.
2. Assess respiratory status and related circulatory compromise:
   - absence or presence of rhonchi, rales, pleural friction rub; evaluation of respiratory effort.
   - cyanosis, spider nevi, distended head and neck veins.
   - history of dyspnea at rest, productive cough, character of sputum.
3. Check for pain, including location, severity, and contributing factors.
4. Assess for malnutrition and dehydration (poor skin turgor, muscle wasting).
5. Evaluate need for home health services and supportive equipment.

Nursing Interventions

1. See Nursing Interventions, Level 2.
2. Maintain a patent airway:
   - provide humidification and suction as needed.
   - provide tracheostomy care as needed.
3. Monitor cardiac output.

4. Place patient in a position that allows for maximum chest expansion (e.g., orthopneic position).
5. Plan activities to allow minimum energy expenditure with adequate periods of rest:
   - assist patient during meals as needed.
   - provide assistance for bathing as needed.
   - provide passive range-of-motion exercises.
   - change patient's position q2–4h to prevent pressure sores as needed.
6. Assist patient in dealing with anticipatory grief, fear of dying, fear of suffocation.
7. Encourage optimal hydration and nutritional status.
8. Prevent aspiration pneumonia by placing patient in semi-Fowler position during and for 1 hour after meals.
9. Provide adequate pain relief, especially before nursing interventions.
10. Refer to home health agency for home care services including respiratory services, supportive equipment, speech and language therapy, home health aide.
11. Refer to speech and language therapy for effective communication as needed (e.g., laryngeal assistance devices, esophageal speech).

Patient Teaching

1. See Patient Teaching, Levels 1 and 2.
2. Teach importance of and procedures for maintaining continuous oxygen therapy and clear airway (e.g., tracheostomy care).
3. Explain rationale and measures for emergency treatment (chemotherapy, radiation therapy).
4. Instruct patient/caregiver to keep emergency telephone numbers readily available at home.
5. Instruct patient/caregiver in energy-saving techniques:
   - small, frequent meals.
   - activities planned to allow periods of rest between.
   - activity levels maintained within limits imposed by disease process.

- assistance obtained with activities of daily living as needed.
- patient positioned to promote maximum aeration of lungs, prevention of pressure sores, prevention of aspiration pneumonia.
6. Teach management of home care equipment, cleaning, and maintenance:
   - home tracheostomy care as needed.
7. Teach signs and symptoms of respiratory distress, including those to be reported to health care team:
   - air hunger.
   - cyanosis.
   - dyspnea at rest.
   - respiratory stridor.
   - spider nevi.
   - head/neck edema.

SUGGESTED READINGS

Bouchard, R., and Owens, N.F.: Nursing Care of the Cancer Patient. St. Louis, C.V. Mosby, 1981.

Canellos, G.P., Cohen, C., and Posner, M.: Pulmonary emergencies in neoplastic disease. *In* Yarbro, J.W., and Bornstein, R.S. (Eds.): Oncologic Emergencies. New York, Grune & Statton, 1981.

Carter, S., Crooke, S.T., and Umezawa, H.: Bleomycin: Current Status and New Developments. New York, Academic Press, 1978.

Haylock, P.J.: Breathing difficulty: Changes in respiratory function. Seminars in Oncology Nursing 3(4):293–298, 1987.

Nogeire, C., Mincer, F., and Botstein, C.: Long survival in patients with bronchogenic carcinoma complicated by superior vena caval obstruction. Chest 75:325–329, 1979.

Norton, L.C.: Oxygenation and ventilation. *In* Johnson, B.L., and Gross, J.: Handbook of Oncology Nursing. New York, Wiley Medical, 1985.

Perez, C., Presant, C.A., and Van Amberg, A.L. III: Management of superior vena cava obstruction syndrome. Seminars in Oncology 5:123–134, 1978.

Spross, J., and Stern, R.: Nursing management of oncology patients with superior vena cava syndrome. Oncology Nursing Forum 6:3–5, 1979.

Wood, H.: Developments in the support of patients with malignant pleural effusion. *In* Tiffany, R. (Ed.): Cancer Nursing Update. London: Bailliere Tindall, 1981.

Yarbro, C.H. (Ed.): Head and neck cancer. Seminars in Oncology Nursing 5(3):1–219, 1989.

Yasko, J.: Guidelines for Cancer Care—Symptom Management. Reston, VA, Reston Publishing, 1982.

Impaired Gas Exchange

Judith A. Schreiber

Population at Risk

- Individuals who have tumors of the lung, mediastinum, or neck, or CNS tumors involving the respiratory center
- Individuals who have received radiation therapy to chest or neck region
- Individuals who have received chemotherapeutic agents with known pulmonary toxicities
- Individuals with pleural effusion, pneumonia, pulmonary emboli, pulmonary edema, concurrent chronic obstructive pulmonary disease, and superior vena cava obstruction
- Individuals who have had surgery involving head, neck, trachea, chest, or a portion of lung
- Individuals with history of tuberculosis, lung infections, or smoking
- Individuals with increased risk from occupational or environmental hazards
- Individuals with reduced hemoglobin

LEVEL 1: Potential

EXPECTED OUTCOME

1. Patient demonstrates knowledge of risk factors and prevention of impaired gas exchange:
   - identifies occupational and environmental hazards.
   - identifies early signs and symptoms of impaired gas exchange.
   - identifies strategies for optimal pulmonary health.
   - develops plan for behavioral and life style changes.
2. Patient maintains adequate pulmonary function:
   - vital signs remain within normal limits for patient.
   - respirations remain within normal limits for patient.
   - breath sounds clear.
   - activity tolerance remains within normal limits for patient.

NURSING MANAGEMENT

Assessment

1. Obtain patient history:
   - Preexisting or past pulmonary diseases.
   - previous radiation treatment to the thorax.
   - smoking habits.
   - exposure to irritants–chemicals, dust, asbestos.
   - previous treatment with chemotherapeutic agents with known pulmonary toxicities.

2. Assess history of symptoms of respiratory difficulty:
   - type of onset–acute or gradual.
   - dyspnea.
   - tachypnea.
   - sputum production.
   - hemoptysis.
   - shoulder or arm pain.
   - change in activity level.
   - headache.
   - change in mental status.
3. Assess ventilatory abilities:
   - respiratory movements–depth, rate, rhythm.
   - use of accessory muscles.
   - anterior-posterior diameter.
   - patency of airway via nares.
   - fingertip clubbing.
   - nail bed, skin, mucous membrane color.
4. Palpate chest region for abnormalities:
   - crepitation.
   - fremitus.
   - nonsymmetrical chest expansion.
   - deviation of trachea.
5. Percuss chest region for density:
   - consolidation.
   - displacement of organs.
   - other densities.
6. Auscultate lung and airway regions for absent, diminished, or adventitious sounds.
7. Assess activity level.

Patient Teaching

1. Explain function of lungs:
   - anatomy and physiology.
   - purpose.
   - specific alteration in patient's lung tissue.
2. Discuss relationship between occupational and environmental hazards and current physical status.
3. Identify signs and symptoms to report to health care team:
   - increased sputum production.
   - unusual shortness of breath.
   - chest pain or tightness.
   - change in sputum color.
   - inability to maintain normal activity.
   - bloody sputum.
   - persistent cough.
4. Define measures to maintain adequate ventilatory abilities:
   - keep workplace and living areas well ventilated.
   - use masks in areas of high pollution.
   - get pneumococcal vaccine.
   - avoid contact with individuals with upper respiratory infections.
   - do not smoke.
5. Alert patient to local resources–support groups, American Lung Association, American Cancer Society.

LEVEL 2: Moderate

EXPECTED OUTCOME

1. Patient demonstrates knowledge related to altered ventilation:
   - verbalizes signs and symptoms of impaired gas exchange.
   - identifies factors that influence impairment and maintenance of gas exchange.
   - identifies potential sequelae/complications.
   - identifies relationship between emotional status and ventilatory abilities.
2. Patient identifies/demonstrates measures to promote gas exchange:
   - performs necessary treatments and procedures.
   - demonstrates proper knowledge and administration of medication and oxygen.

- identifies signs and symptoms to report to health care team.
- states ways to conserve ventilatory abilities.
3. Patient achieves or maintains adequate pulmonary function:
   - vital signs within normal limits for patient.
   - respiration within normal limits for patient.
   - breath sounds remain at patient's baseline.

NURSING MANAGEMENT

Assessment

1. See Assessment, Level 1.
2. Determine psychosocial and emotional status:
   - coping style.
   - support systems.
   - patient outlook regarding present health, and prognosis.
   - social activities.
   - reactions of significant others.
   - financial situation.
   - home environment.
3. Monitor results of laboratory and diagnostic testing:
   - arterial blood gases.
   - CBC.
   - electrolytes.
   - cytology.
   - cultures.
   - bacteriology tests.
   - biopsy.
   - pulmonary function studies.
   - chest x-rays.
   - scans.
4. Treatment history:
   - head, neck, chest radiation therapy; treatment field, number of treatments, dosage.
   - chemotherapy with specific cytotoxic agents.
5. Assess for pain:
   - presence or absence of pain.
   - intensity.
   - duration.
   - precipitating factors.
   - relief measures.
   - location.

Nursing Interventions

1. Provide an environmentally beneficial atmosphere:
   - multipositional bed.
   - humidification.
   - adequate ventilation.
2. Promote optimum patient activity:
   - adequate tubing length or portable oxygen.
   - appropriate pain or anxiety medications proper to activity.
   - plan rest periods between activities.
3. Maintain hydration and nutritional status:
   - oxygen use with meals if necessary.
   - 2 to 3 l of fluid per daily unless contraindicated.
4. Administer oxygen to maintain respiratory status:
   - maintain prescribed level of oxygen flow.
   - humidification with continuous oxygen.
   - appropriate set-up of low-flow (trach collar, nasal cannula, face mask, or partial rebreather) or high-flow (nonrebreather Venturi mask) system.
5. Administer medications to enhance respiratory status (e.g., terbutaline sulfate [Brethine], aminophylline, Aarane, codeine, Romilar, terpin hydrate, or nasal congestants).
6. Assist in breathing and posturing techniques as appropriate:
   - elevate HOB.
   - pursed-lip breathing.
   - forced abdominal breathing.

- percussion and vibration.
- postural drainage.
- effective coughing techniques.
7. Promote patient comfort:
    - scheduled use of medications.
    - transcutaneous nerve stimulation.
    - splinting techniques.
    - posturing for comfort.
8. Provide measures to decrease anxiety and stress:
    - decrease in noxious environmental stimuli.
    - antianxiety medications.
    - relaxation techniques.
    - emotional support.
9. Make referrals to other professionals as necessary.
10. Coordinate plans for home care with patient and family and with home nursing agency and respiratory care company.

Patient Teaching

1. See Patient Teaching, Level 1.
2. Explain purpose, administration, and side effects of medications.
3. Discuss use of oxygen:
    - importance of maintaining correct system parameters (e.g., flow rate–prn or continuous).

- safety precautions (e.g., no aerosols, no petroleum products, no open flames, only approved grounded electrical equipment).
- dose-related toxicities (e.g., CO_2 narcosis).
4. Outline measures to maximize ventilatory abilities:
    - oxygen-sparing techniques.
    - rest periods.
    - humidification.
    - adequate hydration.
    - adequate nutrition.
    - use of incentive spirometer.
5. Teach signs and symptoms to report to the health care team:
    - fever.
    - increased sputum production.
    - increased shortness of breath.
    - chest pain or tightness.
    - change in mental status.
6. Teach relaxation techniques:
    - controlled breathing.
    - diversion.
    - use of imagery or similar methods.
    - use of touch.
    - massage.
7. Discuss relationship between ventilatory abilities and related diagnoses pertinent to the patient.
8. Discuss management of dyspneic episodes.

LEVEL 3: Severe

EXPECTED OUTCOME

1. Patient/caregiver demonstrate knowledge related to severely altered ventilation:
    - identify signs and symptoms to report to health care team.
    - identify signs and symptoms of complications/sequelae.
    - identify purpose and ramifications of medical interventions.
2. Patient/caregiver demonstrate measures to manage severely impaired ventilation:
    - perform necessary treatments and procedures.
    - demonstrate proper knowledge and administration of medication and oxygen.

- verbalize/demonstrate adequate fluid and nutritional intake.
- identify/demonstrate emergency treatments for management of acute ventilatory distress.
- plan daily activities with attention to ways to conserve ventilatory abilities.
3. Patient achieves/maintains adequate pulmonary function:
    - vital signs stable per patient's baseline.
    - respirations stable per patient's baseline.
    - breath sounds stable or improved.
    - activity tolerance stable per patient's parameters.

NURSING MANAGEMENT

Assessment

1. See Assessment, Levels 1 and 2.
2. Inspect chest drainage system if present:
    - patency of tubes.
    - drainage: fluctuation, amount, color, consistency, character, odor.
    - air leak.
3. Note conditions associated with acute respiratory change:
    - cyanosis.
    - chest pain.
    - increase in pulse.
    - decrease in blood pressure.
    - change in level of consciousness.
    - air hunger.
    - sternal retractions.
    - absence or presence of rhonchi, rales, pleural friction rub.
4. Inspect ventilator system if present:
    - proper connections and routing.
    - unobstructed airflow.
5. Observe for complications related to mechanical ventilation if present:
    - pulmonary trauma.
    - fluid retention.
    - gastric air retention.

Nursing Interventions

1. See Nursing Interventions, Level 2.
2. Monitor chest drainage system:
    - keep tubes free of kinks and dependent loops.
    - keep drainage system lower than patient.
    - keep connections airtight.
    - check insertion site.
    - check q4h for drainage amount and notify physician if volume greater than 200 ml/hr or if dramatic change in fluid volume develops over a short period of time.
    - keep hemostats and occlusive dressing near patient.
3. Pleuredesis may be ordered. Normal procedure is to instill 250 mg of tetracycline in 50 ml normal saline into pleural cavity via chest tube:
    - explain procedure to patient.
    - administer analgesics as ordered.
    - turn and position patient as ordered.
4. Assist with breathing efforts:
    - pulmonary hygiene.
    - use of assistive devices.
    - suctioning as appropriate.
5. Monitor ventilator system:
    - accurate settings of controls.
    - placement of endotracheal tube.
    - alarms functioning correctly.
    - endotracheal tube care (e.g., placement, cuff management, pressure sores).
6. Assist with hydration.

Patient Teaching

1. See Patient Teaching, Levels 1 and 2.
2. Teach signs and symptoms to report to the health care team.

3. Discuss pulmonary hygiene methods:
   - suctioning.
   - oral care.
   - use of assistive devices.
4. Explain rationale for treatment, procedures, and assistive devices.
5. Instruct in tracheotomy care if applicable.
6. Discuss rehabilitation service that may be found within many hospital settings:
   - support groups, assistance with financial concerns, assistance with obtaining equipment are offered by the American Lung Association.
   - Breathers Club, HOPE Club, The Smoking Phone are available through the American Cancer Society.

SUGGESTED READINGS

Bates, B.: A Guide to Physical Examination. Philadelphia, J.B. Lippincott, 1974, pp. 73–90.

Brown, M.L., Carrie, V., Jenson-Bjerklie, S., et al.: Lung cancer and dyspnea: The patient's perception. Oncology Nursing Forum 13(5):19–24, 1986.

Cockcroft, A., and Guz, A.: Breathlessness. Postgraduate Medical Journal 63:637–641, 1987.

Haylock, P.J.: Breathing difficulty: Changes in respiratory function. Seminars in Oncology Nursing 3(4):293–298, 1986.

Lareau, S., and Largon, J.L.: Ineffective breathing pattern related to airflow limitation. Nursing Clinics of North America 22(1):179–191, 1987.

Mahler, D.A.: Dyspnea: Diagnosis and management. Clinics in Chest Medicine 8(2):215–230, 1987.

Mayo, J.M., and Hammer, J.B.: A nurses's guide to mechanical ventilation. RN 50(8):18–23, 1987.

Mimms, B.C.: The risks of oxygen therapy. RN 50(7):20–25, 1987.

Openbrier, D.R., and Covey, M.: Ineffective breathing pattern related to malnutrition. Nursing Clinics of North America 22(1):225–247, 1987.

Varricchio, C.G., and Jassak, P.F.: Acute pulmonary disorders associated with cancer. Seminars in Oncology Nursing 1(4):269–277, 1987.

Williams, S.M.: Pulmonary system. In Alspach, J.G., and Williams, S.M. (Eds.): Core Curriculum for Critical Care Nursing (3rd ed.). Philadelphia, W.B. Saunders, 1985, pp. 2–101.

Altered Breathing Patterns: Diversional Methods

Laura M. Benson and Maureen Larkin

Population at Risk

- Individuals with cancer of oropharynx or larynx
- Individuals who have undergone surgery to head and neck, laryngectomies (total and partial supraglottic), radical neck dissection, tracheotomy

LEVEL 1:   Potential

EXPECTED OUTCOME

1. Patient demonstrates knowledge related to potential alteration in respiratory function:
   - identifies signs and symptoms of alteration.
   - identifies predisposing factors.
   - identifies potential need for diversional method.
2. Patient maintains adequate respiratory function:
   - laboratory values within normal limits.
   - breath sounds clear.
   - respiratory efforts and rates within normal limits.
   - sputum clear.

NURSING MANAGEMENT

Assessment

1. Obtain history of risk factors:
   - smoking.
   - alcohol consumption.
   - radiation therapy to head and neck area.
   - poor nutritional status.
   - poor oral hygiene.
2. Assess for symptoms of respiratory difficulty:
   - dyspnea.
   - stridor.
   - sputum production.
   - hoarseness.
   - cough.
   - shortness of breath.
   - increased respiratory rate.
   - use of accessory muscles of respiration.
3. Auscultate lungs and tracheobronchial airway for absent or diminished breath sounds or adventitious sounds.
4. Assess for a change in the amount and consistency of respiratory tract secretions.
5. Assess oral cavity.
6. Evaluate pertinent laboratory values.

7. Assess patient's understanding of proposed surgery.
8. Assess patient's knowledge of a tracheotomy.

Nursing Interventions

1. Arrange for preoperative evaluation for prosthesis use and reconstruction (functional and cosmetic).
2. Refer for preoperative consultation with speech pathology.
3. Arrange preoperative visits from lay laryngectomy volunteer through American Cancer Society.

Patient Teaching

1. Explain relationship between head and neck cancer risk factors and health.
2. Provide patient with information on available resources (e.g., smoking cessation clinics, American Cancer Society, lung associations, Alcoholics Anonymous).

3. Describe signs and symptoms to report to health care team:
   • increased sputum production/changes in color or consistency.
   • cough.
   • shortness of breath.
   • increased respirations.
   • painful or noisy respirations (stridor).
   • bleeding.
   • hoarseness.
4. Explain importance of good oral hygiene.
5. Emphasize importance of balanced diet and increased fluid intake.
6. Explain importance of coughing and deep breathing q2h if pulmonary secretions are present.
7. Teach need to minimize exposure to pathogens (e.g., avoid people with infections, avoid contaminated equipment, tissue).
8. Explain proposed surgical procedure (e.g., radical neck dissection, laryngectomy, tracheotomy) and postoperative considerations.
9. Provide information concerning self-help and support groups (e.g., International Association of Laryngectomy).

LEVEL 2: *Diversional Method*

EXPECTED OUTCOME

1. Patient identifies/demonstrates respiratory hygiene measures:
   • performs coughing, deep breathing exercises.
   • complies with oxygen and chest therapy measures if indicated.
   • demonstrates measures to maintain patent airway.
   • makes necessary environmental modifications.
2. Patient demonstrates ability to care for stoma/tracheostomy tube:
   • identifies safety precautions to prevent tracheal aspiration.
   • states first aid measures for neck breathers.
   • identifies signs and symptoms of complications of tracheostomy to report to health care team.
   • performs suctioning techniques correctly.
3. Patient maintains adequate respiratory function:
   • respirations within normal limits.
   • clear, thin sputum.
   • breath sounds clear.

- normal blood gases.
- symmetrical chest expansion.
- absence of fever.

NURSING MANAGEMENT

Assessment

1. See Assessment, Level 1.
2. Evaluate respiratory effort for effectiveness (e.g., rate, depth, effort, symmetrical chest expansion).
3. Assess for signs and symptoms of respiratory difficulty:
   - dyspnea.
   - shortness of breath.
   - cyanosis.
   - anxiety.
   - laryngospasms.
   - stridor.
   - retraction of soft tissue around neck.
   - presence of bubbly, noisy respiration.
   - use of accessory muscles of respiration.
4. Observe stoma and note health of tissue.
5. Assess tracheostomy secretions (amount, color, odor, consistency).
6. Monitor arterial blood gases if respiratory difficulties develop.
7. Assess patient's coping and self-care management:
   - changes in facial movements, body movements, composure.
   - handling of secretions and stoma care.
   - measures used to seek assistance if indicated.
8. Monitor vital signs q4h or prn.
9. Assess skin color, temperature, and moisture.
10. Monitor intake and output.
11. Monitor nutritional status.

Nursing Interventions

1. Assist patient in coughing and deep breathing q4h or prn.
2. Suction tracheostomy every hour or prn using sterile technique postoperatively. Decrease to q4h or prn as secretions decrease.
3. If patient has cuffed tracheostomy tube, deflate cuff slowly before suctioning; inflate after suctioning.
4. Instill 3 to 5 ml of normal saline into tracheostomy tube before suctioning if patient's secretions are tenacious.
5. Clean and care for tracheostomy tube and site as needed (e.g., tracheostomy care q4–8h or prn. Change tracheostomy ties prn).
6. Provide patient with humidified air:
   - high humidity oxygen collar for at least 24 to 72 hours postoperatively.
   - humidifier in patient's home.
7. Elevate head of bed 30 degrees.
8. Encourage adequate fluid intake of 3000 ml/day unless contraindicated.
9. Have extra tracheostomy tube at bedside for emergency insertion.
10. Have Trousseau dilator or Kelly hemostat at bedside to hold tracheostomy open until new tracheostomy tube is inserted.
11. Provide frequent oral hygiene.
12. Have call bell accessible.
13. Provide a form of communication for patient (e.g., magic slate, letter board, pen and paper).
14. Provide sexual counseling for patient and spouse.
15. Encourage vocational counseling (American Cancer Society provides job placement for recovering patients. State office of vocational rehabilitation will also assist in job rehabilitation).

Patient Teaching

1. See Patient Teaching, Level 1.
2. Discuss rationale, procedure, and function of tracheostomy and laryngectomy.

3. Describe effective coughing and deep breathing exercises.
4. Explain self-care of tracheostomy (e.g., independent tracheal tube or stoma care and sterile suctioning technique used in hospital, clean technique used at home).
5. Discuss importance of maintaining proper humidity.
6. Discuss importance of adequate nutrition.
7. Teach signs and symptoms of altered respiratory status to report to health care team.
8. Inform patient of signs and symptoms of complications of tracheostomy insertion (e.g., subcutaneous emphysema; thick, crusty secretions; bleeding; difficulty with removal or insertion of tracheostomy tube).
9. Explain safety precautions to prevent tracheal aspiration through stoma:
   • avoid using loose cotton applicators or any fluffy material.

   • protect stoma from dust or dirt with stoma cover.
   • wear protective tracheal shield when showering.
   • caution barber or beautician to use special care with loose hairs, powders, sprays.
10. Discuss rationale for carrying identification and information that states that patient is neck breather, and instructions for resuscitation in event of an accident.
11. Teach family resuscitation techniques for neck breathers.
12. Teach rationale for continuation of vocational rehabilitation using various available resources.
13. Inform patient and spouse of resources available for sexual counseling.
14. Provide information on support groups for patient and family.

LEVEL 3: Complications Related to Diversional Methods of Ventilation

Tracheoesophageal Fistula Formation

EXPECTED OUTCOME

Patient/caregiver demonstrate knowledge of fistula formation:
• report increased secretions, especially after eating.
• report presence of liquid or food particles among tracheal secretions after eating.
• identify proper techniques to use while eating.

NURSING MANAGEMENT

Assessment

1. See Assessment, Levels 1 and 2.
2. Observe closely for leakage of secretions around neck incision.
3. Assess for fistula using grape juice or methylene blue before first oral feeding. Observe closely for leakage from esophagus into trachea.
4. Assess for signs of respiratory difficulty.

5. Auscultate lungs for signs of aspiration.
6. Watch for increased tracheal secretions secondary to gradual tracheal aspiration of secretions.
7. Monitor vital signs and observe for signs of infection.

Nursing Interventions

1. See Nursing Interventions, Levels 1 and 2.
2. Ensure that patient maintains appropriate position of head and torso while eating and drinking:
   - flexion of head.
   - torso elevated 60 to 75 degrees.
3. Withhold oral intake if fistula is suspected; notify physician.
4. Monitor hydration status.
5. Administer grape juice or methylene blue orally before first oral feeding and before subsequent feedings if fistula is suspected.
6. Suction patient promptly in event of aspiration.

7. Provide oxygen therapy as needed.
8. Keep tracheal cuff deflated at all times, except when patient is eating.

Patient Teaching

1. See Patient Teaching, Levels 1 and 2.
2. Describe fistula information and rationale for care.
3. Explain to patient with fistula why npo is necessary.
4. If patient is allowed to eat, teach proper head positioning.
5. If npo, teach alternate feeding methods.
6. Explain signs and symptoms to report to health care team:
   - leakage of liquids or food from trachea.
   - fever.
   - respiratory difficulty.
   - excessive coughing.
7. Note importance of adequate nutrition, hydration, and moderate activity.

Excoriation of Neck Wound

EXPECTED OUTCOME

1. Patient/caregiver demonstrate measures to improve or maintain stomal skin integrity:
   - perform proper stomal tracheostomy care.
   - patient maintains intake of sufficient calories, high-protein, balanced diet either orally or per feeding tube to maintain positive nitrogen balance.
   - identify signs and symptoms of excoriation of neck wound to report to health care team.

NURSING MANAGEMENT

Assessment

1. Inspect stomal borders for:
   - erythema.
   - skin breakdown.
   - drainage.
   - odor.
   - swelling.
2. Assess patient for complaints of pain, tenderness, tightness.
3. Monitor vital signs q4h.
4. Monitor CBC for elevated WBC.

5. Assess nutritional status.
6. Evaluate history of radiation therapy to neck region.

Nursing Interventions

1. Keep skin around stoma dry and free of irritants.
2. Cleanse skin around stoma q4h (may use small amount of hydrogen peroxide followed by normal saline).
3. Maintain sterile technique with tracheostomy care and suctioning.
4. Apply small amount of antibiotic ointment (e.g., bacitracin) per physician order.
5. If drainage present, send for culture.
6. Administer analgesics as needed.
7. Administer antibiotics for positive cultures per physician order.
8. Avoid skin irritation from tracheostomy ties:
   • leave space for 1 finger to pass between ties and neck.
   • change daily or prn.
9. Maintain proper humidity.

Patient Teaching

1. Teach importance of reporting signs and symptoms of excoriation to health care team:
   • redness.
   • tenderness.
   • pain.
   • irritation.
   • odor.
   • swelling at site.
   • fever.
   • bleeding.
   • purulent drainage.
   • lesions.
2. Discuss maintenance of skin integrity through proper stoma or tracheostomy care.
3. Describe use of lubricant or bland ointment around stoma if skin becomes irritated.
4. Explain risk factors that potentiate skin breakdown.

Stomal Stenosis

EXPECTED OUTCOME

1. Patient maintains patent airway:
   • normal respiratory rate.
   • effective removal of secretions.
2. Patient/caregiver demonstrate knowledge of measures to prevent stomal stenosis:
   • identify signs and symptoms to report to health care team.
   • state rationale for prompt replacement of outer cannula.

NURSING MANAGEMENT

Assessment

1. See Assessment, Levels 1 and 2.
2. Assess stoma for changes in size during postoperative course.
3. Check airway for patency.

Nursing Interventions

1. Replace tracheostomy or laryngectomy tube promptly when exchanged or cleansed.
2. Notify health care team of respiratory distress or change in stoma diameter.
3. Deflate tracheostomy tube cuff frequently to avoid ischemia of tracheal mucosa.
4. Keep tracheostomy tube secured to prevent excessive movement.

Patient Teaching

1. Explain importance of reporting early signs of respiratory distress and constriction of stomal opening.
2. Note importance of replacing outer cannula as soon as cleaning is complete.
3. Reinforce correct tracheostomy tube care and cuff care.

Mucous Plug Obstructing Tracheobronchial Tree

EXPECTED OUTCOME

1. Patient maintains patent airway:
   - normal respiratory rate.
   - effective removal of secretions.
2. Patient/caregiver demonstrate measures to prevent tracheobronchial plug:
   - run humidifier constantly.
   - instill saline before suctioning.
   - maintain adequate hydration.

NURSING MANAGEMENT

Assessment

1. See Assessment, Levels 1 and 2.
2. Evaluate characteristics of secretions for consistency and excessive tenacity.

Nursing interventions

1. Provide adequate humidity for maintenance of thin secretions.
2. Suction patient as needed.
3. Instill 3 to 5 ml of sterile normal saline into tracheostomy while patient takes deep breath before suctioning to loosen secretions.
4. Encourage intake of at least 3000 ml of fluid per day unless contraindicated.

Patient Teaching

1. Explain importance of humidification at home as well as during hospitalization.
2. Teach coughing, deep breathing techniques, and suctioning if appropriate.
3. Describe signs and symptoms of tracheobronchial obstruction to report to health care team:
   - respiratory difficulties.
   - air hunger.
   - shortness of breath.
   - dyspnea.
   - thick and tenacious secretions.
   - inability to clear airway by coughing/suctioning.

SUGGESTED READINGS

Chernecky, C.C., and Ramsey, P.W.: Critical Nursing Care of the Client with Cancer. Norwalk, CT, Appleton-Century-Crofts, 1984, pp. 114–117.

Dietz, J.H. Jr.: Rehabilitation Oncology. New York, John Wiley & Sons 1981, pp. 59–72.

Groenwald, S.L. (Ed.): Cancer Nursing: Principles and Practices. Monterey, CA, Jones & Bartlett 1987, pp. 634–653.

Gunn, A.E. (Ed.): Cancer Rehabilitation. New York, Raven Press, 1984.

Johnson, B.L., and Gross, J. (Eds.): Handbook of Oncology Nursing. New York, John Wiley & Sons, 1985.

Myers, E., Stool, S., and Johnson, J.T.: Tracheostomy. New York, Churchill Livingstone, 1985.

Shekleton, M.E., and Neild, M.: Ineffective airway clearance related to artificial airway. Nursing Clinics of North America 22(1):167–177, 1987.

Zagars, G., and Norante, J.D.: Head and neck tumors. In Rubin, P. (Ed.): Clinical Oncology: A Multidisciplinary Approach, Sixth Edition. New York, American Cancer Society, 1983.

Alteration in Breathing Patterns: Mechanical Ventilation

Catherine Panouryas

Population at Risk

- Individuals with history of cardiac disease (chronic heart failure, left heart failure), lung disease (chronic obstructive pulmonary disease, asthma, chronic bronchitis, history of adult respiratory distress syndrome [ARDS])
- Individuals who have experienced a surgical intervention including anesthesia and thoracic pain resulting in splinting of rib cage
- Individuals with cancer of the head and neck region, including thyroid and laryngeal cancers
- Individuals with primary or metastatic tumors (including lymphoma, mammary, pulmonary, leukemia, mesothelioma, ovarian, prostatic) compressing or occluding the primary or segmental bronchi
- Individuals with pulmonary fibrosis resulting from the administration of chemotherapeutic agents, including bleomycin, busulfan, Actinomycin D, BCNU, chlorambucil, Adriamycin
- Individuals with an alteration in the immune process resulting in viral, bacterial, or fungal pneumonias, graft-versus-host reactions involving the lungs, or acquired immunodeficiency syndrome
- Individuals experiencing complications of cancer treatment: superior vena cava syndrome, pulmonary embolus, pleural effusions, radiation pneumonitis, fluid overload resulting from chemotherapy hydration, intravenous antibiotics, kidney failure blood transfusions; anaphylaxis
- Individuals experiencing drug toxicities of opiates or sedatives.

LEVEL 1:   Potential

EXPECTED OUTCOME

1. Patient demonstrates knowledge of potential alteration in respiratory function:
   - identifies basic lung anatomy.
   - identifies underlying lung disease.
   - describes potential alterations in respiratory status related to cancer treatment protocols.
   - identifies measures to prevent alteration in respiratory function.
2. Patient identifies early signs and symptoms of an alteration in respiratory status and functioning.
3. Patient maintains adequate pulmonary function:
   - vital signs within normal limits.
   - respirations within normal limits.

- breath sounds clear.
- activity tolerance within normal limits.

NURSING MANAGEMENT

Assessment

1. Auscultate breath sounds bilaterally, assessing for:
   - rales.
   - rhonchi.
   - wheezing.
   - stridor.
   - snoring.
   - friction rubs.
2. Observe patient for potential signs of respiratory compromise:
   - tachypnea.
   - retractions.
   - use of accessory muscles for breathing.
   - inability to swallow.
3. Assess history of symptoms of respiratory difficulty:
   - shortness of breath.
   - dyspnea on exertion.
   - orthopnea.
4. Assess integumentary system for:
   - color.
   - temperature.
   - moisture.
   - clubbing of fingers.
5. Assess for pain in the thoracic area.
6. Assess vital signs including:
   - heart rate and rhythm.
   - blood pressure.
   - respiratory rate and rhythm.
   - oxygen saturation.
   - temperature.
   - level of consciousness.
7. Obtain an arterial blood gas level to serve as a baseline value.

Nursing Interventions

1. Monitor serial pulmonary function tests on patients at risk for developing respiratory compromise.
2. Monitor chest x-rays for patients with primary and metastatic lung tumors.
3. Administer adequate pain medication following surgical procedures and in the patient with bone metastases.
4. Supply humidified oxygen via nasal cannula or face mask if needed.
5. Elevate head of bed 45 to 60 degrees as needed.
6. Perform respiratory physical therapy to aid in removal of secretions.
7. Obtain sputum cultures if productive cough is present.

Patient Teaching

1. Teach patient basic lung anatomy.
2. Discuss the importance of reporting any alterations in respiratory status.
3. Teach patient medication administration including drug name, dosage, time schedule, action, and side effects.
4. Teach patient early signs and symptoms of respiratory compromise.
5. Discuss with the patient the need to report a temperature greater than 100°F.

LEVEL 2: Moderate

EXPECTED OUTCOME

1. Patient demonstrates knowledge related to alteration in breathing patterns:
   - identifies need for immediate hospitalization if symptoms of airway obstruction occur.

- identifies measures to control altered breathing patterns.
- recognizes signs and symptoms of imminent airway obstruction or impairment in gas exchange.
2. Patient achieves or maintains adequate pulmonary function:
   - vital signs within normal limits.
   - respirations stable for age and condition.
   - breath sounds stable.
   - activity tolerance stable.

NURSING MANAGEMENT

Assessment

1. See Assessment, Level 1.
2. Monitor chest x-rays to identify areas of pulmonary dysfunction.
3. Obtain serial arterial blood gases and monitor results. Respiratory failure is defined as the retention of $pCO_2 > 50$ mm Hg, hypoxemia with $pO_2 < 50$ mm Hg, and evidence of muscle fatigue.
4. Assess for signs and symptoms of imminent airway obstruction or impairment of gas exchange:
   - breath sounds every 15 to 30 minutes in the unstable patient.
   - difficulty swallowing.
   - hoarseness.
   - stridor.
   - increasing dyspnea.
   - confusion.
   - fatigue.
5. Monitor patient to determine if criteria for intubation are met including:
   - arterial pH < 7.3.
   - increasing retention of pCO_2 despite aggressive therapy.
   - increasing hypoxemia despite maximum oxygen therapy.
   - increasing muscle fatigue with vital capacity < 10 ml/kg.

Nursing Interventions

1. See Nursing Interventions, Level 1.
2. Continuously monitor oxygen, set alarms appropriately.

3. Continuously monitor heart rate and rhythm, and set alarms appropriately.
4. Obtain intravenous access.
5. Administer aerosolized nebulizer medications for symptoms management as ordered:
   - bronchodilator–sympathomimetics that relax the smooth muscles of the bronchi:
     - epinephrine.
     - isoproterenol (Isuprel).
     - isoetharine (Bronchosol).
     - metaproterenol (Metaprel, Alupent).
     - terbutaline (Bucanyl).
   - anticholinergics–inhibit parasympathetic stimulation resulting in decreased secretions, inhibition of laryngeal spasms, relaxation of smooth muscle of the bronchi (e.g., Atropine 1 per cent solution).
   - vasoconstrictors–used for extubation to decrease edema caused by intubation (e.g., racemic epinephrine [Vaponefrin, Micronefrin]) that stimulates α-adrenergic receptors of the blood vessels of the upper airway mucosa resulting in vasoconstriction.
   - corticosteroids–decrease inflammation, enhance action of bronchodilators:
     - beclomethasone depropionate (Vanceril).
     - betamethasone valerate (Bentasol).
   - mucolytics–thins secretions, (e.g., acetylcysteine [Mucomyst] is given with bronchodilator to decrease bronchospasm).

6. Perform respiratory physical therapy to aid in mobilization of secretions.
7. Keep suction equipment at bedside.
8. Keep intubation equipment at bedside if respiratory status deteriorates.
9. Keep tracheostomy insertion equipment at bedside if upper airway obstruction is evident.
10. Support the patient/caregiver emotionally and psychologically, and encourage patient/caregiver to ask questions.
11. Encourage caregiver to participate in patient's care.

Patient Teaching

1. Explain all policies, procedures, and scheduled tests to patient/caregiver.
2. Review with patient/caregiver signs and symptoms of airway obstruction and impaired gas exchange and the need for immediate medical intervention.
3. Review with patient/caregiver signs and symptoms of respiratory failure.
4. Explain to patient/caregiver need for aggressive medical therapy requiring hospitalization.
5. Review all medications that the patient receives including actions and side effects.

LEVEL 3: Severe, Necessitating Mechanical Ventilation

EXPECTED OUTCOME

1. Caregiver demonstrates knowledge of treatment for severely altered breathing patterns with mechanical ventilation:
   - identifies mechanical ventilation.
   - describes protocols and care routines in the intensive care unit.
   - cooperates with regimens involved with ventilator care.
   - demonstrates operation of equipment needed for home discharge.
   - identifies discharge medications that control alteration in breathing pattern including actions, dosage, side effects.
   - identifies side effects of mechanical ventilation.

NURSING MANAGEMENT

Assessment

1. See Assessment, Levels 1 and 2.
2. Assess for proper positioning of the endotracheal tube:
   - breath sounds equal bilaterally.
   - chest rises equal bilaterally.
   - arterial blood gases.
   - continuous oxygen saturations.
   - normal color of nail beds and mucosa.
3. Assess for signs and symptoms of infection:
   - consistency, color, odor, amount of respiratory secretions.
   - temperature.
   - WBC count.
4. Observe for side effects of mechanical ventilation:
   - infection.
   - increased intracranial pressure, altered neurologic status, lethargy, change in mental status.
   - pneumothorax or pneumomediastinum.
     - auscultate breath sounds for equality.
     - monitor arterial blood gases and oxygen saturations.

- ○ monitor chest x-rays.
- ○ palpate for subcutaneous emphysema.
- atelectasis.
- stress ulcers (test all stools and emesis for blood).
5. Assess readiness for weaning:
  - FIO_2 < 40 per cent.
  - spontaneous respiratory rate > 20 breaths per minute.
  - low compliance.
  - arterial blood gases within normal limits for patient.
  - adequate nutritional status.
  - adequate rest and sleep.
6. When extubated:
  - continuously assess oxygen saturations.
  - continuously assess respiratory rate and rhythm.
  - assess serial arterial blood gases until stable.
  - auscultate breath sounds every 15 minutes until stable.

Nursing Interventions

1. See Nursing Intervention, Levels 1 and 2.
2. Check ventilator settings every hour.
3. Check functioning and settings of ventilator alarms every hour.
4. Practice frequent, thorough handwashing.
5. Suction patient through endotracheal tube q4h or prn, using aseptic technique.
6. Provide rest periods for patient.
7. Administer antacids through nasogastric tube.
8. Assess pressure of endotracheal tube cuff q4h and correct if necessary.
9. Turn and position patient q2–3h.
10. Implement appropriate mode of weaning patient from ventilator:
    - synchronized intermittent mandatory ventilation (SIMV)–ventilatory rate slowly decreased.
    - T-piece–patient intermittently placed on T-piece for increased periods of time, and placed on ventilator for rest.
    - Continuous positive airway pressure (CPAP)–no ventilatory rate delivered by respirator, only pressure.
11. Raise side rails; pad rails if patient is confused or disoriented. Restrain patient as necessary to maintain patient safety.
12. At time of extubation, have appropriate oxygen and reintubation equipment at bedside until patient is stable.
13. Perform mouth care q3–4h.
14. Refer to home health services at time of discharge for home care services.
15. Refer to respiratory therapy for respiratory physical therapy.
16. Refer to community agencies for information, out-patient resources (e.g., American Lung Association, American Cancer Society, Cancer Care).

Patient Teaching

1. Explain all protocols and procedures to patient/caregiver including management of equipment and alarms.
2. Explain all tests to patient/caregiver.
3. Encourage caregiver's participation in patient's care whenever appropriate, including suctioning, turning and positioning, medication administration, oral hygiene, weaning procedures, extubation.
4. Explain need for intubation and mechanical ventilation.
5. Explain sensitivity of alarm settings.
6. Answer any questions in terms patient/caregiver can understand.
7. Teach patient/caregiver infection control measures:
   - need for frequent, thorough handwashing.
   - avoid patient contact with ill individuals.
8. Review all medications with patient/caregiver including actions and side effects.
9. Instruct patient and caregiver regarding preparations for discharge to home:
   - management of equipment:
     - ○ home oxygen equipment can in-

clude either portable compressed gas or O_2 concentrator.
- home nebulizer equipment.
- information regarding diagnosis, treatments, prognosis, complications of disease.
- medication names, dosage, actions, side effects.
- signs and symptoms of respiratory compromise.
- measures to control infection:
  - influenza vaccine each fall.
  - thorough handwashing techniques.
  - importance of reporting signs and symptoms of infection.

10. Teach patient and caregiver methods of respiratory physical therapy including:
- principles of postural drainage if needed.
- pursed lip breathing.
- energy conservation.
- activities of daily living to be performed during time of day of maximum energy.

SUGGESTED READINGS

Carlon, G.C.: Acute respiratory failure in the cancer patient. *In* Howland, W.S., and Carlon, G.C., (Eds.): Critical Care of the Cancer Patient. Chicago, Year Book Medical Publishers, 1985, pp. 39–90.

Ewer, M.S., Ali, M.K., Atta, M.S. et al.: Outcome of lung cancer patients requiring mechanical ventilation for pulmonary failure. Journal of the American Medical Association *256*(24):3364–3366, 1986.

Hauser, M.J., Tabak, J., and Baier, H.: Survival of patients with cancer in a medical critical care unit. Archives of Internal Medicine *142*:527–529, 1982.

Holt, T.B.O.: Assessment-Based Respiratory Care. New York, John Wiley & Sons, 1986.

Reuben, D.B., and Mor, V.: Dyspnea in terminally ill cancer patients. Chest *89*(2):234–236, 1986.

Venus, B., Smith, R.A., and Mathru, M.: National survey of methods and criteria used for weaning from mechanical ventilation. Critical Care Medicine *15*(5):530–533, 1987.

CIRCULATION

The nurse assesses the patient's alterations in tissue perfusion and alterations in cardiac output to formulate actual or potential nursing diagnoses.

Appropriate patient outcomes to consider in planning nursing interventions will specify the patient's ability to:

1. identify signs and symptoms of alteration in circulation.
2. contact an appropriate health care team member when initial signs and symptoms of alteration in circulation occur.
3. describe measures to manage an alteration in circulation.

Evaluation of the patient's responses to nursing care is based on whether the patient recognizes signs and symptoms of impaired circulation and takes appropriate action.

Excerpted from the ANA/ONS Standards of Cancer Nursing Practice.

Altered Tissue Perfusion, Peripheral, Related to Lymphedema

60

Linda Fauth Kennelly and Carol A. Yurkovic

Population at Risk

- Individuals who have undergone surgical resection of lymph channels (radical mastectomy, modified radical mastectomy, simple mastectomy, axillary node dissection, groin dissection)
- Individuals who experience increasing tumor burden resulting in pressure/blockage of lymphatic system
- Individuals who have undergone radiation therapy to lymphatic channels
- Individuals with prolonged immobility/dependency of an extremity
- Individuals who have had recurrent infections with lymphangitis
- Individuals who are overweight
- Individuals who have history of cardiovascular disease

LEVEL 1: Potential

EXPECTED OUTCOME

1. Patient demonstrates knowledge related to potential lymphedema:
   - describes measures to prevent or minimize lymphedema.
   - identifies factors that place patient at high risk.
   - identifies signs and symptoms of lymphedema and importance of reporting to health care team.
2. Patient achieves or maintains mobility within own normal limits as evidenced by
   - complete range of motion of extremities.
   - independence in ambulation and self-care activities of daily living.
   - absence of lymphedema.

NURSING MANAGEMENT

Assessment

1. Perform subjective assessment:
   - discomfort of extremity.
   - change in size of extremity.
   - change in fit of clothing and jewelry.
   - change in extremity sensation.
2. Perform objective assessments:
   - range of movement.
   - circumference of extremity.

387

- color of extremity.
- peripheral pulses.
- edema (e.g., cyclical changes with humidity, menstrual cycle, time of day).

Nursing Interventions

1. Protect affected extremity from potential trauma (e.g., venipuncture, fingerstick, IV, fluid administration, blood pressure determination).
2. Avoid prolonged dependent positioning of affected extremity; position postmastectomy arm on a pillow in slight abduction and elevation; elevate legs as needed for patients with groin dissection.
3. Avoid trauma and infection to affected extremity.
4. Demonstrate postmastectomy arm care and exercises. To prevent increased blood flow to axillary area (causing swelling), do not exercise affected arm until healing occurs.
5. Encourage gradual return to normal activity.

Patient Teaching

1. Explain general measures for prevention of internal and external pressure on lymphatic system:
   - wear clothing that does not constrict limb (avoid elastic sleeves, tight wristbands, tight jewelry).
   - avoid constrictive tourniquet dressings.
   - avoid prolonged dependent positioning of limb.
   - elevate upper extremity 45 degrees abduction, 60 to 90 degrees flexion, so that distal end is higher than proximal end.
   - use pillows, blankets, foam padding for support.
   - prevent injury and infection to affected extremity.
   - clean breaks in skin with soap and water.
   - seek immediate treatment in cases of tissue injury.
   - maintain good nail care, manicure carefully, seek professional assistance for toenail care.
   - clean and lubricate skin of affected extremity regularly.
   - avoid prolonged sun exposure to affected extremity.
   - avoid rapid or strenuous movement of extremity.
   - avoid extremes of temperature (e.g., heating pads, ice packs).
   - begin gradual exercise as indicated in treatment plan.
   - return to normal activity level as tolerated.
2. Explain measures to prevent internal and external pressure on lymphatic system if upper extremity is affected:
   - avoid wearing shoulder bag on affected side.
   - avoid carrying heavy objects with affected extremity.
   - blood pressure should not be taken on affected extremity.
   - use protective gloves when gardening.
3. Explain measures to prevent internal and external pressure if lower extremity is involved:
   - do not cross legs when sitting.
   - avoid restrictive clothing to waist, leg, or groin area (e.g., garter, tight-fitting socks).
   - check shoes for areas of irritation.
   - inspect feet carefully and maintain good foot care regimens.
4. Explain dietary measures to prevent increased potential for fluid retention and weight gain:
   - dietary consultation regarding current nutritional intake and practices.
   - review current medications that may affect fluid load and retention.
5. Review use of isometric exercises for patients unable to do isotonic exercises.

EXPECTED OUTCOME

1. Patient achieves resolution or control of lymphedema as evidenced by:
   - maintenance of mobility/independence.
   - decrease or stabilization in size of extremity (moderate, 21 per cent increase in volume).
   - absence of superimposed infection.
   - maintenance of adequate circulation.
   - maintenance of adequate comfort.
2. Patient identifies measures to decrease or control mild to moderate lymphedema:
   - states signs of superimposed infection, indicating those to report to health care team.
   - states signs of impairment of limb circulation, indicating those to report to health care team.
   - verbalizes/demonstrates proper positioning and exercises.
   - verbalizes/demonstrates measures to prevent infection.
   - demonstrates proper use of assistive devices.
   - verbalizes dietary measures to control fluid retention.
   - overweight patients verbalize dietary changes to control caloric intake.

NURSING MANAGEMENT

Assessment

1. See Assessment, Level 1.
2. Evaluate for existing versus newly developing mobility problem.
3. Check for signs of infection (e.g., tenderness, changes in temperature, pain, redness).
4. Observe for impairment of circulation (e.g., skin color, temperature, sensation, turgor).

Nursing Interventions

1. See Nursing Interventions, Level 1.
2. Elevate upper extremity 45 degrees abduction, 60 to 90 degrees flexion so that distal end is higher than proximal end, a minimum of 30 minutes several times throughout the day.
3. Encourage range-of-motion exercises while awake, isometric exercises qid.
4. Consult with physician/physical therapist to develop exercise plan.
5. Alert health care team, patient, and family to avoid trauma to affected limb.
6. Apply stockinette or antiembolism stocking when indicated.
7. Use assistive devices when indicated (e.g., intermittent pressure pump to prevent venous stasis).
8. If elastic wraps are used, reapply often to maintain constant pressure.
9. Use stretch gauze wrapping rather than tape.
10. Review needs for change in types of clothing.
11. Review current life style practices that may require adjustment (e.g., physical demands of home and occupation).

Altered Tissue Perfusion, Peripheral, Related to Lymphedema

Patient Teaching

1. See Patient Teaching, Level 1.
2. Remove stockinette or antiembolism stocking or sleeve q8h.
3. Demonstrate use of assistive devices.
4. Review exercise plan.
5. Describe proper positioning of extremity.
6. Educate patient regarding utilization of medications to control pain and edema.
7. Review patient's specific dietary plan including dietary changes for overweight patients.

LEVEL 3: Severe

EXPECTED OUTCOME

1. Patient demonstrates control of severe lymphedema (41 per cent increase in volume) as evidenced by:
   - optimal mobility and independence.
   - maintenance of circulation.
   - maintenance of skin integrity.
2. Patient and caregiver identify/demonstrate measures to control lymphedema and complications:
   - identify/demonstrate measures to avoid infection.
   - identify/demonstrate measures to maintain circulation.
   - state signs and symptoms to report to health care team.
   - verbalize/demonstrate proper positioning and exercises.
   - demonstrate proper knowledge and administration of medications.
   - perform necessary treatments and procedures.
   - demonstrate proper use of assistive devices.

NURSING MANAGEMENT

Assessment

1. See Assessment, Levels 1 and 2.
2. Document evidence of pitting edema.
3. Assess intensity and location of pain.
4. Check for systemic reactions (e.g., fever, chills).
5. Evaluate laboratory data (e.g., CBC, sedimentation rate, cultures).
6. Observe fluid and nutritional status.
7. Assess for change of sensation in site of absent limb.
8. Measure limb daily to evaluate efficacy of treatment (15 cm distal to the acromion and 15 cm distal to the olecranon are convenient sites; measure also 15 cm proximal and distal to elbow).

Nursing Interventions

1. See Nursing Interventions, Levels 1 and 2.
2. Administer albumin, diuretics, and benzopyrodones per physician order; monitor intake and output.
3. Medicate for pain and evaluate effectiveness.
4. Position and support affected extremity.

5. Utilize loose-fitting clothing on affected extremity.
6. Utilize measures to prevent skin breakdown (e.g., air mattress, turning prn, skin care).
7. Incorporate measures to prevent hazards of immobility (e.g., coughing, deep breathing).
8. Avoid extremes in temperature to affected extremity.
9. Implement passive range of motion.
10. Allow patient to express feelings regarding potential alteration to body image.
11. Use assistive devices to promote mobility.

Patient Teaching

1. See Patient Teaching, Levels 1 and 2.
2. Instruct patient in meticulous skin and nail care.
3. Describe signs and symptoms of impaired circulation.
4. Provide pre- and postoperative teaching if LeVeen or Denver shunt used (for patients with ascites as well as lower extremity edema).
5. Review principles of medication use with fluid retention (e.g., diuretics; review potential side effects).

SUGGESTED READINGS

DeLisa, J.A., Miller, R.M., Melnick, R.P., et al.: Rehabilitation of the cancer patient. *In* DeVita, V.T., Hellman, S., and Rosenberg, A.: Cancer Principles and Practice of Oncology. Philadelphia, J.B. Lippincott, 1989, pp. 2344–2346.
Donegan, W., and Spratt, J.: Cancer of the Breast. Philadelphia, W.B. Saunders, 1988, pp. 32–33, 442–447, 601.
Getz, D.H.: The primary, secondary, and tertiary nursing interventions of lymphedema. Cancer Nursing 8(3):177–184, 1985.
Jungi, W.F.: The prevention and management of lymphedema after treatment for breast cancer. International Rehabilitation Medicine 3(3):129–134, 1981.
Lippman, E., Lichter, S., and Danforth, N. Jr.: Diagnosis and Management of Breast Cancer. Philadelphia, W.B. Saunders, pp. 458–496, 1988.
Ruschhaupt, W.F., and Graor, R.A.: Evaluation of the patient with leg edema. Postgraduate Medicine 78(2):132–139, 1985.
Ruschhaupt, W.F. III: Differential diagnosis of edema of the lower extremities. Clinics in Cardiology 13(2):307–320, 1983.
Schirger, A.: Lymphedema. Clinics in Cardiology 13(2):293–305, 1983.
Stillwell, G.K.: Treatment of postmastectomy lymphedema. Modern Treatment 6:396, 1959.
Strombeck, R. (Ed.): Surgery of the Breast: Diagnosis and Treatment of the Breast. New York, Thieme, 1986, pp. 225–234.

PATIENT EDUCATION MATERIALS AND COMMUNITY RESOURCES

American Cancer Society: Reach to Recovery: An Ounce of Prevention. Suggestions for Hand and Arm Care [n.d.].

American Cancer Society: Reach to Recovery: Exercises After Mastectomy, Patient Guide [n.d.].

U.S. Department of Health and Human Services: After Breast Cancer: A Guide to Followup Care. U.S. Government Printing Office, 1986.

U.S. Department of Health and Human Services: Mastectomy: A Treatment for Breast Cancer [n.d.].

U.S. Department of Health and Human Services: Radiation Therapy: A Treatment of Early Stage Breast Cancer [n.d.].

61

Fluid Volume Deficit Related to Disease Process and Treatment

Carol A. Zabinski

Population at Risk

- Individuals experiencing difficulties ingesting fluids (mucositis, dysphagia, nausea, vomiting, altered mental status, anorexia, surgical procedures, especially head and neck and gastrointestinal surgery)
- Individuals experiencing fluid loss (diarrhea, draining wound, electrolyte imbalance, fever)

LEVEL 1: Potential

EXPECTED OUTCOME

1. Patient demonstrates knowledge of the potential for fluid volume deficit:
   - identifies early signs and symptoms of fluid volume deficit.
   - identifies factors that influence alterations in fluid intake.
2. Patient relates measures to maintain adequate fluid volume:
   - verbalizes appropriate volume of fluid intake required for good hydration.
   - verbalizes self-care measures to manage side effects of the disease or treatment that alters ability to take in adequate amounts of fluids.
3. Patient maintains adequate fluid volume as evidenced by:
   - serum electrolytes within normal limits.
   - serum osmolality within normal limits.
   - blood urea nitrogen and creatinine within normal limits.
   - skin turgor normal and mucous membranes moist.
   - daily intake and output balanced within patient's norms.
   - hematocrit within normal limits.
   - specific gravity of urine within normal limits.
   - absence of thirst or dry mouth.

NURSING MANAGEMENT

Assessment

1. Assess pattern and amount of fluid intake and output.

2. Assess fluid preferences: type, temperature, frequency, and amount.
3. Inspect skin and tongue for turgor and integrity.

4. Inspect mucous membranes for moistness and integrity.
5. Evaluate treatment program for potential side effects related to fluid balance:
   - chemotherapy (nausea, vomiting, diarrhea, dysphagia, mucositis).
   - radiation therapy (nausea, vomiting, diarrhea, dysphagia, mucositis).
   - surgery (draining wound, nasogastric tubes, aspiration, dysphagia, fistulas).
   - biotherapy (nausea, vomiting, diarrhea, flu-like syndrome).
6. Assess weight and vital signs.
7. Evaluate appropriate laboratory values (e.g., blood urea nitrogen, creatinine, hematocrit, electrolytes, serum osmolality).
8. Assess medications the patient is taking for their potential to cause dehydration.
9. Assess vital signs. Fever can precipitate fluid volume deficit if extra fluids are not supplied as indicated.

Patient Teaching

1. Teach early signs and symptoms of fluid volume deficit (e.g., thirst, dry skin, dry mucous membranes, lethargy, lassitude, constipation).
2. Note factors that influence maintenance and disruption of fluid volume (e.g., nausea, vomiting, diarrhea, fever, diaphoresis, fluid intake, drainage, diureses associated with chemotherapy).
3. Discuss appropriate level of fluid intake to maintain adequate hydration. Give specific amounts of fluid to be ingested (e.g., 6 glasses of water as well as other fluids).
4. Discuss self-care measures to minimize the effect of the disease and treatment on fluid intake (e.g., take antiemetic around-the-clock to control emesis, drink fluids in small amounts, eat frozen juices in popsicles, use ice chips, drink with a straw).
5. Discuss self-care measures to minimize fluid loss (e.g., antidiarrheal medications around-the-clock to control diarrhea, antipyretic medications as instructed).
6. Discuss when the health care team should be notified regarding disease effects or side effects of treatment (e.g., diarrhea or vomiting lasting longer than 24 hours).

LEVEL 2:   Mild to Moderate

EXPECTED OUTCOME

1. Patient demonstrates knowledge of alterations in fluid balance:
   - identifies signs and symptoms of fluid volume deficit to report to health care team.
   - identifies disease process or treatment factors that influence fluid volume balance.
   - identifies potential complications related to fluid volume deficit.
2. Patient relates measures to correct fluid volume deficit:
   - identifies fluid preferences.
   - identifies factors that promote fluid intake.
   - identifies factors that prevent fluid loss.
   - identifies recommended 24-hour fluid intake.
   - recognizes that good oral hygiene promotes fluid intake.
3. Patient maintains adequate fluid volume as evidenced by:
   - stable daily weights.
   - balance between fluid intake and output.

- skin turgor and mucous membrane integrity return to normal.
- return to normal range of laboratory values (e.g., electrolytes, blood urea nitrogen, creatinine, serum and osmolality).
- absence of complaints of thirst, dry mouth.

NURSING MANAGEMENT

Assessment

1. See Assessment, Level 1.
2. Assess for type and amount of fluid intake and output. Assess for excessive perspiration.
3. Check daily weight (weight loss of > 5 per cent can indicate fluid volume deficit).
4. Evaluate appropriate laboratory values (e.g., electrolytes, blood urea nitrogen, creatinine, serum osmolality, hematocrit, hemoglobin).
5. Monitor vital signs for changes (e.g., postural hypotension, fever).
6. Assess skin turgor and moistness of mucous membranes.
7. Assess hand vein filling, neck vein filling.

Nursing Interventions

1. Offer small amounts of patient's favorite fluids frequently.
2. Assist patient to use appropriate equipment to take fluids as indicated.
3. Identify treatment and disease effects that may compromise fluid intake.
4. Identify treatment and disease effects that

may contribute to fluid loss (e.g., diarrhea, wound drainage, electrolyte imbalance, fever, diaphoresis).
5. Maintain skin integrity and oral hygiene (e.g., brush teeth after all meals, keep lips moist, rinse mouth with alcohol-free mouthwash or saline, use artificial saliva).

Patient Teaching

1. See Patient Teaching, Level 1.
2. Teach signs and symptoms of fluid volume deficit to report to the health care team (e.g., scanty output, dry skin and mucous membranes, acute weight loss of > 5 per cent, lethargy, or lassitude).
3. Demonstrate/describe techniques for good oral hygiene and skin care.
4. Discuss factors related to disease process and treatment that influence fluid volume balance.
5. Note potential complications related to fluid deficit (e.g., abdominal cramps, shock symptoms, shortness of breath, cardiac failure, convulsions, constipation, tachycardia, arrhythmias).

LEVEL 3: Severe

EXPECTED OUTCOME

1. Patient/caregiver demonstrate knowledge of severe fluid volume deficit:
   - identify results or complications of severe fluid volume deficit.
   - identify when health care team should be notified regarding signs and symptoms of severe fluid volume deficit.

2. Patient/caregiver identify/demonstrate measures to manage severe alterations in fluid volume balance:
   - relate understanding of action and scheduling of antiemetic drugs.
   - verbalize rationale for feeding tube.
   - perform feeding procedure under supervision.
   - identify type, temperature, amount of tolerated fluids.
   - fluid intake equals 1 liter per day.
   - verbalize rationale for intravenous fluids.
   - report signs and symptoms of complications to report to health care team.
3. Patient's severe fluid volume deficit is stabilized:
   - excessive fluid volume loss controlled or decreased.
   - adequate skin turgor and moist mucous membranes maintained.
   - vital signs stable.
   - laboratory values stable.

NURSING MANAGEMENT

Assessment

1. See Assessment, Levels 1 and 2.
2. Assess for cause of fluid volume deficit.
3. Observe for diarrhea with tube feedings.
4. Observe for signs of inflammation, infection, infiltration, or rate change with intravenous fluids.

Nursing Interventions

1. See Interventions, Level 2.
2. Maintain integrity of intravenous line to supply necessary fluids.
3. Follow recommended institutional infection control measures to prevent contamination of intravenous line.
4. Observe for complications related to intravenous fluids.
5. Select appropriate tube for tube feedings. Maintain integrity of tube by following recommended flushing and maintenance procedures.
6. Maintain fluid intake when a nutritional supplement is used for tube feedings.
7. Maintain skin integrity around tube.
8. Maintain accurate recordings of fluid intake and output.

Patient Teaching

1. See Patient Teaching, Levels 1 and 2.
2. Explain tube feedings:
   - rationale for external feeding tubes.
   - demonstrate skills necessary to perform daily care and feeding.
   - indicate signs and symptoms to report to health care team (e.g., choking, lack of gag reflex, gagging, nausea, diarrhea).
3. Discuss intravenous fluids:
   - rationale.
   - daily care and protection of insertion site.
   - signs and symptoms to report to health care team (e.g., redness, swelling, pain at site).
4. Discuss community resources for assistance such as nutritional support team, support groups, American Cancer Society, home care coordinator, home care nurse.

SUGGESTED READINGS

Aker, S.N.: Oral feedings in the cancer patient. Cancer 43:2103–2107, 1979.
Boylan, A., and Marbach, B.: Dehydration: Subtle, sinister, preventable. RN 42:36–44, 1979.

Fields, A.L., Jasse, R.G., and Bergsagel, R.E.: Metabolic emergencies. *In* DeVita, V.T., Hellman, S., and Rosenberg, S.A. (Eds.): Principles and Practices of Oncology: Philadelphia, J.B. Lippincott, 1985, 1866–1877.

Groenwald, S.: Cancer Nursing: Principles and Practice. Boston, Jones & Bartlett, 1987, pp. 144, 147, 161.

Metheny, N.: Oncologic Conditions in Fluid and Electrolyte Balance, Nursing Considerations. Philadelphia, J.B. Lippincott, 1987, pp. 310–320.

Metheny, N.: Fluid Volume Deficit in Fluid and Electrolyte Balance, Nursing Considerations. Philadelphia, J.B. Lippincott, 1987, pp. 40–45.

Schrier, R.: Renal and Electrolyte Disorders. Boston, Little, Brown, & Co., 1986, pp. 96, 235.

Shils, M.E.: Principles of nutritional therapy. Cancer *43*:2093–2102, 1979.

Body Fluid Composition, Alteration in: Hypercalcemia

Anne Calafato and Ann L. Jessup

Population at Risk

- Individuals with bone metastases
- Individuals with squamous cell cancer of lung, breast, cervix, head and neck, or esophagus
- Individuals with multiple myeloma, hypernephroma, lymphoma, or leukemia
- Individuals with breast cancer who are receiving hormones
- Individuals with intercurrent disease resulting in dehydration and immobilization
- Individuals receiving thiazide diuretics

LEVEL 1: Potential (Serum Level: 9 to 11 mg/100 ml)

EXPECTED OUTCOME

1. Patient demonstrates knowledge related to potential hypercalcemia:
   - identifies predisposing factors.
   - identifies signs and symptoms of hypercalcemia.
2. Patient identifies/demonstrates measures to prevent hypercalcemia:
   - maintains adequate activity level.
   - maintains adequate fluid intake.
   - complies with treatment schedule.
   - identifies signs and symptoms of hypercalcemia to report to health care team.
3. Patient maintains serum calcium within normal limits.

NURSING MANAGEMENT

Assessment

1. Evaluate laboratory studies:
   - serum calcium level.
   - blood urea nitrogen, creatinine (renal function).
   - albumin (low albumin may give false normal serum calcium).

2. Assess potential clinical manifestations of hypercalcemia by systematic review of all systems:
   - neuromuscular:
     - muscle weakness and fatigue.
     - hypotonia.
     - apathy.
     - depression.

397

- confusion.
- decreased deep-tendon reflexes.
- restlessness.
- cardiovascular:
  - hypertension.
  - shortened S–T interval on ECG.
  - arrhythmias.
  - digitalis toxicity (e.g., nausea, arrhythmias, visual disturbances).
- renal:
  - polyuria.
  - nocturia.
  - glucosuria.
  - polydipsia.
- gastrointestinal:
  - anorexia.
  - nausea.
  - vague abdominal pain.
  - constipation.
  - decreased bowel sounds.
  - abdominal distention.
- miscellaneous:
  - musculoskeletal pain.
  - pruritus.
3. Determine if patient is taking digitalis (patients on digitalis are more susceptible to effects of increased serum calcium).
4. Monitor cardiovascular status.
5. Evaluate mobility status and activity level.
6. Monitor bowel status.
7. Monitor neurologic status.

Patient Teaching

1. Discuss rationale and need for adequate fluid intake (3 to 4 liter per day if not contraindicated).

2. Teach signs and symptoms of hypercalcemia:
   - weight loss.
   - anorexia.
   - fatigue.
   - muscle weakness.
   - pruritus.
   - polydipsia.
   - nausea and vomiting.
   - constipation.
   - polyuria.
   - lethargy.
3. Teach signs and symptoms of digitalis toxicity:
   - nausea.
   - arrhythmias.
   - visual disturbances.
4. Instruct in physical exercise program appropriate to patient's condition and underlying disease:
   - erect position decreases bone resorption of calcium.
   - encourage walking.
5. Review with patient drugs that may potentiate hypercalcemia:
   - thiazide diuretics.
   - lithium carbonate.
   - antihypertensives.
   - vitamin supplements, especially vitamin D
6. Review signs and symptoms of hypercalcemia.
7. Explain rationale and schedule for monitoring serum calcium.
8. Discuss importance of complying with treatment program.

LEVEL 2: Mild to Moderate (12 to 15 mg/100 ml)

EXPECTED OUTCOME

1. Patient/caregiver demonstrate knowledge related to hypercalcemia:
   - identify signs and symptoms of hypercalcemia.

- identify factors that influence serum calcium levels.
- identify potential sequelae/complications of hypercalcemia.
2. Patient identifies/demonstrates measures to enhance and maintain normal serum calcium level:
   - maintains adequate hydration status.
   - maintains activity and mobilization appropriate to physical status.
   - avoids calcium, vitamin D antacids, vitamin A and retinoids.
   - complies with treatment program.
   - identifies signs and symptoms to report to heath care team.
3. Patient achieves serum calcium level within normal limits.

NURSING MANAGEMENT

Assessment

1. See Assessment, Level 1.
2. Monitor intake and output.
3. Weigh patient daily.
4. Monitor vital signs.
5. Monitor laboratory tests:
   - albumin.
   - serum calcium.
   - urine calcium.
   - blood urea nitrogen, creatinine.
   - electrolytes.
6. Evaluate symptoms by system:
   - neuromuscular:
     - depression.
     - aggravation.
     - anxiety.
     - muscle weakness.
     - fatigue.
     - decreased deep-tendon reflexes.
     - lethargy.
     - confusion.
   - cardiovascular:
     - ECG changes (shortening of Q–T interval; configuration of S–T junction and T wave have concave appearance).
   - renal:
     - polyuria.
     - nocturia.
     - polydipsia.
     - dehydration.
     - glucosuria.
   - gastrointestinal:
     - signs and symptoms of paralytic ileus (decreased bowel sounds, distension).
     - constipation.
     - anorexia.
     - nausea.
     - abdominal pain.
   - miscellaneous:
     - bone pain.
     - pruritus.
7. Assess if patient is taking nonsteroidal antiinflammatory agents or H_2-receptor antagonists (cimetidine or ranitidine).

Nursing Interventions

1. Implement medical regimen as prescribed by physician and monitor side effects:
   - hydrate with normal saline, 200 to 400 ml per hour.
   - may administer oral phosphates (e.g., Phospho-Soda): observe for diarrhea; monitor blood pressure. Long-term use of phosphates may cause hypotension.
   - administer diuretics (furosemide or ethacrynic acid).
   - monitor serum sodium and potassium. Thiazide diuretics are contraindicated as they may potentiate hypercalcemia.
   - administer steroids; monitor for possible hyperglycemia.

- administer etidronate disodium (Didronel); monitor renal function.
- administer mithramycin; monitor CBC, renal function.
- administer calcitonin; monitor serum calcium closely as it may precipitate hypocalcemia; may cause nausea.
- administer prostaglandin inhibitors (e.g., indomethacin, ibuprofen); not recommended for hospitalized patients or those with compromised renal function.

2. Implement comfort measures.
3. Notify physician of patient's use of nonsteroidal antiinflammatory agents or H_2-receptor antagonists that decrease renal flow.
4. Provide support during chemotherapy or radiation treatment for primary disease.

Patient Teaching

1. See Patient Teaching, Level 1.
2. Instruct patient regarding medical treatment regimen and possible side effects.

3. Teach rationale and measures to maintain normal serum calcium level:
   - increase fluid intake to prescribed level to obtain adequate hydration.
   - avoid excessive intake of calcium, vitamin D, vitamin A and retinoids (e.g., antacids, calcium, multivitamin supplements).
   - comply with treatment program.
   - report signs and symptoms to health care team.
4. Define exercise and activity program to maintain muscle tone and promote resorption of calcium:
   - active resistive, active, passive range-of-motion exercises.
   - isometric exercises.
   - use of walker, cane to promote mobility.
5. Teach sequelae of untreated hypercalcemia:
   - severe hypertension.
   - renal calculi, azotemia.
   - constipation.
   - stupor, coma, death.

LEVEL 3: Severe (Greater than 15 mg/100 ml)

EXPECTED OUTCOME

1. Patient/caregiver demonstrate knowledge related to hypercalcemia:
   - identify signs and symptoms of hypercalcemia.
   - identify factors that influence serum calcium levels.
   - identify potential sequelae/complications of hypercalcemia.
2. Patient identifies/demonstrates measures to enhance and maintain normal serum calcium level:
   - maintains adequate hydration status.
   - maintains activity and mobility appropriate to physical status.
   - avoids excess amounts of calcium, vitamin D, antacids.
   - complies with treatment program.
   - identifies signs and symptoms to report to health care team.
3. Patient achieves serum calcium level within normal limits.

NURSING MANAGEMENT

Assessment

1. See Assessment, Levels 1 and 2.
2. Do diagnostic studies:
   - ECG: arrhythmias, widened T-wave.
   - cardiac: systolic ejection time interval: left ventricular ejection fraction and S-T interval shortened.
3. Check for:
   - profound muscle weakness.
   - level of consciousness (obtund, comatose).
   - signs and symptoms of hypokalemia.
   - signs of renal failure.

Nursing Interventions

1. See Nursing Interventions, Level 2.
2. Take hourly intake and output.
3. Monitor neurologic signs q2h.
4. Implement medical regimen as ordered by physician:
   - hydrate with normal saline 6 to 10 liter per day.
   - titrate closely according to output.
   - maintain central venous pressure at 10 cm H_2O.
   - monitor for signs of complications of medical interventions (e.g., congestive heart failure, respiratory distress).
5. Administer etidronate disodium (Didronel) as prescribed:
   - monitor for renal dysfunction.
6. Administer mithramycin as prescribed:
   - monitor for side effects (renal, hepatic, hematologic toxicities).
   - medicate patient with antiemetic before administering IV bolus mithramycin.
   - monitor serum calcium level. Stabiliza-

tion of calcium occurs approximately 12 hours postinjection, followed by a decrease in 36 to 48 hours.

7. Administer gallium citrate as continuous infusion as ordered.
   - monitor blood urea nitrogen, creatinine, electrolytes.
   - aminoglycoside antibiotics should not be administered concomitantly.
   - may not be available in certain institutions.

Patient Teaching

1. See Patient Teaching, Levels 1 and 2.
2. Teach rationale and procedures for all treatment interventions.

SUGGESTED READINGS

Bockman, R.S.: Hypercalcemia in malignancy. Clinics in Endocrinology & Metabolism, 9:317–331, 1980.

Brown, E.M.: When you suspect hypercalcemia. Patient Care 16:14–37, 1982.

DeVita, V., Hellman, S., and Rosenberg, S.A.: Cancer Principles and Practice of Oncology, Vol 2, (3rd Ed). Philadelphia, J.B. Lippincott, 1989.

Doogan, R.A.: Hypercalcemia of malignancy. Cancer Nursing 4:299–304, 1981.

Krause, M.: Metastatic carcinoma of the breast. Nursing Mirror 146:20–24, 1978.

O'Dorisio, T.M.: Hypercalcemic crisis. Heart and Lung 7:425–434, 1978.

Seyburth, H.W., Segre, G.U., Morgan, J.C., et al.: Prostaglandins as mediators of hypercalcemia associated with certain types of cancer. New England Journal of Medicine 293:1278–1283, 1975.

Yarbro, J.W., and Bornstein, R.S.: Oncologic Emergencies. New York, Grune & Stratton, 1981.

Zeluf, F.: Hypercalcemia: Etiology, manifestations, and management. Heart and Lung 9:146, 1980.

63 Body Fluid Composition, Alteration in: Syndrome of Inappropriate Antidiuretic Hormone (SIADH)

Linda Kratcha-Sveningson

Population at Risk

- Individuals with neoplasms, especially small cell carcinoma of the lung
- Individuals with CNS disorders, pulmonary diseases, infections, and inflammatory diseases
- Individuals receiving certain pharmacologic agents
- Individuals experiencing limbic stimulation as a result of pain, stress, fear, or trauma

LEVEL 1: Potential (Serum Sodium > 135 mEq/l)

EXPECTED OUTCOME

1. Patient demonstrates knowledge related to potential SIADH:
   - identifies factors that influence antidiuretic hormone (ADH) secretion.
   - verbalizes signs and symptoms of SIADH to report to health care team.
2. Patient demonstrates absence of SIADH:
   - serum sodium range within normal limits.
   - serum osmolality within normal limits.
   - normal urine output of at least 1500 ml/24 hr.
   - normal weight for patient.
   - urine osmolality within normal limits.

NURSING MANAGEMENT

Assessment

1. Monitor laboratory studies:
   - serum sodium level.
   - serum osmolality.
   - urine osmolality.
2. Monitor:
   - intake and output q24h.
   - weight.
   - vital signs.
3. Monitor for signs and symptoms of SIADH:
   - alteration in sensorium (lethargy, drowsiness).
   - personality changes (e.g., irritability/hostility).
   - headache.
   - anorexia.
   - muscle cramps.
   - abdominal cramps.

- weakness.
- fatigue.
- nausea and vomiting.
- weight gain.
- oliguria or anuria.
4. Identify factors that may alter ADH secretion and predispose patient to SIADH:
   - surgery.
   - severe pain.
   - physical or emotional stress.
   - nausea.
   - administration of chemotherapy associated with water-retaining properties (cisplatin, vincristine, cyclophosphamide).
   - positive pressure ventilation.
   - malignant tumors (e.g., primarily small cell carcinoma of lung, but can also involve cancers of duodenum, pancreas, prostate, bladder, brain; lymphosarcomas, Ewing's sarcoma, acute and chronic leukemia, thymoma, Hodgkin's disease).
   - CNS disorders (e.g., head injury, skull fracture, subarachnoid hemorrhage, subdural hematoma, cerebral vascular thrombosis, encephalitis, meningitis, Guillain-Barré syndrome).
   - endocrine disorders (adrenal insufficiency, hypothyroidism).
   - lung disorders (e.g., pneumonia, lung abscess, status asthmaticus, fungal and tuberculous cavitary lesions).
5. Identify drugs that alter ADH secretion and consult physician regarding their use:
   - vincristine.
   - vinblastine.
   - cyclophosphamide.
   - cisplatin.
   - melphalan (high dose: 2 mg/kg).
   - morphine.
   - meperidine HCl.
   - acetaminophen.
   - chlorpropamide.
   - carbamazepine.
   - tricyclic depressants.
   - Diabinese.
   - oxytocin.
   - thiazide diuretics.
   - general anesthesia.
   - nicotine.

Patient Teaching

1. Emphasize need to comply with treatment program to control tumor.
2. Teach signs and symptoms to report to health care team:
   - mental confusion.
   - drowsiness.
   - weakness.
   - muscle cramps.
   - fatigue.
   - anorexia.
   - nausea and vomiting.
   - weight gain.
3. Explain rationale and correct technique for daily weight measurement.
   - weigh daily at the same time, with same type of clothing and with same scale.
4. Explain rationale and schedule for monitoring serum sodium.
5. Discuss factors that influence ADH secretion and predispose to SIADH.

LEVEL 2: Mild to Moderate (Serum Sodium > 120 mEq/l)

EXPECTED OUTCOME

1. Patient demonstrates knowledge related to altered body fluid composition related to SIADH:
   - identifies signs and symptoms of SIADH.

- identifies factors that influence ADH secretion.
- identifies potential sequela/complications of SIADH.
2. Patient demonstrates measures to correct or control altered body fluid composition related to SIADH:
   - performs necessary treatments and procedures.
   - identifies/demonstrates appropriate fluid restriction techniques.
   - identifies/demonstrates measures to relieve symptoms.
   - identifies signs and symptoms to report to health care team.
3. Patient demonstrates resolution of SIADH:
   - serum sodium range within normal limits.
   - serum osmolality within normal limits.
   - urine osmolality within normal limits.
   - normal urine output of at least 1500 ml/24 hr.
   - normal weight for patient.

NURSING MANAGEMENT

Assessment

1. See Assessment, Level 1.
2. Assess neurologic status:
   - level of consciousness.
   - tendon reflexes (e.g., sluggish).
   - muscle strength.

Nursing Interventions

1. Initiate fluid restriction (usually 800 to 1000 ml/24h) or replace fluid equal to the urinary output per physician's order:
   - allocate amount of fluid to be consumed at different times of the day, taking into account medication regimens and IV fluids (e.g., ½ fluids for morning hours, ⅓ for afternoon hours, and the remainder at night).
   - consult with patient regarding fluid allocation (e.g., amounts and types of fluid).
   - administer medications with meals if appropriate, to allow fluid rations to be more flexible.
   - vary fluid secretions, provide fluids high in sodium content (e.g., milk, orange juice, tomato juice, beef and chicken broth).
   - avoid use of IV solutions of 5 per cent dextrose in water.

2. Accurately measure and record intake and output.
3. Weigh the patient daily at the same time, with same type of clothing and with the same scale (when fluid restriction is adequate, there should be a steady decline in body weight with concurrent elevation of serum sodium. Serum sodium should begin to return to normal within 7 to 10 days).
4. Provide oral hygiene q2–4h or prn:
   - brush teeth, gums, tongue.
   - avoid all commercial mouthwash preparations containing alcohol, which creates a drying effect; avoid lemon-glycerine swabs.
   - use artificial saliva as needed.
5. Monitor closely patients receiving parenteral fluids to avoid unintentional fluid overload:
   - use IV regulator.
   - discontinue positional IV infusions and restart in another site.
6. Provide safety measures for confused or disoriented patient:
   - orient to time and place.
   - employ soft restraints as necessary.
   - keep side rails up on bed and bed at its lowest position.
   - assist with ambulation.

7. Initiate measures to control nausea and vomiting:
   - administer antiemetic 30 minutes before meals.
   - administer antiemetic before, during, or after chemotherapy and radiation therapy prn or around-the-clock if indicated.
   - administer antiemetic via alternate route during episode of nausea and vomiting.
8. Provide pain relief.
9. Reduce stressful factors for the patient.
10. Provide emotional support and reassurance.
11. Administer chemotherapeutic agents as ordered and monitor for side effects.
12. Monitor response to treatment.

Patient Teaching

1. See Patient Teaching, Level 1.
2. Teach rationale and measures to maintain fluid restriction.

3. Outline measures to control thirst:
   - avoid foods that increase thirst (e.g., salty foods).
   - avoid commercial mouthwashes containing alcohol and lemon-glycerine swabs.
   - stimulate salivation with sugar-free gum or sugar-free lemon drops or artificial saliva preparations.
   - rinse mouth with normal saline q2h.
4. Discuss measures to control nausea and vomiting:
   - take antiemetic as prescribed by physician (e.g., around-the-clock).
   - eat foods that do not upset the stomach.
5. Teach avoidance of stressful situations and methods to decrease stress:
   - relaxation techniques.
   - cancer support groups.
6. Discuss complications/sequelae of SIADH (e.g., seizures, coma, changes in sensorium).

LEVEL 3: Severe (Serum Sodium < 110 mEq/l)

EXPECTED OUTCOME

1. Patient and caregiver demonstrate knowledge of altered body fluid composition related to SIADH:
   - identify factors that influence ADH secretion.
   - identify signs and symptoms of SIADH.
   - identify sequelae/complications of SIADH.
2. Patient and caregiver identify/demonstrate measures to correct or manage altered fluid composition related to SIADH:
   - perform necessary treatments and procedures.
   - identify/demonstrate appropriate fluid restriction techniques.
   - identify/demonstrate measures to relieve symptoms.
   - identify signs and symptoms to report to health care team.
   - demonstrate safety-related behaviors.
3. Patient demonstrates resolution of SIADH and a stable composition of body fluids consistent with disease process.
   - laboratory values normal or improved.
   - decreased or absent signs or symptoms of SIADH.

Body Fluid Composition, Alteration in: Syndrome of Inappropriate Antidiuretic Hormone (SIADH)

NURSING MANAGEMENT

Assessment

1. See Assessment, Levels 1 and 2.
2. Check for neurologic signs:
   - gross change in sensorium.
   - muscular twitching.
   - seizure activity (e.g., frequency, level of consciousness, body parts involved, length of activity).
   - coma.
3. Monitor:
   - blood pressure.
   - pulse.
   - bowel sounds.
   - lung sounds.
   - mucous membrane status.
   - skin turgor.
4. Monitor for hypernatremia as a result of overcorrection of low sodium level:
   - thirst.
   - dry, sticky mucous membrane.
   - lethargy.
   - irritability.
   - seizures.
5. Monitor for side effects of drug toxicity that may occur while receiving drug therapy for SIADH:
   - lithium toxicity (digestive upset, cardiac irritability, drowsiness, tremor, muscle twitching).
   - demeclocycline toxicity (nausea, photosensitivity, superinfections, azotemia, hematologic changes).
   - demeclocycline predisposes patient to dehydration and volume depletion since urine is not appropriately concentrated.
   - for lithium use, monitor daily serum lithium level (if greater than 1.5 mEq/l, notify physician before continuing therapy).

Nursing Interventions

1. See Nursing Interventions, Level 2.
2. Initiate fluid restrictions per physician's orders (usually limited to 500 to 700 ml/24hr).
3. Administer hypertonic saline (200 to 300 ml of 3 to 5 per cent NaCl) with furosemide as ordered (rate of serum sodium rise should be limited to 1 to 2 mEq/l/hr):
   - monitor output (hourly urine).
   - monitor for signs and symptoms of pulmonary edema.
   - monitor electrolyte imbalance (e.g., potassium, calcium, magnesium loss).
4. Impose seizure precautions:
   - use padded side rails.
   - keep bed in lowest position.
   - avoid oral temperature.
   - prevent injury during seizure activity (support and protect head and turn to side if possible; avoid restraining limbs; do not attempt to force jaws open).
5. Administer medications as ordered (e.g., lithium carbonate, demeclocycline, urea).
6. Note factors that affect drug therapy effectiveness:
   - demeclocycline must be administered no less than 1 hour before or no sooner than 2 hours after meals (milk and other calcium-containing products may impair drug absorption).
   - concurrent use of aminophylline or acetazolamide decreases lithium effectiveness.
   - current use of methyldopa enhances lithium toxicity.
   - fluid restriction may not be required with drug therapy.

Patient Teaching

1. See Patient Teaching, Levels 1 and 2.
2. Teach signs and symptoms of drug toxicity to report to health care team.
3. Explain drug action and proper administration:
   - demeclocycline must not be taken with meals.
   - chronic users of demeclocycline should

avoid sunlight and sunlamps to prevent severe sunburn.

- take lithium carbonate with meals to minimize gastrointestinal symptoms.

SUGGESTED READINGS

Bunn, P., and Ridgeway, E.: Paraneoplastic syndromes. *In* DeVita, V.T., Hellman, S., and Rosenberg, S. (Eds.): Cancer: Principles and Practice of Oncology. Philadelphia, J.B. Lippincott, 1989.

Cunningham, S.: Fluid and electrolyte disturbances associated with cancer and its treatment. Nursing Clinics of North America *17*(4):579–583, 1982.

Glover, D., and Glick, J.: Oncologic emergencies and special complications. *In* Calabresi, P., Schein, P., Rosenberg, S., et al. (Eds.): Medical Oncology: Basic Principles and Clinical Management of Cancer. New York, MacMillan, 1987.

Marcus, S., and Fuks, J.: Syndrome of inappropriate antidiuretic hormone secretion and hyponatremia. *In* Dutcher, J.P., and Wiernik, P.H. (Eds.): Handbook of Hematologic and Oncologic Emergencies. New York, Plenum, 1987.

Poe, C., and Taylor, L.: Syndrome of inappropriate antidiuretic hormone: Assessment and nursing implications. Oncology Nursing Forum *16*(3):373–381, 1989.

Rice, V.: Problems of water regulation: Diabetes insipidus and syndrome of inappropriate anti-diuretic hormone. Critical Care Nurse *3*(1):64–82, 1983.

Schrieber, N.: Abnormal hormone secretion. *In* Groenwald, S. (Ed.): Cancer: Principles and Practice of Oncology. Boston, Jones & Bartlett, 1987.

Silverman, P., and Distelhorst, C.: Metabolic emergencies in clinical oncology. Seminars in Oncology *16*(3):504–515, 1989.

Synder, C.: Oncology Nursing. Boston, Little Brown & Company, 1986.

Trounson, L.: Nursing diagnosis and the syndrome of inappropriate antidiuretic hormone. Journal of Post Anesthesia Nursing *1*(4):244–247, 1986.

Body Fluid Composition, Alteration in: Tumor Lysis Syndrome

Christine Miaskowski

Population at Risk

- Individuals who are receiving treatment for tumors with very high growth rates and rapid cell turnover (e.g., acute leukemia and malignant lymphomas)
- Individuals with the following cancer diagnoses: Burkitt's lymphoma, acute lymphoblastic lymphoma, acute lymphoblastic leukemia, non-Hodgkin's lymphoma, T cell lymphoma, lymphosarcoma, metastatic breast cancer, small cell carcinoma of the lung, and metastatic medulloblastoma
- Individuals receiving the following chemotherapeutic agents: amsacrine, homoharringtonine, etoposide, interferon, or tamoxifen

LEVEL 1: Potential

EXPECTED OUTCOME

1. Patient demonstrates knowledge related to the potential for tumor lysis syndrome (TLS):
   - identifies factors that influence the development of TLS.
   - verbalizes signs and symptoms of TLS to report to health care team.
2. Patient demonstrates an absence of TLS as evidenced by:
   - uric acid levels within normal limits.
   - potassium levels within normal limits.
   - phosphate levels within normal limits.
   - calcium levels within normal limits.

NURSING MANAGEMENT

Assessment

1. Identify patients at risk for the development of TLS.
2. Identify risk factors for the development of TLS:
   - stage of disease: in patients with aggressive lymphomas, the presence of stage C (abdominal tumor) or stage D lymphoma (abdominal tumor with one or more extraabdominal sites).
   - pretreatment elevations in serum lactic acid dehydrogenase levels.

- parenchymal infiltration of tumor with lymphoma.
- mechanical ureteral obstruction by enlarged lymph nodes.
- sepsis.
3. Monitor laboratory studies q12h:
   - serum electrolytes.
   - blood urea nitrogen.
   - creatinine.
   - uric acid.
   - calcium.
   - phosphorus.
4. Monitor for signs and symptoms of hyperkalemia:
   - nausea.
   - diarrhea.
   - ECG changes: wide-to-absent T wave; depressed S–T segment; tall, peaked T wave; prolonged Q–T interval.
   - irritability, restlessness.
   - paresthesias.
   - difficult speech.
   - spastic-to-flaccid muscle tone.
5. Monitor for signs and symptoms of hypocalcemia and hyperphosphatemia:
   - tetany.
   - seizures.
   - laryngeal spasm.
   - positive Chvostek's sign or Trousseau's sign.
   - papilledema.
   - psychiatric disorders.
   - ECG changes: prolongation of the Q–T and S–T intervals.
6. Monitor for signs and symptoms of hyperuricemia:
   - nausea.
   - vomiting.
   - diarrhea.
   - lethargy.
   - edema.
   - flank pain.
   - hematuria.
   - crystaluria.
   - azotemia.
   - oliguria.
7. Monitor intake and output.
8. Monitor urine pH.

Nursing Interventions

1. Administer intravenous hydration at a rate of approximately 3 l/m^2 body surface area for 24 to 48 hours before and during cytotoxic chemotherapy.
2. Administer allopurinol 500 mg/m2 per day. This dosage may be reduced to 200 mg/m^2 per day, 3 days after beginning cytotoxic chemotherapy.
3. Administer diuretics as prescribed.
4. Administer sodium bicarbonate (50 mEq/l) to maintain a urine pH of 7 or greater, if the patient is hyperuricemic.

Patient Teaching

1. Explain that TLS occurs when large numbers of cells are destroyed by chemotherapeutic agents releasing intracellular minerals, potassium, phosphorus, and nucleic acids into the blood stream. This then results in hyperuricemia, hyperkalemia, hyperphosphatemia, and hypocalcemia.
2. Teach signs and symptoms to report to the health care team:
   - nausea.
   - diarrhea.
   - difficult speech.
   - muscle twitching.
3. Explain the rationale and measures to prevent TLS:
   - assessment of baseline renal function before initiation of aggressive antineoplastic chemotherapy.
   - treatment of prerenal azotemia and hyperphosphatemia before initiation of chemotherapy.
   - intravenous hydration and diuresis.
   - importance of monitoring intake and urine output and blood values.
   - administration of allopurinol to decrease uric acid levels.
   - use of sodium bicarbonate to alkalinize urine.

LEVEL 2: *Acute*

EXPECTED OUTCOME

1. Patient demonstrates knowledge related to the development of TLS:
   - identifies signs and symptoms of TLS.
   - identifies sequelae/complications of TLS.
2. Patient demonstrates measures to correct or control the signs and symptoms of TLS.
3. Patient demonstrates resolution of TLS:
   - uric acid levels within normal limits.
   - potassium levels within normal limits.
   - phosphate levels within normal limits.
   - calcium levels within normal limits.

NURSING MANAGEMENT

Assessment

1. See Assessment, Level 1.
2. Assess for signs and symptoms of hypervolemia and congestive heart failure.
   - changes in vital signs (e.g., blood pressure, pulse, respiratory rate).
   - jugular venous distention.
   - dyspnea.
   - pulmonary congestion.
   - presence of S3 or S4 gallop rhythm.
3. Assess for signs and symptoms of acute renal failure:
   - change in mental status.
   - anorexia.
   - nausea and vomiting.
   - diarrhea.
   - decreased urine output (usually less than 400 to 600 ml in 24 hr).
   - increased serum levels of urea, creatinine, uric acid, magnesium, potassium.
   - decreased urine specific gravity.
   - elevated urine sodium ($>$ 40 mEq/l).
4. Monitor laboratory studies q6–12h:
   - serum electrolytes.
   - blood urea nitrogen.
   - creatinine.
   - uric acid.
   - calcium.
   - phosphorus.

Nursing Interventions

1. See Nursing Interventions, Level 1.
2. Implement measures to decrease serum potassium:
   - intravenous hydration and diuresis.
   - intravenous administration of 50 per cent glucose with insulin coverage.
   - administration of an ion exchange resin (e.g., Kayexalate) orally or rectally.
3. Implement measures to control hyperphosphatemia and hypocalcemia.
   - intravenous hydration and diuresis.
   - administration of phosphate-binding antacids (e.g., Amphogel, Basaljel).
   - administration of calcium supplements.
4. Prepare patient for hemodialysis if the following indications are present:
   - serum potassium $\geq$ 6 mEq/l.
   - serum uric acid $\geq$ 10 mg/dl.
   - serum creatinine $\geq$ 10 mg/dl.
   - serum phosphorus $\geq$ 10 mg/dl.
   - symptomatic hypocalcemia (e.g., positive Chvostek's sign, hyperreflexia, tetany).
   - fluid overload.
5. Encourage patient/caregiver to verbalize fears and feelings and offer psychosocial support.

Patient Teaching

1. See Patient Teaching, Level 1.
2. Teach signs and symptoms to report to health care team:
   - sudden decrease in urinary output.
   - change in mental status.
   - dyspnea.
   - edema.

3. Teach patient/caregiver the rationale for early initiation of hemodialysis:
   - effective in decreasing uric acid, potassium, calcium, phosphate levels.
   - effective in reversing acute renal failure caused by hyperphosphatemia.
   - aggressive treatment required to prevent fatal consequences.
4. Discuss procedures for implementation of hemodialysis.

LEVEL 3: Severe

EXPECTED OUTCOME

1. Patient/caregiver demonstrate knowledge related to severe TLS:
   - identify signs and symptoms of complications of TLS.
   - verbalize that complications are potentially fatal.
2. Patient/caregiver demonstrate knowledge of measures to control complications of TLS.

NURSING MANAGEMENT

Assessment

1. See Assessment, Levels 1 and 2.
2. Assess for signs and symptoms of ventricular arrhythmias:
   - feelings of palpitations.
   - pale to cyanotic skin.
   - diaphoresis.
   - decreased blood pressure.
   - rapid, irregular heart beat.
   - precordial pain.
   - severe weakness.
   - dyspnea.
   - widened and bizarre-shaped QRS complexes.
3. Monitor for signs and symptoms of chronic renal failure:
   - anorexia.
   - hypertension.
   - lethargy progressing to coma.
   - seizures.
   - anemia.

Nursing Interventions

1. See Nursing Interventions, Levels 1 and 2.
2. Administer medications and blood products as prescribed (e.g., antiarrhythmics, oxygen).
3. Monitor cardiac status frequently.

Patient Teaching

1. See Patient Teaching, Levels 1 and 2.
2. Inform patient/family of rapid progression of TLS.
3. Teach patient/caregiver signs and symptoms to report to health care team:
   - feelings of palpitations.
   - precordial chest pain.
   - dyspnea.
   - severe weakness.
   - lethargy.
   - seizures.

4. Reinforce importance of compliance with medical regimen.

SUGGESTED READINGS

Barton, J.C.: Tumor lysis syndrome in nonhematopoietic neoplasms. Cancer *64*:738–740, 1989.

D'Elia, J.A., Aslani, M., Schermer, S., et al.: Hemolytic-uremic syndrome and acute renal failure in metastatic adenocarcinoma treated with mitomycin: Case report and literature review. Renal Failure *10*(2):107–113, 1987.

Dietz, K.A., and Flaherty, A.M.: Tumor lysis syndrome. *In* Groenwald, S.L., Frogge, M.H., Goodman, M., and Yarbro, C.H. (Eds.): Cancer Nursing: Principles and Practices. Boston, Jones & Bartlett, 1990, pp. 658–660.

Fields, A., Josse, R.G., and Bergsagel, D.E.: Tumor lysis syndrome. *In* DeVita, V.T., Hellman, S. and Rosenberg, S.A. (Eds.): Cancer: Principles and Practice of Oncology. Philadelphia, J.B. Lippincott, 1985, pp. 1874–1875.

Hussein, A.M., and Feun, L.G.: Tumor lysis syndrome after induction chemotherapy in small-cell lung carcinoma. American Journal of Clinical Oncology *13*(1):10–13, 1990.

Marcus, S.L., and Einzig, A.I.: Acute tumor lysis syndrome: Prevention and management. *In* Dutcher, J.P., and Wiernik, P.H. (Eds.): Handbook of Hematologic and Oncologic Emergencies. New York, Plenum, 1987.

O'Connor, N.T.J., Prentice, H.G., and Hoffbrand, A.V.: Prevention of urate nephropathy in the tumor lysis syndrome. Clinical Laboratory and Haematology *11*:97–100, 1989.

Stark, M.E., Dyer, M.C.D., and Coonley, C.J.: Fatal acute tumor lysis syndrome with metastatic breast carcinoma. Cancer, *60*:762–764, 1987.

Stokes, D.N.: The tumor lysis syndrome. Anaesthesia, *44*:133–136, 1989.

Warrell, R.P., and Bockman, R.S.: Tumor lysis syndrome. *In* DeVita, V.T., Hellman, S., and Rosenberg, S.A. (Eds.): Cancer: Principles and Practice of Oncology. Philadelphia, J.B. Lippincott, 1989, pp. 1996–1997.

Alteration in Cardiac Output, Decreased: Related to Third Space Syndrome

Carol A. Zabinski

Population at Risk

- Individuals with malignant effusions into the peritoneal, pericardial, or pleural compartments
- Individuals with obstruction of lymphatic drainage or venous return secondary to tumor pressure (e.g., bowel obstruction)
- Individuals diagnosed with neoplastic disease and having a nonmalignant cause for an effusion such as cirrhosis, congestive heart failure, peritonitis, nephrosis, pancreatitis, pneumonia, pulmonary embolism, atelectasis, pericarditis, previous irradiation, connective tissue disease, anemia, rheumatic fever

LEVEL 1: Potential

EXPECTED OUTCOME

1. Patient demonstrates knowledge of the potential for third space syndrome:
   - identifies early signs and symptoms.
   - identifies factors that influence maintenance and disruption of fluid.
2. Patient maintains adequate fluid volume as evidenced by:
   - serum electrolytes within normal limits.
   - blood urea nitrogen/creatinine ratio 10:1, hematocrit within normal limits.
   - skin turgor, mucous membrane and tongue hydration normal.
   - daily intake and output balanced and adequate.
   - absence of thirst or dry mouth.
   - vital signs within patient's baseline.
   - urine specific gravity within normal limits.
3. Patient demonstrates knowledge of measures to conserve energy and maintain adequate fluid volume:
   - verbalizes volume of fluid intake needed for adequate hydration.
   - verbalizes signs and symptoms of cardiovascular changes (e.g., decreased blood pressure, increased pulse rate, postural hypotension [dizziness or lightheadedness upon rising], decreased pulse volume and pressure).
   - implements safety measures to prevent injury in the presence of weakness or postural hypotension.

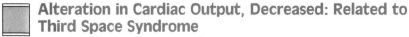

Alteration in Cardiac Output, Decreased: Related to Third Space Syndrome

NURSING MANAGEMENT

Assessment

1. Identify risk factors.
2. Assess energy level.
3. Assess pattern and amount of fluid intake and output.
4. Assess skin for turgor and integrity. Inspect tongue for size and additional longitudinal furrows. Inspect mucous membranes for moistness and integrity.
5. Assess weight for baseline data. Body weight change is not significant for third space losses.
6. Evaluate appropriate laboratory values (e.g., blood urea nitrogen/creatinine ratio 10:1).
7. Assess medications patient is taking for potential to cause fluid loss (e.g., diuretics, laxatives, antibiotics, tranquilizers, antiepileptics).
8. Assess vital signs including symptoms of hypotension.
9. Assess appearance and behavior of patient.

Patient Teaching

1. Discuss risk factors with the patient.
2. Identify and discuss/demonstrate energy conservation measures as appropriate to the patient's individual energy profile.
3. Discuss/demonstrate safety measures to prevent injury in the presence of postural hypotension or weakness.
4. Teach signs and symptoms of fluid volume deficit (e.g., thirst, dry mucous membranes, lethargy, decreased urine volume).
5. Discuss appropriate amounts of fluid intake as indicated by the individual patient's treatment plan.
6. Discuss when the health care team should be notified regarding disease signs and symptoms (e.g., progressive dyspnea, increasing abdominal girth, palpitations).
7. Discuss self-care measures to minimize fluid loss (e.g., antidiarrheal medications around-the-clock or as instructed).

LEVEL 2: Mild to Moderate

EXPECTED OUTCOME

1. Patient demonstrates understanding of third space syndrome:
   - identifies signs and symptoms of fluid volume deficit and third space syndrome to report to health care team.
   - identifies factors related to third space fluid retention that influence fluid volume balance.
2. Patient identifies measures to compensate for third space syndrome:
   - identifies nutritional measures necessary to achieve medical stability (e.g., high-protein diet, tube feedings, total parenteral nutrition and intravenous fat emulsions).
   - identifies recommended amount of fluid intake as indicated in the individual patient's treatment plan.

NURSING MANAGEMENT

Assessment

1. See Assessment, Level 1.
2. Monitor and evaluate appropriate laboratory values (e.g., electrolytes, serum albumin, ferritin, blood urea nitrogen/creatinine ratio, serum osmolality).
3. Monitor vital signs. Assess for postural hypotension, fullness of pulses.
4. Assess nutritional status.
5. Assess fluid intake patterns.

Nursing Interventions

1. Institute measures to prevent decreased fluid intake (e.g., encourage small amounts of fluids at frequent intervals, provide assistance as needed with oral intake).
2. Evaluate patient's energy level. Demonstrate energy conservation measures (e.g., prioritize activities of daily living and pace them to allow for frequent rest periods). Monitor sleep patterns and disturbances.
3. Institute measures to protect the patient from injury in the presence of postural hypotension or weakness (e.g., sit on the side of the bed for five minutes before standing, request assistance before getting out of bed).
4. Discuss nutritional interventions to restore fluids and electrolytes, and enhance protein intake.
5. Monitor intravenous fluids and maintain skin integrity around intravenous lines. Observe for signs of inflammation or infection around the intravenous insertion site.

Patient Teaching

1. See Patient Teaching, Level 1.
2. Teach patient recommended fluid intake for particular situation.
3. Discuss/demonstrate energy conservation measures and how to prioritize activities of daily living.
4. Discuss/demonstrate safety measures to prevent falls and injury.
5. Identify nutrition necessary to maintain activity and energy. Discuss dietary modifications appropriate to patient's situation.
6. Discuss/demonstrate intravenous line care and maintenance.

LEVEL 3: Severe

EXPECTED OUTCOME

1. Patient/caregiver demonstrate knowledge related to severe third space syndrome:
   - identify potential sequelae/complications of third space syndrome.
   - identify signs and symptoms to report to health care team.
2. Patient/caregiver identify measures to manage severe third space syndrome:
   - verbalize rationale for nutritional support.
   - verbalize rationale for monitoring abdominal girth, leg edema, dyspnea, peritoneovenous shunt, thoracostomy at home.
   - identify risk factors, when to report signs and symptoms of complications to health care team.

3. Patient exhibits stabilization of severe third space syndrome:
   • stability in vital signs.
   • stability in laboratory values.

NURSING MANAGEMENT

Assessment

1. See Assessment, Levels 1 and 2.
2. Assess for cause of decreased cardiac output by assessing for risk factors.
3. If the patient is receiving radiation or chemotherapy, monitor for and treat side effects.
4. Assess patient for peritoneovenous shunt if intractable malignant ascites is the etiology of the third space syndrome.
5. Assess patient for chest tube, paracentesis, or pericardial drainage systems.
6. Monitor for response to diuretics if these are used to control malignant ascites. Fluid volume deficit may occur with high dosages of diuretics used to treat malignant ascites; do not give potassium supplements with spironolactone (which is potassium sparing) because hyperkalemia may occur.
7. Assess for need for pain medication. Discomfort and feelings of tightness may occur with ascites. These respond well to low-dose analgesics.
8. Monitor laboratory values.
9. Assess for nutritional deficits.

Interventions

1. See Interventions, Level 2.
2. Ensure that the patient is medically stable, particularly regarding nutrition (this may take 4 to 5 days). If the patient cannot tolerate oral feedings, provide total parenteral nutrition and intravenous fat emulsions to correct deficiencies and maintain a positive nitrogen balance.
3. Monitor serum electrolytes, albumin, serum osmolality, blood urea nitrogen/creatinine ratio.

4. Monitor abdominal girth, vital signs, respiratory status, intake and output, weight, chest tube drainage, pericardial drainage, and paracentesis drainage as indicated.
5. Maintain skin integrity around drainage tubes.
6. If pleurodesis is recommended administer a narcotic analgesic before the procedure. Assist patient with position changes as ordered.
7. If total parenteral nutrition is required, follow institutional policies for monitoring and infection control.
8. Assist patient with self-care to manage activities of daily living and conserve energy.
9. Contact community support agencies for required supplies.

Patient Teaching

1. See Patient Teaching, Levels 1 and 2.
2. Explain technology pertinent to the individual patient's situation (e.g., peritoneovenous shunt, chest tubes, paracentesis drainage).
3. Discuss/demonstrate care measures to maintain function/potency of equipment.
4. Demonstrate skin care necessary to maintain skin integrity.
5. Explain procedure for managing homegoing total parenteral nutrition following institutional recommendations for infection control and trouble shooting.
6. Discuss energy conservation measures applicable to the individual patient's situation.
7. Discuss community resources for assistance such as nutritional support team, support groups, American Cancer Society, home care coordinator, home care nurse.

SUGGESTED READINGS

Gobel, B.H., and Lawler, P.E.: Malignant pleural effusions. Oncology Nursing Forum *12*(4):49–54, 1985.

Hewitt, J., and Janssen, R.: A management strategy for malignancy-induced pleural effusion: Long-term thoracostomy drainage. Oncology Nursing Forum *14*(5):17–22, 1987.

Horton, J.: Malignant effusions. *In* Moossa, A.R., Robson, M., and Schimpff, S. (Eds.): Comprehensive Textbook of Oncology. Baltimore, Williams & Wilkins, 1986, p. 403.

Klopp, A.: Shunting malignant acites. American Journal of Nursing *84*(2):212–213, 1984.

Metheny, N.: Fluid and Electrolyte Balance, Nursing Considerations. Philadelphia, J.B. Lippincott, 1987, pp. 201–202, 312–313.

Miller, N., and Pazdur, M.: Serous effusions. *In* Groenwald, S., et al. (Eds.): Cancer Nursing Principles and Practice. Boston, Jones & Bartlett, 1987, pp. 269–277.

Rosetti, A.C.: Nursing care of patients treated with intrapleural tetracycline for control of malignant pleural effusion. Cancer Nursing *8*(3):103–109, 1985.

Wegman, J.A., and Forshee, T.: Malignant pleural effusions: Pertinent issues. Heart and Lung *12*(5):533–543, 1983.

Zehner, L.C., and Hoogstraten, B.: Malignant effusions and their management. Seminars in Oncology Nursing *1*(4):259–268, 1985.

66 Alteration in Cardiac Output, Decreased: Related to Superior Vena Cava Syndrome

Margaret M. Cawley

Population at Risk

- Individuals with lung cancer especially central or right-sided tumors and small cell carcinoma
- Individuals with lymphoma
- Individuals with metastatic mediastinal tumors
- Individuals with radiation-induced fibrosis
- Individuals with thyroid goiter
- Individuals with tuberculosis, aneurysms
- Individuals who have thrombosis from central venous catheters

LEVEL 1: Potential

EXPECTED OUTCOME

1. Patient demonstrates knowledge of decreased cardiac output related to potential superior vena cava syndrome (SVC):
   - identifies early signs and symptoms of SVC syndrome.
   - verbalizes importance of communicating early signs and symptoms to health care team.
2. Patient maintains adequate cardiac function:
   - pulse regular and not rapid.
   - respirations regular and nonlabored.
   - laboratory values within normal limits.
   - chest x-ray absent of mediastinal mass.

NURSING MANAGEMENT

Assessment

1. Obtain history of risk factors.
2. Assess current circulatory status:
   - baseline pulse.
   - respiration rate.
   - blood pressure.
   - level of activity.
   - mental status.
   - color of skin, lips.

Patient Teaching

1. Describe early signs and symptoms to report to health care team:
   - fullness in head that increases when bending over.
   - tightness of collar.
   - weight gain.
   - periorbital edema in AM.
   - shortness of breath.

2. Discuss importance of reporting early signs and symptoms to health care team as soon as they occur.
3. Explain measures to promote circulatory output and increase comfort:
   - loosen clothing around neck, waist.
   - restrict fluids as ordered.
   - sleep in elevated position with pillows for support.

LEVEL 2: Mild

EXPECTED OUTCOME

1. Patient demonstrates knowledge of decreased cardiac output related to SVC syndrome:
   - verbalizes signs and symptoms related to SVC syndrome.
   - identifies potential sequelae related to progressive SVC syndrome.
2. Patient demonstrates strategies to promote optimal circulation.

NURSING MANAGEMENT

Assessment

1. See Assessment, Level 1.
2. Assess symptoms of SVC syndrome related to venous hypertension:
   - dyspnea.
   - upper body swelling.
   - fullness in head, headache.
   - neck vein distention.
   - periorbital edema.
   - dilation of hand veins that do not collapse when hand is elevated.
   - substernal chest pain.
   - dysphagia.
   - cough.
   - change in mental status.

Nursing Interventions

1. Include family members in plan of care.
2. Implement medical regimen as prescribed by physician:
   - administer diuretics.
   - administer steroids as indicated.
3. Facilitate comfort by placing patient in upright position in bed or chair. Elevate head of bed 60 degrees.
4. Elevate arms to reduce swelling.
5. Provide emotional support.

Patient Teaching

1. See Patient Teaching, Level 1.
2. Explain to patient anatomy and physiology related to SVC syndrome.
3. Teach patient progressive signs and symptoms to report to health care team:
   - increased shortness of breath.
   - tachycardia.
   - changes in mental status.
   - distended veins on anterior chest or neck.
4. Teach patient how to minimize symptoms:
   - conserve energy, pace activities.

419

Alteration in Cardiac Output, Decreased: Related to Superior Vena Cava Syndrome

- positioning measures.
- relaxation techniques.
5. Explain rationale of oxygen therapy when applicable.

6. Teach patient measures to manage the side effects of radiation therapy to the anterior chest (see Chapter 12).

LEVEL 3: Moderate to Severe

EXPECTED OUTCOME

1. Patient/caregiver demonstrate knowledge of decreased cardiac output related to SVC syndrome:
   - identify signs and symptoms of acute SVC syndrome.
   - identify complications related to acute SVC syndrome.
   - identify rationale of emergency therapy.
2. Patient/caregiver demonstrate strategies to manage or alleviate SVC syndrome:
   - identify purpose for diagnostic workup.
   - compliance with emergency treatment regimen.
   - demonstrate strategies to provide comfort.
   - demonstrate knowledge of administering medications and oxygen.
3. Patient maintains optimal circulatory status:
   - alleviated or absent signs and symptoms of SVC syndrome.
   - blood gases within normal limits.
   - vital signs stable.

NURSING MANAGEMENT

Assessment

1. See Assessment, Levels 1 and 2.
2. Assess for circulatory compromise:
   - cyanosis.
   - tachycardia.
   - tachypnea.
   - respiratory distress.
3. Monitor for CNS involvement related to cardiac compromise:
   - headache.
   - lethargy.
   - dizziness.
   - visual changes.
   - loss of consciousness.
   - convulsions.
4. Monitor for increased blood pressure in upper extremities while blood pressure in lower extremities will be in a range close to normal.
5. Assess whether veins of hands collapse when hand is elevated above the heart level.
6. Monitor arterial blood gases PO_2, PCO_2.

Nursing Interventions

1. See Nursing Interventions, Level 2.
2. Monitor blood pressure, heart rate, and respirations every 15 minutes during acute phase.
3. Monitor pulsus alternans q4h (unpalpable pulse during inspiration).
4. Monitor urine output hourly; calculate input and output for fluid balance q8h.

5. Measure central venous pressure or Swan-Ganz catheter as indicated.
6. Administer oxygen therapy as ordered.
7. Administer low-sodium diet as ordered; assist with meal planning related to decreased sodium intake.
8. Administer medications as ordered:
   - diuretics.
   - steroids.
   - anticoagulants/fibrinolytics.
   - chemotherapy.
9. Assist patient to conserve activity (e.g., assist with personal care).
10. Implement measures to maintain tissue perfusion:
    - place patient on air mattress.
    - position q2h.
    - utilize pillows to elevate upper extremities to reduce edema.
    - keep head of bed at 60 degrees.
11. Implement measures to control anxiety:
    - maintain frequent physical and eye contact with patient.
    - encourage caregiver to remain with patient if beneficial.
    - administer tranquilizers, as prescribed.

Patient Teaching

1. See Patient Teaching, Levels 1 and 2.
2. Explain rationale for diagnostic workup:
   - thoracotomy/biopsy.
   - mediastinoscopy/biopsy.
   - bronchoscopy/biopsy.
   - lump node biopsy (supraclavicular).
   - sputum cytology.
   - bronchial washing.
3. Explain rationale for emergency treatment regimen (radiation, chemotherapy).

4. Teach patient/caregiver side effects related to therapeutic procedures.
5. Explain change in body image due to venous congestion ("purple frog" is temporary).
6. Encourage patient/caregiver to verbalize fears and concerns.
7. Refer patient/caregiver to appropriate resource for:
   - assistance with transportation to and from therapy.
   - patient/caregiver support groups.
   - patient/caregiver educational programs (e.g., American Cancer Society I Can Cope).

SUGGESTED READINGS

American Cancer Society: Managing oncologic emergencies involving structural dysfunction. CA: A Cancer Journal for Clinicians 35:7–10, 1985.

Carabell, S.C., and Goodman, R.L.: Oncologic emergencies. In DeVita, V.T., Hellman, S., and Rosenberg, S., (Eds.): Cancer: Principles and Practice of Oncology. Philadelphia, J.B. Lippincott, 1982, pp. 1582–1586.

Donoghue, M.: Superior vena caval syndrome. In Yasko, J.M. (Ed.): Guidelines for Cancer Care: Symptom Management. Reston, VA, Reston Publishing, 1983, pp. 358–361.

Miller, S.E.: Superior vena cava syndrome. In Polomamo, R.C., and Miller, S.E. (Eds.): Understanding and Managing Oncologic Emergencies. Adria Laboratories, 1987, pp. 27–31.

Perez, C., Presant, C.A., and Van Ambert A.L. III: Management of superior vena cava syndrome. Seminars in Oncology 5:123–134, 1978.

Stuckey, P.A., and Waters, H.: Oncology alert for the home care nurse: Superior vena cava syndrome. Home Health Nurse 5:34–37, 1987.

Varricchio, C.G., and Jassek, P.F.: Acute pulmonary disorders associated with cancer. Seminars in Oncology Nursing 1:269–277, 1985.

67

Alteration in Cardiac Output, Decreased: Related to Cardiac Tamponade

Catherine A. Hydzik

Population at Risk

- Individuals with metastatic disease of the pericardium; primary cancers of the lung, breast, and gastrointestinal tract, leukemia, Hodgkin's and non-Hodgkin's lymphoma, melanoma
- Individuals with primary tumors of pericardium; mestholiomas, sarcomas, teratomas, fibromas, and angiomas
- Individuals who receive radiation of 4000 rads or more to the mediastinal area
- Individuals who have central venous catheters
- Individuals with infusions or trauma to the chest

LEVEL 1: Potential

EXPECTED OUTCOME

1. Patient demonstrates knowledge related to potential for decreased cardiac output related to cardiac tamponade:
   - identifies risk factors for cardiac tamponade.
   - verbalizes signs and symptoms of cardiac tamponade.
   - identifies signs and symptoms to report to health care team.
2. Patient maintains a normal cardiac output and demonstrates absence of cardiac tamponade.

NURSING MANAGEMENT

Assessment

1. Identify patients at risk for cardiac tamponade.
2. Assess patient's present ventilatory and circulatory status:
   - mental status.
   - cardiac status (blood pressure, pulse).
   - respiratory rate.
   - skin assessment (color, texture, temperature, turgor).
3. Perform neurologic assessment.
4. Perform cardiac assessment.
5. Perform respiratory assessment.
6. Perform skin assessment.

Patient Teaching

1. Teach signs and symptoms to report to health care team:
   - clinical picture varies depending on rate of onset (slow or rapid) and degree of intrapericardial pressure.
   - changes in mental status.
   - restless or agitated.
   - chest pain.
   - shortness of breath.
   - skin cool, pale, clammy.

LEVEL 2: Mild to Moderate

EXPECTED OUTCOME

1. Patient/caregiver demonstrate knowledge of decreased cardiac output related to cardiac tamponade:
   - verbalize signs and symptoms of cardiac tamponade.
   - identify sequelae/complications of cardiac tamponade.
2. Patient/caregiver identify/demonstrate interventions to correct or manage decreased cardiac output related to cardiac tamponade:
   - explain purpose for diagnostic workup.
   - comply with treatment plan.
   - verbalize/demonstrate strategies to relieve symptoms and promote comfort.
3. Patient maintains optimal cardiac output.

NURSING MANAGEMENT

Assessment

1. See Assessment, Level 1.
2. Assess patient for clinical manifestation of cardiac tamponade:
   - neurologic:
     - change in level of consciousness.
     - increased level of anxiety or apprehension.
   - cardiovascular:
     - retrosternal chest pain.
     - heart sounds (muffled or distant).
     - cardiac friction rub.
     - changes in venous pressure (jugular venous distention, increase in central venous pressure).
     - palpate peripheral pulses.
   - respiratory:
     - increased rate (assess for dyspnea/tachypnea).
     - cough, hoarseness.
   - integumentary:
     - change in color (pale, ashen, cyanotic).
     - texture (diaphoretic, clammy).
     - temperature (cool).
     - decreased turgor.
   - genitourinary:
     - decreased urinary output.
   - gastrointestinal:
     - nausea, vomiting, abdominal pain.

Nursing Interventions

1. Implement medical regimen as prescribed by physician and monitor side effects:
   - administer diuretics as indicated.
   - administer steroids as indicated.
   - administer humidified oxygen by nasal cannula as ordered.
2. Monitor intake and output.

423

3. Monitor cardiac rhythm and rate.
4. Provide emotional support to the patient/caregiver.
5. Have emergency equipment available
6. Provide a safe environment.
7. Place call bell within patient's reach.
8. Make referral to community agencies as appropriate for home care nursing, and support groups.

Patient Teaching

1. See Patient Teaching, Level 1.
2. Explain all tests and procedures to patient/caregiver:
   - chest x-ray.
   - electrocardiogram.
   - echocardiogram.
   - computerized tomography scan.
   - cardiac catheterization.
   - cardiac monitor.
3. Explain to patient/caregiver pathophysiology related to cardiac tamponade.
4. Teach patient/caregiver to report any changes in symptoms to the health care team.
5. Teach patient passive range-of-motion exercises to extremities.
6. Teach patient measures to promote respiratory function (e.g., turning, coughing, deep breathing).
7. Teach patient/caregiver need to verbalize fears and concerns.
8. Inform patient/caregiver of appropriate resources:
   - patient/caregiver support groups if appropriate.
   - clergy support if appropriate.
   - volunteer to provide additional support.

LEVEL 3: Severe

EXPECTED OUTCOME

1. Patient/caregiver demonstrate knowledge of decreased cardiac output related to cardiac tamponade:
   - verbalize signs and symptoms of cardiac tamponade.
   - identify sequelae/complications of cardiac tamponade.
2. Patient/caregiver identify/demonstrate interventions to correct or manage altered cardiac output related to cardiac tamponade:
   - explain purpose for diagnostic workup.
   - comply with treatment plan.
   - verbalize/demonstrate strategies to relieve symptoms and promote comfort.
3. Patient maintains optimal cardiac output.

NURSING MANAGEMENT

Assessment

1. See Assessment, Levels 1 and 2.
2. Assess patient for clinical manifestation of cardiac tamponade:
   - neurologic:
     - impending sense of doom.
     - confusion.
     - coma.
     - seizures may be present.
   - cardiovascular:
     - ECG changes (electrical alterations, decreased QRS voltage, T wave changes, elevated S–T segment).

- narrowing pulse pressure.
- decreased systolic and increased diastolic blood pressure.
- decreased cardiac output.
- murmur.
- precordial oppressive feeling or retrosternal chest pain.
- nailbed color.
- absent PMI (point of maximal impulse).
- Beck's triad (includes arterial hypotension, muffled heart sounds, elevated central venous pressure).
- respiratory:
  - pulsus paradoxus.
  - respiratory alkalosis.
  - hypoxemia.
  - Kussmaul's respirations.
- gastrointestinal:
  - increased abdominal girth.
  - hepatomegaly with hepatojugular reflux.

Nursing Interventions

1. See Nursing Interventions, Level 2.
2. Monitor blood pressure, heart rate, and respirations every 15 minutes if condition is acute.
3. Assess for pulsus paradoxus with each blood pressure measurement.
4. Assess hemodynamic pressure by a Swan-Ganz catheter or central venous pressure as indicated.
5. Assess laboratory data (arterial blood gases, CBC, serum chemistries, prothrombin time, partial thromboplastin time).
6. Administer medications as ordered:
   - unloading medication (Nipride, Dopamine)
   - medication for pain, anxiety, nausea and vomiting.
7. Administer blood, saline, plasma, or dextran as ordered.
8. Minimize activity and maintain bedrest.
9. Maintain thromboembolic disease hose until ambulatory.

10. Elevate head of bed 45 to 60 degrees or to position of greatest comfort.
11. Maintain patient npo.
12. Administer oral hygiene q3–4h.
13. Provide patient with tepid water sponge baths after diaphoretic episodes if stable.
14. Reorient patient if necessary.
15. Alleviate anxiety:
   - maintain frequent contact with patient.
   - identify validity of feelings.
   - provide reassurance.
   - encourage caregiver to participate in care if mutually therapeutic.
16. Assist with pericardiocentesis and monitor patient.

Patient Teaching

1. See Patient Teaching, Levels 1 and 2.
2. Explain rationale for emergency treatment regimen:
   - pericardiocentesis.
3. Explain rationale for chronic treatment regimen:
   - pericardial window.
   - insertion of an indwelling pericardial catheter.
   - intrapericardiac installation of chemotherapeutic agent or radioisotopes.
   - radiation therapy to control pericardial effusion.
   - pericardiotomy.
4. Explain rationale for nursing care.
5. Teach signs and symptoms of infection or complications postchronic treatment regimen.

SUGGESTED READINGS

Chernecky, C.C., and Ramsey, P.W.: Critical nursing care of the client with cancer. Norwalk, CT, Appleton-Century-Crofts, 1984, pp. 88–94.
Concilus, E.M., and Bohachick, P.A.: Cancer: Pericardial effusion and tamponade. Cancer Nursing, *1:*391–398, 1984.

Alteration in Cardiac Output, Decreased: Related to Cardiac Tamponade

Estes, M.E.: Management of the cardiac tamponade patient: A nursing framework. Critical Care Nurse *5:*17–26, 1985.

Gilbert, I., and Henning, R.J.: Adenocarcinoma of the lung presenting with pericardial tamponade: Report of a case and review of the literature. Heart and Lung *14:*83–87, 1985.

Glover, D.J., and Glick, J.H.: Managing oncologic emergencies involving structural dysfunction. CA: A Cancer Journal for Clinicians *35:*238–251, 1985.

Hiller, G.: Cardiac tamponade in the oncology patient. Focus on Critical Care *14:*19–23, 1987.

Karnauchow, P.N.: Cardiac tamponade from central venous catheterization. Canadian Medical Association Journal *135:*1145–1147, 1986.

King, D.E.: Assessment and evaluation of the paradoxical pulse. Dimensions of Critical Care Nursing *1:*266–274, 1982.

Miller, S.E., and Campbell, D.B.: Malignant pericardial effusions. *In* Polomano, R.C., and Miller S.E. (Eds.): Understanding and Managing Oncology Emergencies. Columbus, OH, Adria Laboratories, 1987, pp. 19–26.

Missri, J., and Schechter, D.: When pericardial effusion complicates cancer. Hospital Practice *23:*277–281, 284–286, 1988.

Press, O.W., and Livingston, R.: Management of malignant pericardial effusion and tamponade. Journal of the American Medical Association *257:*1088–1092, 1987.

Pursley, P.: Acute cardiac tamponade. American Journal of Nursing *83:*1414–1418, 1983.

Spodick, D.H.: Acute pericardial disease. Heart and Lung *14:*599–604, 1985.

Theologides, A.: Neoplastic cardiac tamponade. Seminars in Oncology *5:*181–191, 1978.

Wojciechowicz, V.: Pericardial window surgery for cardiac tamponade. Critical Care Nurse *5:*28–33, 1985.

Yasko, J.M., and Schafer, S.L.: Neoplastic pericardial tamponade. *In* Yasko, J.M. (Ed.): Guidelines for Cancer Care: Symptom Management. Reston, VA, Reston Publishing, 1983, pp. 343–346.

Index

427

439